CULTURE CARE DIVERSITY AND UNIVERSALITY: A THEORY OF NURSING

Madeleine M. Leininger, Editor

JONES AND BARTLETT PUBLISHERS
Sudbury, Massachusetts
BOSTON   TORONTO   LONDON   SINGAPORE

RT
86.54
.C85
2001

World Headquarters
Jones and Bartlett Publishers
40 Tall Pine Drive
Sudbury, MA 01776
978-443-5000
www.jbpub.com
info@jbpub.com

Jones and Bartlett Publishers International
Barb House, Barb Mews
London W6 7PA
UK

Jones and Bartlett Publishers Canada
2406 Nikanna Road
Mississauga, ON L5C 2W6
CANADA

ISBN 0-7637-1825-4

This book is a rerelease of a book previously published in 1991 by the National League for Nursing, ISBN 0887375197.

Library of Congress Cataloging-in-Publication Data
Culture care diversity and universality : a theory of nursing / Madeleine M.
    Leininger, editor.
    p. cm.
Includes index.
ISBN 0-7637-1825-4
    1. Transcultural nursing. 2. Nursing—Cross-cultural studies. 3. Nursing—
Philosophy. I. Leininger, Madeleine M.

RT86.54 .C85 2001
610.73'01—dc21
                           2001020234

Production Credits
Acquisitions Editor: Penny M. Glynn
Associate Editor: Christine Tridente
Production Editor: AnnMarie Lemoine
Editorial Assistant: Thomas Prindle
Manufacturing Buyer: Amy Duddridge
Cover Design: AnnMarie Lemoine
Printing and Binding: Malloy Lithographing

Printed in the United States of America
05 04 03 02   10 9 8 7 6 5 4 3 2

Contributors

Irene Zwaycz Bohay, MSN, RN, Maternal Child Clinical Specialist and Consultant, Detroit, Michigan

Marie F. Gates, PhD, RN, Associate Professor, Eastern Michigan University, Department of Nursing Education, Ypsilanti, Michigan

Madeline M. Leininger, PhD, RN, CTN, LHD, DS, Ph.DNSc, FAAN, Professor of Nursing and Anthropology and Human Care Research, Colleges of Nursing and Liberal Arts, Wayne State University, Detroit Michigan, Founder of Transcultural Nursing and Leader in Human Care Research

Janet Rosenbaum, PhD, RN, Profesor, University of Windsor, School of Nursing, Windsor, Ontario, Canada

Zenaida Spangler, PhD, RN, Director of Nursing Education and Research, Robert Packer Hospital, Sayre, Pennsylvania

David B. Statiak, MEd, MSN, CRNA, Assistant Professor and Director, Graduate Program of Nursing Anesthesiology, University of Detroit Mercy, Detroit, Michigan

Anna Frances Wenger, PhD, RN, Associate Professor and Director, Center for Transcultural and International Nursing, Nell Hodgsen Woodruff School of Nursing, Atlanta, Georgia

Foreword

This book, *Culture Care Diversity and Universality: A Theory of Nursing*, remains the primary, definitive, and comprehensive source on the Culture Care Theory with the Sunrise Model, the ethnonursing method, and enablers. Several early and classic transcultural nursing studies by transcultural nursing experts are included with the Culture Care Theory and the ethnonursing research method. These studies demonstrate the use of the theory with the Sunrise Model as a conceptual guide to discover culture care phenomena from a holistic perspective. In addition, these are the first research findings of culture-specific care meanings and actions of 22 Western and non-Western cultures to guide nurses' practices. There are also chapters on nursing administration and the future of transcultural nursing.

Dr. Madeleine Leininger was visionary as she saw the need in the 1950s to prepare nurses for an increasingly multicultural world related to health and nursing care. The Culture Care Theory has been conceptualized from a worldwide comparative and holistic perspective to study many cultures in the world focused on discovering commonalities (universals) and differences (diversities) in order to establish a body of transcultural nursing care knowledge. The Culture Care Theory was also conceptualized within the qualitative discover paradigm with largely inductive emic (or people-centered) data from diverse and similar cultures (Western and non-Western) for in-depth and meaningful knowledge of cultures.

This historical book presents the philosophical, theoretical, and epistemic foundations of the Culture Care Theory with three creative new modalities to guide nurses in arriving at and to plan for culturally congruent care. The theorist predicted that both generic (referring to folk, lay, or indigenous nonprofessional care) and professional care were essential to help people remain well, face handicaps, or face death within a cultural context. This prediction has been well confirmed today with the discovery of complementary care practices which are presented in this book with generic and professional care findings as essential for professional care. Today the Culture Care Theory remains one of the most important, unique, comprehensive, and holistic theories in nursing. It is a theory that continues to be ahead of its time, and yet it is so imperative for nursing and health care. Since the 1990s medicine, pharmacy, mortuary science, and other disciplines have begun to discover and use the Culture Care Theory in research, teaching, and clinical practice to meet the mandate for culturally-based care practices. Nursing practitioners and other health-related disciplines are not only using the theory but also the research findings to provide "culturally congruent care"—the term first coined by Leininger in the early 1960s with the theory.

Professor Leininger, a renowned scholar, teacher, and futurist also predicted that nursing would become quite different in the 21st century. This has come true as nursing has become intensely multicultural and is seeing the critical need for a distinct holistic body of transcultural nursing knowledge to guide practice. The Culture Care Theory has become known worldwide as one of the most comprehensive theories with specific ways to care for clients, families, communities, and institutions of diverse and similar cultures. Unquestionably, the Culture Care Theory will continue to be more important and meaningful in this Third Millennium in teaching, clinical practices, curricula, consultation, and research within nursing but also in other health disciplines and public services. The theory has been developed soundly to discover sensitive, competent, and culturally-based care knowledge for individuals, families, communities, subcultures, and cultural institutions of many diverse cultures. The Culture Care Theory also accommodates relevant medical, nursing, and social sciences along with other areas depicted in the Sunrise Model. But it is a new paradigm different from nursing's traditional views and medical treatment practices that is being used in nursing curricula and practice arenas worldwide.

From this definitive theory and method book, many new research-theory articles have been generated and published in transcultural nursing books, articles, and other publications. This book, however, remains the primary and fundamental source on the theory and method with definitive guides for the use of the theory with the valuable research enablers to tease out embedded or covert data. Nurses and other health professionals as well as health care institutions worldwide will continue to find this breakthrough theory book one of their most reliable to provide congruent, competent, and safe care for a growing multicultural world.

Before closing this Foreword, a few major and unique features of the theory and method can be stated. They are: 1) The theory remains the oldest theory in nursing since launched in the 1950s; 2) It is the only theory explicitly focused on the interrelationships of culture and care linked with health, well-being, illness and dying; 3) The theory and method focus on holistic, comprehensive and yet very specific comparative care phenomena; 4) Both the theory and the ethnonursing method are focused on discovering cultural care diversities (differences) and universalities (commonalities to arrive at meaningful, safe, and congruent care; 5) The theory has both abstract and yet, specific practical features to discover culture care knowledge; 6) the three decision and section modes of the theory are unique and different than the symptom-management present-day nursing focus; 7) It is the first theory and method to discover in-depth generic (emic) and professional (etic) care data; and 8) The theory can be used by other disciplines if modified to fit their interests or goals. These unique features should stimulate the reader to study and reflect thoughtfully on learning the theory and method, and then applying available research findings for culturally congruent and safe care to people.

Marilyn R. McFarland Ph.d, RN, CTN

Faculty Member, Saginaw Valley State University, Michigan USA

Former Editor, Jr. of Transcultural Nursing & Worldwide Transcultural Consult

DEDICATION

This book is dedicated to nursing students, faculty and multidisciplinary colleagues whom I have taught or known over the past 50 years in academe and clinical nursing and anthropology. It is also dedicated to many cultural informants who have shared their rich cultural and care heritage with me and others to discover culturally-based health care needs and practices. It has been a great joy and most rewarding to see users of the theory of Culture Care Diversity and Universality value and reaffirm the importance of theoretically-based research knowledge and findings to establish or improve care to people of diverse cultures. Although the field of transcultural nursing was launched almost fifty years ago, the theory and ethnonursing method have become essential to develop new knowledge and practices. Transcultural nursing has been one of the most significant and creative breakthroughs in nursing and health care services the past century. It has been the enthusiastic users of this theory that have made this important development possible.

I am appreciative of many leaders and followers who have made this Culture Care theory relevant to the discipline and practice of transcultural nursing. I am particularly grateful to several outstanding and persistent theory teachers and researchers such as Drs. Marilyn McFarland, Elizabeth Cameron-Traub, Akram Omeri, Fran Wenger, Gennie Kenny, Kristin Gebru, Rhoda Gelazis, Joan MacNeil, Beverly Horn, Joanne Ehrman, Linda Luna, Margaret Andrews, Cheryl Leuning, Anita Berry, and Rick Zoucha. These transcultural nurse leaders and others have given leadership nationally and transnationally to the theory and method. I am grateful to Penny Glynn of Jones and Bartlett for making a few important update revisions for this reprinting and to Dr. Marilyn McFarland for her assistance. This book is dedicated to my transcultural colleagues and my family.

Preface

A decade has passed since this book was published. The theory of Culture Care Diversity and Universality has markedly grown in use, meaning, and relevance to many users worldwide. Theories and methods that are thoughtfully developed to discover new or reaffirm existing knowledge are always valued and stand the test of time for many years and even centuries. This theory has been unique to advance humanistic scientific transcultural nursing care knowledge in order to provide culturally competent and responsible service to people of diverse cultures.

This book remains the primary and definitive source of the theory of Cultural Care Diversity. This hallmark publication is an explication of the theory with the philosophical base, tenents, assumptions, purpose, and goal of the theory. It is followed by the ethnonursing qualitative research method which has been uniquely designed with enablers and with rigorous phases of data analysis to fit the theory tenets. The book also contains classic transcultural nursing studies to show how the theory and the ethnonursing research method with findings are used to arrive at culturally congruent nursing care. An additional feature is that research findings from 22 Western and non-Western cultures are presented showing the dominant culture core meanings and actions to guide nurses in providing culturally congruent care. Other special interest chapters are included such as transcultural nursing administration and the future directions of transcultural nursing.

During the past decade, it has been most rewarding to see the theory and some research findings are now being used worldwide to provide culturally congruent care (the term I coined in the 1960s). Most importantly, the concept of culturally congruent care, and often the theory, is now being used by national and international disciplines to meet the growing demand for meaningful and safe health care to a rapidly growing multicultural world to transform health care and educational systems in multicultural institutions.

It has been a joy to hear nursing students share their comments with me such as, "This theory is highly relevant and long overdue in nursing as we have been caring for clients of diverse cultures and desperately need cultural care knowledge to help us;" "Your theory is truly holistic, comparative and yet very specific to guide my practice in meaningful ways;" "I am baffled why it took so long for nursing to provide formal educational courses and programs on human care and culture until you gave leadership to it;" "I love the Sunrise Model as it guides my thinking and actions as I care for cultural strangers every day and now I can practice care that fits clients' needs;" "The theory and the ethnonursing research method make sense and have opened a whole new way to discover knowledge and use it." These statements and many others reveal how important the Culture Care theory and the ethonursing research method have been to help nurses discover transcultural nursing knowledge and use the findings to care for people of different cultures.

The theory, which was conceptualized in the mid-1950s, has become known and valued. It has several noteworthy and distinct hallmark features. First, it is the oldest nursing theory focused explicitly on discovering human care and culture to advance nursing science. Second, the theory was conceptualized to discover what is universal and diverse about cultures and human care and the explanatory dimensions. Third, the goal of the theory was to generate and disseminate knowledge relevant to providing culturally congruent, responsible, and safe care to people of diverse cultures. Fourth, the theory is one of the most comprehensive and holistic to discover many potential influences on human care focus on worldview, social structure, ethnohistory, language use and environmental and generic and professional factors. Fifth, the ethnonursing research method was the first nursing research method explicitly designed to fit the theory in order to examine systematically the tenets, purpose, and goal of the theory. Sixth, the theory is unique as it has three theoretical modes to provide culturally congruent care for nursing decisions and actions. Finally, the theory was developed to help shift nurses from traditional unicultural to multicultural transcultural nursing in order to provide sensitive, compassionate, and therapeutic care to people of diverse cultures.

In this Third Millennium theory will, of necessity, continue to grow in much relevance in a rapidly growing and intense multicultural world. The demand for therapeutic care to minorities, poor, and all cultures will increase to reduce cultural clashes, pain, racism, conflicts, and imposition practices. It should move all of nursing to become a truly transcultural nursing discipline and profession to benefit humanity. Research findings from over 200 cultures are already providing a wealth of new knowledge to transform nursing education and health care practices. And as all of nursing and health care becomes transculturally based, it will be extremely important to improve human caring services worldwide.

Since this book was published in 1991, it is most encouraging that a number of credible research studies and general articles have been publised using the theory in Western and non-Western cultures. These publications reveal the great interest and relevance of the theory with the Sunrise Enabler and other methodological features. The reader is recommended to use this primary source and read publications that continue to use the theory. Hopefully someday soon all people from diverse or similar cultures will receive culturally congruent, responsible, and meaningful care worldwide that has largely been derived from the theory of Culture Care Diversity and Univerality or related theories.

Madeleine Leininger, PhD, LHD, DS, CTN, RN, FAAN, FRCNA
Author; Professor Emeritus of Nursing and Founder of Transcultural Nursing and Human Care Research
May 2002

Part

I

CULTURE CARE DIVERSITY AND UNIVERSALITY THEORY

PHILOSOPHIC, EPISTEMIC, AND OTHER DIMENSIONS OF THE THEORY

In this book, the author presents the philosophy, historical developments, nature, purpose, significance of the theory, along with the assumptive premises, major tenets, orientational definitions, Sunrise Model, and predictions with the theory of Culture Care Diversity and Universality. The evolutionary developments and refinements of the theory over nearly five decades provide insights about the need and importance of developing a relevant and comprehensive nursing theory with use worldwide. As one of the earliest theories in nursing designed to be used in Western and non-Western cultures, the theory is essential to advance nursing knowledge transculturally.

The theory focuses on describing, explaining, and predicting nursing similarities and differences focused primarily on human care and caring in human cultures. For nearly five decades, the theorist held that care is the essence of nursing and the central, dominant, and unifying focus of nursing. Accordingly, the theory of Culture Care was constructed to discover the universal and diverse features of care as the major and central component of nursing. This theory reflects a significant and bold new approach to establish knowledge for the discipline. The theory's relevance has grown more significant only as the world of nursing and health care becomes increasingly multicultural and nurses find it is imperative to understand the cultural values and lifeways of many different people. Moreover, nursing decisions and actions require such knowledge to serve people of diverse backgrounds in any typical day or night of work.

The first chapter has been written from the theorist's lived experiences and lifelong career in developing a theory that could be used worldwide. The theorist presents her creative efforts to develop a theory that was not culture-bound, narrow or ethnocentric, and one that could be used in all cultures to discover universal and diverse aspects of human care.[1] The reader will be presented with the major concepts, theoretical framework, the Sunrise Model, and the importance of the theory. The use of the worldview, social structure, language, ethnohistory, environmental context, and the generic and professional system is discussed to provide a comprehensive and holistic view of influencers in culture care and well being. The three modes of nursing decisions and actions focused on culture care preservation and/or maintenance, culture care accommodation and/or negotiation, and culture care repatterning and/or restructuring are presented to

3

show ways to provide culturally congruent care. In Part II, the ethnonursing method and eight major research studies are presented by
nurse researchers who have used the theory. These studies provide
valuable information of the use of the theory with the ethnonursing
method.

At the outset, the reader will discover that this theory is constructed
differently from traditional nursing theories and it moves beyond
nurse–client interaction or transactions to that of focusing on care for
families, groups, communities, cultures, and institutions. Although the
theorist developed and used the ethnonursing qualitative research
method to study the theory, the method remains open to other research methods to obtain the epistemics of nursing knowledge. The
Sunrise Model is the conceptual guide or the cognitive map to guide
nurses in the systematic study of all dimensions of the theory. Finally,
the theorist presents the importance of using qualitative criteria as
essential in examining a qualitative and inductively derived study as
ethnonursing. In Part III, the theorist shares her research findings of
culture-specific care constructs from a number of Western and non-
Western cultures. These findings are some of the "golden nuggets" of
part of the total findings from the use of a theory which can help
nurses realize that different cultures tend to have specific meanings,
expressions, and structures of care transculturally. Such knowledge is
essential to understand and guide the nurse in entering clients' worlds
and their normative expectations.

1

The Theory of Culture Care Diversity and Universality

Madeleine M. Leininger

What the people need most to grow, remain well, avoid illnesses and survive or to face death is human caring; Care is the essence of nursing and the distinct, dominant, central, and unifying, focus of nursing; Caring is the "heart and soul" of nursing and what people seek most from professional nurses and in health care services; Nurses are therefore challenged to gain knowledge about cultural care values, beliefs, and practices, and to use this knowledge to care for well and sick people; Cultural Care theory and the use of research findings from many different cultures constitutes the new challenge for nurses in providing meaningful and congruent care to people in the world. (selected excerpts from Leininger's writing and public addresses 1950–1991)

Over the past four decades, the above statements and other writings by Leininger have challenged nurses worldwide to reflect on the importance and centrality of human care to the discipline and profession of nursing. As such, care has become the essence and central focus

5

of nursing and a major theoretical and research interest for nurse scholars, clinicians, researchers, and other theoreticians in nursing. Although the uniqueness of nursing has long been care, it was not until the early 1960s that the phenomena was studied rigorously and systematically. Around 1978, a cadre of nurses became interested in care phenomena as revealed in the unfolding work of Bevis and Murray (1979), Gaut (1984), Larson (1987), Leininger (1978, 1980, 1984a,b, 1988a,b,c), Ray (1981), Reiman (1986), Roach (1984, 1987), and Watson (1985a). These nurses joined in the author's efforts to explicate care as the essence of nursing and to initiate the National Research Care Conferences.

It has been encouraging to find culture care a dominant topic with many nurses today who are interested in studying care. Such interest has led to a significant increase in the number of nursing articles on human care and caring phenomena. It also is encouraging to see the humanistic, scientific, ethical, and moral dimensions of human care become a major research focus for nursing after a long dormant period through the 1960s and 1970s. During that period, human caring had become largely invisible, devalued, and of limited interest with some researchers contending that care was a phenomena impossible to study and measure. Spearheading the systematic and rigorous study of care in the mid-1950s when "high-tech" was a predominant focus in nursing was extremely difficult. Yet through persistence and commitment, more nurses began to realize the importance of human care to nursing knowledge. As a result, nurses in the United States and other places in the world are now studying human care as essential to nursing knowledge, teaching, and curricular work, along with the focus on cultural care differences and similarities (Benner & Wrubel, 1989; Colliere, 1986; Gaut, 1981; Larson, 1987; Leininger, 1978, 1984a, 1988a; Ray, 1981, 1987; Roach, 1984; Watson, 1985a). This worldwide cultural movement is giving nurses new hope for establishing nursing's discipline knowledge and is providing for other nurses a renewed focus on nursing's traditional legitimacy as a true caring profession.

Especially important now to nurses worldwide who work with so many different people in so many different places and nursing circumstances is the theory of Culture Care. Our rapidly growing multicultural world makes it imperative that nurses understand different cultures to work and function effectively with people having different values, beliefs, and ideas about nursing, health, caring, wellness, illness, death, and disabilities. Nursing theories are ways to help nurses discover new perspectives and to use findings to advance nursing practice. The theory of Culture Care was developed particularly to discover the meanings and ways to give care to people who have different values and lifeways. It is a theory designed ultimately to guide nurses to provide nursing care that fits or is congruent with the people being helped. In this sense, Culture Care theory differs from theories that are focused on medical symptoms, disease entities, and treatments. Instead, the focus is on cultural care factors and ways people expect nursing care that is meaningful to them. As nurses feel or experience clients as culture strangers who show signs of frustration, confusion, anger, or of being misunderstood, the theory gains relevance. These indicators and others are clues that both nurses and clients of different cultures need to examine factors that influence their way of functioning together. The theory of Culture Care encourages nurses to study and discover these factors so that the client benefits from nursing services, and the nurse does not feel so helpless and ineffective with the culturally different.

DISCOVERING THE NEED FOR CULTURE CARE THEORY: AN EVOLUTIONARY DEVELOPMENT

When I first realized the need for culture care as essential to nursing practices in the mid-1940s, I was caring for several patients on a medical-surgical unit of a large general hospital as a staff nurse. During that time, the patients (term used in the 1940s) with a variety of health problems and medical treatments frequently made comments to the nurses on the unit such as: "It is you nurses that are helping me to get well"; "Nurses who give good care really can make the difference of how I feel and whether I get well or die"; "You give good care by listening, comforting, and talking to me, it helps me get well"; "I could have never left this hospital without your good nursing care"; "While I think the doctor's work is important, what nurses do is more important—I will always remember this." These patient statements and others made me realize that caring and nursing activities were extremely important to help people get well and to prevent illnesses and, possibly, death. I was a young graduate nurse, and these ideas expressed by patients were powerful incentives—they challenged me to focus on caring practices and to value what nurses do and how nurses can help the patient recover. Such caring values remained with me. I also could see differences among patients in the way they responded to the nurses and her caregiving practices. Such diversities and commonalities in the way nursing care was perceived by patients and nurses, and the differences in patient responses to nurses, signified, again, the importance of human care.

During the mid-1940s, high technologies were sparse and had not yet invaded our nursing lifeways and work environments. Nurses were busy caring for patients, and there were only a few medications and virtually no machines to monitor or tend. There were few assembly line procedures to prepare patients for laboratory tests, special surgeries, or high-tech therapies. Instead, the nurse functioned in the hospital at a regularized pace to give "good and complete nursing care to patients"—the recurrent phrase and its several variations then used in the large general hospital. Nurses were highly motivated and committed to comprehensive quality care and to make the patient as comfortable and satisfied as possible. It was the nurse's caring skills that seemed to be the focus of nursing. Nurses were expected to be compassionate caregivers and to give "total, complete, and comprehensive care to patients," including spiritual, family, and environmental care. There was a moral commitment "to get patients well and to keep them well."

For many nurses in the 1940s and 1950s, caring meant spending time with patients and listening to their narratives and feelings about themselves, their families, home life, and usually their work situations. There usually were signs of respect for patients as human beings and the nurse seemed proud to give "good care" by being attentive, compassionate, and empathic to their needs. Although the concept of humanistic care was not explicitly taught, there were role models and instructors who demonstrated human interest in and respect for patients as individuals and members of some family group. Humanistic care consisted of being fully attentive to the needs of patients and in giving consideration to their ethical, moral, spiritual (or religious) ideas, along with their psychophysical needs. The term *good nurse* and *good nursing care* embodied such humanistic ways of responding to and giving direct care to patients. It was an implicit expectation in clinical practices and demonstrated by humanistic instructors in the classroom and clinical settings.

Even when I did "private duty" (usually several times in the home each week and frequently in the hospital), there was always a normative cultural expectation to be humanistic, compassionate, and ethical in doing "what was best for the patient," and to be morally committed to helping the patient and his or her family. While some of these values derived from my own personal and family orientation, they also found support in my basic nursing education.

During my basic nursing education, I experienced excellent teachers and clinical nurses who demonstrated different ways to give "complete and comprehensive care." Head nurses, supervisors, and clinical instructors often gave feedback on the nursing practices used that came from their direct observations as well as from feedback they had received from clients and families. It was of interest, however, that while such nursing instructors and clinicians expected all nurses to give "good nursing care," they did not teach specific care principles or concepts about human care or caring. Care was a "taken-for-granted" expectation—what was seen and practiced in a favorable way was "good care." While nurses used their personal cultural values in concert with some professional values to give "good care," the very nature of such care remained obscure—it was not really known what helped patients get well. Being grounded in many fundamental principles about physical and emotional care still did not clarify care meanings and practices. In the pre-World War II days, nurses also were challenged to get patients well with their nursing skills and not to rely on "doctor's ideas of cure." Those nurses who demonstrated good nursing care were often rewarded by the staff with positive verbal feedback, new responsibilities, and recognition on the unit as an "excellent nurse" among peers. Receiving "gifts" from patients and family members, and occasionally from physicians who valued good nursing care, was appreciated by nurses as well.

During this time and earlier, before World War II, the nurses' role was largely patient-centered care; there were very few high-tech treatments and only a modest amount of pills to administer. Similarly, there were few clinical nursing research projects. In the absence of research-based nursing knowledge, nurses relied heavily on their experiences and on medical findings and book knowledge to help guide them in their services to patients. I recall a number of confident head nurses and supervisors who were competent caregivers but also quite authoritarian and who would reinforce to novices what they believed to be "good nursing care." Many of these head nurses and supervisors were ideal role models for care and you felt the strength of their words and actions. It also was interesting from my observations and experiences that many of these skilled and trusted head nurses and supervisors could make decisions and take actions without the physician's orders. Accordingly, physicians seemed to respect these nurses and trusted them to do what was best for "their patients." While the patriarchal behavior of physicians was clearly evident and women were supposed to serve them, still many of these strong-willed nursing leaders were directive enough to tell physicians how nurses were going to care for their patients on "their unit or wards." Thus, one felt free to give comfort care measures by listening and talking to patients while applying hot or cold packs on the patient or in selecting foods or drinks that nurses felt needed or preferred. Nurses also counseled, informed, and prescribed what nurses thought could get patients well and keep them healthy. I even delivered mothers as a staff nurse on an obstetrical unit because the mother did not want to wait for hours and endure pain while waiting for the physician to come and "drop the baby in the nurse's hands." Patients knew what nurses could do without physicians. Nurses "took hold" and were responsible for patient's care needs in the broadest sense and from a total care perspective. These nurses were respected by peers and patients and did not feel unduly constrained by most physicians or hospital authorities. Unfortunately, there was little research to document these exemplars of effective, competent, and humanistic nursing care practices, and the benefits to patients' satisfaction and recovery in America.

By the mid and late 1950s and after high technology entered the nursing and hospital world, nursing practices began to change. Nurses soon began to handle many new medications and to administer high-tech treatments under physicians' orders. Nurses spent much time on pouring, measuring, counting, and giving various medications and treatments. More and more, nurses became absorbed in physicians' medical treatments, expectations, and orders. It was of concern to see nurses, who had formerly practiced "good caring," relinquish such caring practices to meet prevailing high-technology and physician demands. Nurses even began to emulate physicians wearing stethoscope and other medical symbols as they become "hooked on" giving new medicines and treatment regimes and watching patients' behavior. As efficiency in giving high-tech treatments, new medicines, and nursing practices gained in prestige, a "cult of efficiency" in nursing took hold without many nurses realizing what had happened. As nurses faithfully and assiduously carried out physicians' orders and medical treatments, they became referred to as "faithful servants," "doers," and "hand-maidens" to physicians. This unfortunate nomenclature persisted until the mid-1970s, continuing even in some places today, until the feminist movement rose to the challenge (Ashley 1976; Kalisch & Kalisch, 1987; Leininger, 1970, 1978).

In general, then, before pre-feminist days and after World War II, nurses devoted most of their time to the classroom and nursing laboratories or units learning how to handle equipment, administer complex treatments, and handle procedures effectively and efficiently. By their strong emulation of physicians, both in practice and appearance, and by taking their cues largely from physicians and hospital administrators, American nurses became less self-directed (Leininger, 1970). In fact, with the burgeoning of medical curing ideologies and practices, the cultural values and art of human care suffered in many high-tech centers to the point of vanishing (Leininger, 1976, 1981).

Having lived through the early and intense eras previous to the introduction of high technology, and as I traveled across America making consultation visits and public addresses, I saw nursing changing significantly. While nurses' recognition for their work and autonomy was evident in hospitals, physicians maintained control of all else, and the strong caring practices of the pre-1950s era seemed to fade away. In the 1960s and early 1970s as well, some nurses stayed at home to raise their children as a felt moral obligation; others were employed in a career trajectory. In the hospital setting, some nurses functioned like "mini" physicians; some nurses were enticed to become "medexs" or physician assistants and work for physicians. Nurses strived to provide "productive," "efficient," and high-tech care and be part of the cult of hospital efficiencies. But where was nursing's moral commitment to practice humanistic care?

Unquestionably, during the intense high-tech era of the 1960s and 1970s, there were some nurses who were deeply committed to humanistic caring. It was this core of nurses who helped to revive and bring care back again into nursing, and at the same time advance the knowledge, art, and science of caring (Bevis & Murray, 1979; Leininger, 1970, 1976 a,b,c, 1984a, 1988a; Ray, 1981, 1987; Reiman, 1986; Roach, 1987; Watson, 1979, 1985 a,b). I well remember a number of public addresses I gave then on the importance of human caring, stressing that caring was the heart of nursing and its unique focus as well as the need for transcultural nursing care concepts and principles. However, while there were older nurses who expressed great interest in this, there were younger nurses who expressed concern about focusing on care. Several of the younger nurses even feared talking about care as the essence of nursing; care was too *feminine*. In fact, I was admonished by some nurses not to talk about care as the essence and central phenomena of nursing; it was far "too negative" an idea for the public to actually think about nursing. Care, for these nurses, was "too soft and feminine," "nonscientific," and would encounter major obstacles in gaining acceptance by nurses and the public. To these nurses, all of whom were women, caring either was too frightening or was simply an ideal whose time had passed. To have nurses reject, devalue, and view care as demeaning for nursing, a domestic lay service, surprised me. Somehow these nurses did not want me to stress care as central to nursing because they believed it would foster a negative image for female nurses and the nursing profession.

As these nurses shared their views, they felt caring had no economic values or gains. They could see many positive images of male physicians as powerful "curers" by ordering treatments and presenting the public with high-tech treatments and cures, as well as making economic gains. These nurses, however, felt "it would be better for nurses to be skilled in the management of medical diseases, symptoms, medications, and treatments, than be a carer." Such comments and others reflected that nurses valued curing rather than caring. They saw very limited public, economic, and professional gains from focusing on care when dramatic cures with high technologies, diagnostic procedures, and treatment regimes reigned in the public image of health services. Rather than express care, they wanted to "ride in on and get some share" of the physicians' positive public image of curing people (Leininger 1970, 1978, 1981). Unquestionably, the dominant cultural values of cure prevailed in nursing with limited perceived benefits in prestige, status, or economic gains from focusing on human caring. Federal money allocations and positive public feedback was focused on great medical achievements and dramatic cures. With many nurses identifying with medical cultural values, normative expectations, and practices, caring was viewed as women's negative work. Caring for children at home and caring for patients in the hospital was "too close for comfort" as domestic labor for medically focused female nurses. With physician patriarchal dominance prevailing perhaps as it never had before, nurses worked not only *for* physicians but *like* them (Ashley 1976; Leininger 1970, 1981).

From 1950 to the late 1970s, nursing education also took its cue from the dominant physician model. Nursing textbooks grew in size and came to resemble medical textbooks. This was especially evident with medical-surgical texts that contained many kinds of medical diseases, symptoms, and treatments. Content on care or caring often was limited to a few paragraphs shuffled to the final, concluding pages where "nursing implications" or "nursing care aspects" were discussed. In this period, *care* and *caring* often were used as cliches in texts and articles. There was limited focus on explicating the meanings, expressions, and patterns of care to the patient or the nurse (Gaut, 1981; Leininger, 1981). There were very few articles and no nursing textbooks explicitly focused on the subject of human care and nursing until the late 1970s and into the 1980s. Most nurse authors generally discussed medical, surgical, psychiatric, and related medical content to help nursing students learn symptoms, diseases, and treatments of diseases. The use of medical knowledge with the phrase "nursing care" seemed to legitimize nursing.

It was, therefore, a major challenge to keep nurses interested in and focused on examining nursing care phenomena for new knowledge until the human caring cultural movement began to take hold in the mid-1970s. I often felt I was working alone and at odds with nurses who held the dominant medical ethos over that of nursing. It was discouraging to see the lack of interest of nurses in care. Nonetheless, there were some nurses of the 1950s who were still hopeful that nurses would focus on care knowledge and develop creative nursing care practices. They were the backup supporters for a "lost generation" of nurses (post-1960s) who had never been taught or barely seen humanistic care practices in nursing. However, to revitalize human caring required more spirited care leaders. With nurses of the 1960s becoming so wed to medical treatment values, care, as a nursing value in and of itself, seemed to fall by the wayside.

DEVELOPING TRANSCULTURAL NURSING
AND CULTURE CARE

The idea of transcultural nursing, the theory of Culture Care, and preserving care as the essence of nursing developed together in the mid-1950s and early 1960s. The close interrelationship of establishing transcultural nursing as a new field of study and practice with a theory to generate knowledge for the field were congruent goals. It was in the mid-1950s while working with disturbed children as a child psychiatric mental health nurse that I discovered the importance of culture in the care of children of different cultural backgrounds (Leininger, 1970, 1978). The behavior and nursing care needs of African, Jewish, Appalachian, German, and Anglo-American children were clearly different except for some physical care needs. In a way, I experienced cultural shock and I felt helpless to assist children who so clearly expressed different cultural patterns and ways they wanted care. These cultural differences were related to playing, eating, sleeping, interaction, and many other areas of their daily care. The children were so expressive and persistent in what they wanted or needed, yet I was unable to respond appropriately to them—I did not understand their behavior. Later, I came to learn that their behavior was culturally constituted and influenced their mental health. Even though I was knowledgeable about psychotherapy and mental health nursing, this was not sufficient to understand and help these children. In addition, the available psychotherapies seemed inappropriate for them.

My curiosity and lack of knowledge of the role cultural factors played in mental and physical health led me to study anthropology, and, later, to develop the field of transcultural nursing with a comparative care focus. Since I had no courses or preparation in anthropology in my nursing program, I soon discovered that anthropology was the discipline primarily focused on human cultures worldwide. This led me to pursue a six-year graduate program in cultural, social, and physical anthropology and to do first-hand field research in New Guinea in the early 1960s. During that time, I found anthropology was fascinating and extremely relevant to nursing, which also focused on people and human conditions. I was shocked why nurses had not been required to study anthropology with the same vigor they studied chemistry, microbiology, anatomy, physiology, and psychology courses.

Clearly, anthropological knowledge was a huge, missing knowledge domain of nursing. The more I studied anthropology, the more I could see the relevance of anthropology to nursing. This led to the first transcultural nursing book, *Nursing and Anthropology: Two Worlds to Blend* (Leininger, 1970). Thinking through the differences and similarities between nursing and anthropology, I became more convinced of their close relationship, the need for the field of transcultural nursing, and for my evolving theory of Culture Care Diversity and Universality (Leininger, 1965, 1966, 1967, 1970). But tremendous leadership work was needed to awaken nurses first to become aware of the concept of culture and then to link this concept with nursing. With no graduate professional nurses prepared in graduate programs in anthropology, however, the idea of bringing anthropological insights to nursing and of developing a Culture Care theory, seemed an almost impossible task. Simply, there were no nurses who had taken steps or interest in conceptualizing the actual or potential relationship between anthropology and nursing in the 1950s. Against such odds, I decided the best way to get nurses to think about linkages between anthropology and nursing would be to establish the field of transcultural nursing (Leininger, 1965, 1966, 1967, 1970, 1978). I predicted that nurses would be unable to provide meaningful, therapeutic quality care, or holistic care, without the inclusion of culturally based transcultural nursing knowledge and skills. Initially quite alone in my efforts and aspirations, I began the long, difficult journey of developing the field of transcultural nursing care to clients. The great challenge also was before me to continue to develop the Culture Care theory that I had envisioned and to help nurses discover new knowledge and different perspectives of nursing (Leininger, 1967, 1969a,b, 1970, 1974, 1976a,b,c, 1978, 1979).

Initially, after formulating and disseminating some theoretical ideas and hunches related to Culture Care theory, there were still very few nurses interested in "such a strange idea in nursing." The idea of linking care to culture to generate substantive knowledge for the discipline of nursing also suffered the same fate. Committed as I was to knowledge development in nursing and to establish the new field of transcultural nursing, I realized that nurses relied too heavily on biophysical and psychological explanations with virtually no awareness of how culture could influence nursing and care. I was troubled that nursing education and clinical practices were too narrow and largely uniculturally focused. In the pre-1950s and during the early 1960s, culture content with a nursing perspective and very little care content in nursing curricula existed. Transcultural nursing and Culture Care theory were missing to establish any relevant discipline and knowledge for nursing's future, which would certainly be multicultural; nurses working with many people from many different foreign cultures within their homeland and overseas. Clearly, nurses without preparation in transcultural nursing would be greatly handicapped when working with people of diverse cultures. My keen sense of urgency increased as I saw more glaring problems in clinical settings related to nurses trying to help culture strangers using the uniculturally focused nursing education provided them. There were some schools of nursing orienting foreign nurses to function in our American hospitals for employment purposes but with no formal programs or culture care courses. Additional concerns of the state of international exposure in those early days I have presented elsewhere (Leininger, 1970, 1978, 1979). What concerned me most was that the world was moving much more rapidly towards multiculturalism than the profession realized and nurses needed cultural knowledge and a theory to build nursing knowledge to guide nursing practices.

However, it was not long before I realized that a theory of Culture Care would have limited meaning and would be misunderstood unless there were nurses prepared in transcultural nursing. As a result, in the mid-1960s, I began to develop and establish transcultural nursing courses, and later several programs of study in the new field. I also encouraged nurses to take foundational courses in anthropology in a way similar to those of anatomy and physiology which supported, for example, physiological or cardiovascular nursing. Although only very few nurses were initially interested in the new field, by the early 1970s I had enticed many nurses into studying anthropology and transcultural nursing as vital and relevant to nursing in its entirety. From 1960 to 1974, I encouraged approximately 45 nurses to take graduate courses (several took doctorates) in anthropology, and many nurses enrolled in my transcultural courses. This cadre of nurses thus helped to establish and support the new field.

By the mid-1970s, the idea of transcultural nursing had gradually taken a firm hold. Writings, public addresses, workshops, conferences, and personal contacts with nurses worldwide facilitated this development. Nurses gradually became intrigued with the idea of the theory of Culture Care as a central focus to transcultural nursing. Some early supporters, students, and leaders included Aamodt, Boyle, DeSantis, Glittenberg, Horn, Morse, Osborne, Ray, and Reiman. Later, of course, there were many nurses who became interested not only in transcultural nursing, but also in the theory.

Publishing a book on the theory itself was another matter, however, and I deliberately held back from that endeavor. Until many more nurses were prepared in transcultural nursing, fundamental misunderstandings were bound to occur. There was still another reason for holding back. During the pre-1975 era, most nurses were deeply involved in professional identity issues, revising nursing curricula, dealing with rapid technological advances, and nurse–physician issues and relationships. Nearly two decades passed before the theory of Culture Care within transcultural nursing seemed ready to be valued and used by nurses. Several workshops and annual summer courses helped to generate interest in the theory and the new field. In addition, in 1968 I initiated and established with the assistance of Hazel Weidman the Committee on Nursing and Anthropology (CONA) through the American Anthropological Association to help nurses and anthropologists communicate ideas and research between the two fields (Leininger, 1967, 1970, 1978). In 1973, I established the Transcultural Nursing Society as a national and international organization for nurses interested in transcultural nursing and human care to share their research and other experiences together. This organization has grown through the years with annual scholarly conventions, and has become a central means for transcultural nurse researchers, teachers, and clinicians to share their ideas. It has been invaluable to discuss research related to the theory of Culture Care, and to share transcultural research findings. In 1978, I initiated with ten colleagues the National Research Care Conferences to stimulate nurses to focus *explicitly on human care* as the central phenomenon of nursing, encouraging nurses to study care from their particular interests. In 1988, this organization had grown considerably and was renamed the International Association of Human Caring with growing worldwide membership. These organizations were all extremely important means to encourage scholarly exchange of ideas, and stimulate research on transcultural nursing with the use of Culture Care theory at annual conferences (Leininger, 1970, 1978, 1981, 1984a,b,c, 1991).

THEORY DEVELOPMENT: AN ENIGMA IN NURSING IN THE EARLY DAYS

In the early 1960s, the idea of developing a Culture Care theory in nursing appeared enigmatic to most nurses. With only few nurse leaders interested in the theory, many other nurses were as reluctant to talk about nursing theory itself. Theories were viewed as "ivory-tower talk," "very impractical," "useless," "irrelevant," and a "waste of time" (Leininger, 1970). In the 1950s and 1960s, the culture of nursing was so strongly oriented to the practical, mundane, and concrete medical or nursing activities that most nurses were generally not interested in nursing theories. It was far more important to teach nursing students about medical diseases, symptoms, and treatments, and to remain "practical in all you did." At most state, national, and international meetings, there was limited interest in nursing theories and virtually no discussions about theories until the mid-1960s and later in the 1970s. Thus it was difficult to attract nurses to consider the idea of nursing theories, let alone a culturally based theory.

Amid this awareness of a lack of interest in theories, I was aware of Nightingale's (1859) ideas on health, the individual, and physical environment, and of Peplau's (1952) pioneering book on interpersonal relationships in psychiatric nursing. Both Nightingale's and Peplau's ideas were important to support theoretical perspectives but were not developed as formal nursing theory. Likewise, Orlando (1961) had written about dynamic nurse–patient relationships and nursing situations, but had not developed her ideas as a theory of nursing. Henderson (1966) had expressed a definition of the nature of nursing, but again, this definition did not constitute a formal theory of nursing. In the mid-1950s, I had coauthored with Hofling (1960) a book entitled *Psychiatric Concepts in Nursing*, which focused on nurse–client therapeutic relationships, therapeutic milieu, and some ideas about nurse caring behaviors. This book was published in 11 languages and used in many countries, but I did not present my ideas about human care and the evolving theory, nor my specific ideas on transcultural nursing, because my coauthor viewed these ideas as "far too advanced for nurses and health personnel in the field, and too premature." Because of such concerns, I withheld my budding new theoretical ideas. Finding no publishers interested in the idea of transcultural nursing or in the theory of Culture Care in those early days also was cause for the delay in sharing my work.

In the mid-1960s, the nurse scientist (PhD) programs for nurses were being established. I took an active leadership role in helping to develop and implement some of these doctoral programs (Leininger, 1976). Retrospectively, some of these programs were important to help nurse scholars gain knowledge of how to develop and analyze formal and informal theories, and ways to conduct systematic research viewed from the many years of experienced scholars, theoreticians, and researchers in other well-established disciplines. Graduates of several of these programs that I mentored attest to how it helped them to become competent theorists, researchers, and scholars in nursing. As director of two of these major early doctoral programs, I found that the programs most successful in developing strong theorists and researchers in nursing were those in which the students had mentors and seminars *in nursing* that were taken concomitantly with their discipline seminars (Leininger, 1974). Several graduates of the nurse-scientist programs gave much support and encouragement for the theory of Culture Care, especially those studying in anthropology with nursing seminars.

Another significant influence to support nursing theories was the movement of nursing education into institutions of higher education. It was just such courses in philosophy, the humanities, and social sciences that liberated nurses' thinking from a tight nursing and logical positivism stance to different ways of discovering and developing ideas. Nurse theorists needed such courses to help them expand their ideas and develop their own philosophical and theoretical perspectives of nursing. It also helped nurses to identify and reflect on major phenomena that could uniquely characterize and legitimize a discipline of nursing and its evolving knowledge and perspectives. In this era, with courses in different disciplines, I philosophized about questions such as: How could human care become central to nursing as a discipline? How could nurses know fully and preserve the nature and meanings of care to people of diverse cultures in the world? What research methods could appropriately be used to explicate the meanings, experiences, and structure of human care to individuals and groups as well as to nurses without reducing the ideas to reductionistic findings, or meaningless numbers treated with statistics? From my field research and doctoral seminars in anthropology, I became aware of the importance of these questions and of the value of qualitative research methods such as ethnography, ethnoscience, ethnology, and other naturalistic methods to discover, in part, these philosophical research questions. I was excited about the idea of naturalistic inquiry and people-centered perspectives to generating theory by inductive methods and to studying multiple factors influencing nursing. This is when I decided to develop the ethnonursing research method as a nursing method to study transcultural human care and other nursing phenomena (see Chapter 2). Again, and along with my own nursing perspectives, several philosophy, social science, and humanities courses helped me to focus and develop ideas related to the theory of Culture Care.

INFLUENCES ON THE THEORY: PERSONAL, PHILOSOPHIC, SOCIOCULTURAL, AND OTHERS

In developing the theory of Culture Care, I am frequently asked what nurses, persons, or ideologies influenced my thinking. I would have to answer, rather candidly, that there was no one person or philosophic school of thought, or ideology *per se* that directly influenced my thinking. I developed the theory by working on the potential interrelationships of *culture* and *care* through creative thinking, and by philosophizing from my past professional nursing experiences and anthropological insights. I pondered on the future of nursing as a discipline, with its distinctive knowledge, and by being a critic of my own thinking and reflections based on extensive readings of the domain of interest to me.

Reading on theories and theoretical perspectives from anthropology and other social sciences, philosophy, and nursing greatly stimulated my thinking about the care theory. Although I had no one person who worked directly or continuously with me as a mentor or peer colleague, there were some outstanding scholars in anthropology, philosophy, and some in nursing whose critical thinking was helpful. Several anthropologists in the Department of Anthropology at the University of Washington, such as Professors Fogelson, Spiro, Read, Watson, and Jacobs, stimulated me to theorize and do self-critiques of initial ideas related to nursing and anthropology (Leininger, 1970). I would add that Margaret Mead, as a visiting professor and woman scholar in the Department of Psychiatry at the University of Cincinnati in the late 1950s, also stimulated my thinking with her keen intellectual abilities, profound cultural knowledge, and with her feminine leadership and role modeling. I remember asking her if she saw any relationship of nursing to anthropology and theoretical notions. She replied: "Well, that is something for you to discover." In those early days, there were no outstanding nurse scholars who directly influenced my thinking related to the development of the Culture Care theory. But as dean and professor of the School of Nursing (1969–1975) at the University of Washington, I always enjoyed my frequent informal scholarly dialogues with faculty and students, but especially with Dorothy Crowley, Oliver Osborne, Delores Little, Beverly Horn, and others, while initiating some major changes in the school's philosophy, curriculum, and organizational structure.

My philosophical interests and conceptual orientations for the theory of Culture Care were primarily derived from a holistic nursing and anthropological perspective of human beings living in different places and contexts. I drew on both anthropological and nursing insights (including clinical experiences) as I conceptualized and developed the theory. My philosophical interests for the theory enthusiastically unfolded as I began to envision a different way for nurses to understand and work with people in the world. I was committed to expanding nurses' limited worldview and knowledge of cultural groups to a worldwide perspective, and to focusing on care as uniquely nursing and culturally constituted. As a nurse futurist, I could envision nursing being quite different in the twenty-first century because of worldwide changes that would bring people closer to each other due to the social, cultural, political, economic, health care, and technological forces at hand. Nursing, I predicted, would be intensely multicultural, and nursing's distinct body of knowledge and contributions to the world would be fulfilled through the use of Culture Care theory leading to a body of transcultural nursing knowledge as the most reliable and meaningful epistemic base of nursing's future as a discipline and profession. In the

1950s, with only a few scholars and futurists in nursing, nursing was far from this perspective. While developing transcultural care theory was a dream, it also seemed relevant to what was happening in the world. Nursing also needed to move from its long dependency on medicine and come into its own as a recognized and legitimate discipline with a unique body of knowledge.

How to move nursing into a humanistic or scientific cultural caring perspective, and to have culture care as the central focus to explain and interpret nursing was a tall order of the day. Human care with a trans-cultural focus had to be systematically studied with a comparative and interpretive focus to help people regain their wellness and to prevent unnecessary illnesses. The explication and discovering of dominant features, nature, and essence of nursing for the epistemic and ontologic bases of nursing needed to be done. I felt that nursing also needed to transcend its primary focus on nurse–patient interactions and dyads to that of conceptualizing nursing as a caring science that could focus on families, groups, communities, total cultures, and institutions. The one-to-one nurse–client relationship perspective had been the major focus of nursing for many decades. There was a critical need to use another perspective to study how communities, cultures, and culture institutions influence or impact on the individual in regard to human care, health, and well being—thus providing rich insights and more predictive findings than when relying solely on dyad relationships. The social sciences and humanities helped me to transcend individualism to think about worldviews, social-cultural institutions, ethnohistory, environmental contexts, and language uses bearing on Culture Care theory and nursing. In those days, however, this was a "too futuristic and impractical" way and too different to be relevant to nursing.

Most assuredly, a body of transcultural knowledge had yet to be envisioned by nurses. In the 1960s, nurses were mainly thinking about and studying particularistic phenomena such as cells, body systems, biophysical functioning systems, mental illnesses, and interpersonal relationships. It was actually this latter narrow view of psychiatric mental health that led me to study cultural phenomena, as culture factors in mental health illness did not exist in psychiatric nursing. In 1973, in my effort to expand nurses' views on culture, I published *Contemporary Issues in Mental Health*, one of the first books on culture factors in mental health. Helping nurses to look at subcultures and societies trying to keep people well by some caring patterns, norms, and practices was important. This philosophic perspective, along with seeing individuals being influenced by social structure factors, was a further challenge for nurses and theory development.

Nurses needed not only a holistic "biopsychosociocultural" view but also a comparative view of cultural differences and similarities as they worked with people in different environmental contexts, and this idea needed to be included in the theory. Most importantly, I did not conceptualize culture care as a compartmentalized or fragmented idea with separate physical, biological, psychological, social, or cultural perspectives. Instead, I theorized culture and human care as a holistic and unified perspective to reflect individuals or groups total caring lifeways or influencers on their well being or illness. Important broad dimensions that needed to be considered by nurses for a full holistic view of people included: worldview; biophysical state; religious (or spiritual) orientation; kinship patterns; material (and nonmaterial) cultural phenomena; the political, economic, legal, educational, technological, and physical environment; language; and folk and professional care practices (Leininger, 1976b, 1978). I conceptualized this holistic stance to reflect human functioning and caring existence in any culture. To know and understand people in their total lifeways and functioning was held important to the theory of Culture Care. To avoid choosing a particular school of thought from psychobiology, anthropology, or nursing, I selectively drew on ideas from anthropology and from nursing with respect to theoretical perspectives about culture and care.

THEORETICAL FRAMEWORK: CONCEPTUALIZING AND DEVELOPING THE THEORY

To develop the theoretical-conceptual framework of the theory of Culture Care, I used selected culture constructs from an anthropological perspective and care constructs from a nursing perspective.[2] These two major constructs were conceptualized as being very broad, integrated, embedded, and nestled into each other like an irreducible whole, a gestalt, or a humanistic orientation to life and living. I envisioned that care was culturally constituted in every culture. All human cultures had some forms, patterns, expressions, and structures of care to know, explain, and predict well being, health, or illness status (Leininger, 1967, 1969a,b, 1976a,b,c, 1978). I held that care was not an isolated activity or act, but was an abstract intellectual phenomenon that connoted more than any isolated activity or act. For a sound epistemic and science of care/caring, I held that *generic* and *professional* care dimensions needed to be fully discovered. The conceptualization of *culture care* as a theoretic phenomenon had to be discovered in its fullest dimensions, and with focus on embedded knowledge dimensions related to nursing.

The scope and broad unifying perspectives of culture with its many definitions by anthropologists also had to be reconceptualized into nursing as meaningful patterned modes that are learned and shared intergenerationally. Culture and care were synthesized as a construct entity that are tightly embedded into each other in order to explain, interpret, and predict phenomena relevant to nursing. Thus culture care was conceptualized and transformed into a nursing perspective to develop a body of new or distinct knowledge in nursing.

The theory of Culture Care, therefore, was not "borrowed" from anthropology, but developed anew and had to be studied within nursing views to discover the epistemic and ontological dimensions of knowledge predicted to influence well being and health. This was a different way of knowing nursing, and a different way to discover nursing knowledge (Brunner, 1962). While the roots of culture were from anthropology and care largely from nursing, a new theoretic perspective was developed to discover knowledge to serve mainly the discipline of nursing (Leininger, 1967, 1970, 1976a, 1978, 1979, 1980, 1981, 1985a, 1988b,c).

While the theory has some features of Walker and Avant's (1983) concept derivation and syntheses, it does not fit well in either of these categories. Nor does Walker and Avant's (1983) levels of theory development and phases of development fit with my theory conceptualization and development. These differences exist largely because the theory was conceptualized within the qualitative discovery paradigm with largely inductive *emic* (people-centered) views and not from the researcher's *a priori* hypotheses. This was a different way to develop a theory than with conventional theories based on logical positivist thinking within the quantitative paradigm and its purposes and goals (Chinn, 1983; Fawcett, 1989; Walker & Avant, 1983). Qualitative inductive theory construction with naturalistic *emic* focus was new to nursing, as most nurse theorists have relied on hypodeductive logical positivism and specific ways to construct or develop theory. It is important to clarify this stance because many nursing students may be led to believe that every theory needs to fit certain prescribed conceptualizations, developmental processes, criteria, rules, and performance models to be a legitimate or "sound" nursing theory. The more one studies theory development from different disciplines and different views, however, the more one discerns considerable creativity and variability in the way theorists can develop and analyze theories. Still, a theory must be able to describe, explain, interpret, and predict certain phenomenon under study.

It may be difficult for students of nursing to realize that, prior to the 1960s, most nurses were not interested in nursing theories or in the idea of developing nursing as a discipline. In contrast, anthropologists, sociologists, psychologists, and so on developed mini and maxi theories and pondered on theoretical hunches, questions, and predictive statements to guide their research in the diligent pursuit for "credible truths" or substantiative knowledge. It is well known that any legitimate discipline has distinct subject matter domains and relative boundaries that are fairly constant but also able to change over time due to a variety of major factors. In the 1950s, when I found that nursing had not declared or claimed any specific focus, I decided to focus on culture care phenomena as a major domain of inquiry to guide future nursing research for the discipline. In addition, I believed that nursing as a profession had a societal charge, a mandate, and a moral expectation to serve society in meaningful and explicit public ways—the same criteria established by other professional scholars of what constituted a profession.

Given the commitment of nursing as a profession, and less reaffirmed as a discipline in the 1950s, it was difficult to imagine how nurses might value discovering transcultural care knowledge for the discipline of nursing and professional knowledge for a societal practice goal. The former could lead to intellectual insights as a discipline that may or may not have direct practice implications as a profession. This reality was supported and was in accord with other disciplines that had profession goals (McGlothlin, 1960; Parson, 1939). Culture care knowledge I held as greatly needed to guide nursing practices, but this knowledge might also serve other disciplines and professions. It was exciting to think that nursing could one day have a body of knowledge to guide practice, but it was also encouraging to think nursing's knowledge could be used by other disciplines. (Parenthetically, this goal conceived in the 1950s is being realized in 1991 as students of other disciplines attend nursing classes today to learn about and use culture care knowledge.)

As I deliberated on culture care, I knew it would be doubtful if nurses would accept and value the idea as central to nursing. Care, we must remember, was not valued as important as high technology at the time. I also questioned if nurses worldwide would accept human or culture care as central to nursing and a unique contribution to humanity due to the heavy emphases worldwide on medical diseases, dealing with medical symptoms, and curing psychopathological conditions. Nonetheless, I felt that if nurses would struggle to explicate and document culture care, nursing would gain a rich and sound base to establish itself as a discipline and profession.

Furthermore, I envisioned the possibility of discovering culture care diversities and universalities. While this was very ambitious theorizing for nursing in the early 1960s, I knew that nursing's myopic view of the world would be broadened and deepened considerably by the theory. I conceptualized nursing as a transcultural human care discipline and profession, and that caring was a universal feature of nursing in all nursing cultures. Human care was held to vary transculturally in meanings, expressions, patterns, symbols, and in other ways. Human care was seen as a universal nursing phenomena, but also with diverse possibilities. With this idea of universal and yet diverse features, in 1960 I searched the anthropological literature in vain; culture care had not been studied by anthropologists. No specific focus on human care or culture caring existed. Human care phenomenon was for nursing to discover.

My anthropological perspective of different cultures helped me to philosophize and to raise transcultural culture care questions, such as:

1. What evidences or expressions of human care existed in prehistorical and modern times?

2. What material or nonmaterial evidences of human care or caring might have existed in the long pre-history record of *homo sapiens*?

3. What human care acts, judgments, or attitudes might have been the major mechanism or explanation for the survival of human beings over time, and from birth to death?

4. Could care be a uniquely human expression belonging only to *homo sapiens?*

5. If care was crucial to human beings for growth, well being, or survival, what meanings and practices were universal and what were diverse among cultures?

6. What were the earliest cultural care expressions, meanings, symbols, functions, rituals, and structures of human caring for specific cultures and how have they changed over time?

7. What care differences or similarities existed transculturally for families, groups, tribes, clans, or other types of human groups and institutions?

8. Was human caring specifically linked to females or males, and if so, what would explain gender differences?

9. In the long history of *homo sapiens,* what was the role of human caregivers and care receivers in different cultures or subcultures and their contexts to facilitate birthing, keep people well, help in sickness or disabilities, or when dying?

10. If human care has been essential to survival of the human race, what is known about care as essential for survival in different cultures?

11. What cultural care values and characteristics have been most evident in the past and today to show how cultural care modalities, symbols, or acts help people to develop and survive in diverse geographic areas or ecologies and in different environmental contexts?

12. What forms of care norms, values, beliefs or practices existed in the pre-history of humans and in early nursing eras?

Most importantly, I was particularly interested to discover how social structure factors such as kinship, politics, religion, legal, technologic, and other specific cultural values influenced or structured care practices of human societies. These weighty philosophical questions made me realize how much there was yet to discover about *universal* and *diverse* features, forms, expressions, structures, and functions of care transculturally.

Some of the more specific questions that I initially raised from a nursing perspective included:

1. What were the ethnohistorical evidences of human care and caring *before* modern nursing or the Nightingale era?
2. Who were the caretakers of the sick, disabled, or well people long before the mid-nineteenth century?
3. How did the pre-Nightingale caregivers or (non-carers) influence today's nursing?
4. What has been universal or diverse about culture care in traditional and modern nursing?
5. What evidence prevails today that knowledgeable and skilled culture care leads to well being, health, or ameliorates the dying experience?
6. What are the meanings, expressions, patterns, and forms of culture care with different and similar cultures?
7. What evidence of caring and non-caring from clients and nurses prevail in different health contexts today?

These philosophical questions and others were, in part, the springboard for developing the theory of Culture Care. Not yet researched before the 1960s, many of these epistemic questions remain unexplored today.

The theoretical position of ultimately discovering in nursing what was universal or that which commonly existed and could be identifiable about human care in all or most cultures worldwide seemed critical if nursing was to be a global or universal profession and discipline. At the same time, it was natural to theorize about the diversities of human care to explain the differences that might prevail within and among cultures. It also was possible to predict that if care existed transculturally, there undoubtedly would be some diverse forms, expressions, structures, patterns, functions, symbols, and rituals that existed among and between cultures. What might explain the diversities or differences as well as the universalities about human care transculturally? The term *transcultural* was deliberately chosen rather than international, as the former referred to across all world cultures, whether a nation or not; whereas international referred to between two nationalized cultures. From a social science position, these definitions were extremely important to recognize and especially since nursing had used the term international, that is, International Council of Nursing. The term universality also was used in the qualitative paradigm to refer to common prevailing patterns within or among cultures and was not conceived in an absolute, statistical, or numerically significant way. Universality was viewed as a dominant commonality, patterned mode (or value), and/or prevailing care patterns seen within the new qualitative naturalistic paradigm that was barely known in the 1960s, and is still slowly emerging in nursing today.

Transcultural nursing had already been conceived as a comparative field of study and practice, but it needed (as did all aspects of nursing) a theoretical and research base to explain and predict nursing as a discipline and to guide nursing practice. The theory of Culture Care Diversity and Universality was viewed as the major theory to explain much of the phenomena related to transcultural nursing, accounting for diverse and similar cultures in the world (Leininger, 1973c, 1977, 1978, 1979, 1983). The idea of caring to serve people worldwide and to help ameliorate and improve human conditions and lifeways was an important direction. It was exciting to think that professional nurses would provide specific care so that healthy patterns, processes, and lifeways could be established and maintained, enabling individuals and groups to function and live through caring.

In considering the theory of Culture Care, I was interested further in explicating culture care from a humanistic viewpoint and in considering what would constitute scientific caring in nursing. Primarily, I viewed caring as a humanistic mode of being with others to assist them in times of need or to help them maintain their well being or health. I believed that caring activities and processes could lead to cure, but especially to healing human ills or conditions (Leininger, 1981). Humanistic expression of compassion, touching, comforting, assisting, supporting, and many other care constructs needed to be fully discovered inductively and understood in diverse naturalistic environmental contexts. I was concerned that these humanistic care expressions could be easily overlooked, devalued, or misinterpreted. Or, if studied from a logical positivist perspective with a statistical or measurement view, these care features would be reduced to numbers without meanings and especially in deductive theory development. I held to the sayings: "You do not have to measure everything to know it" and "You don't have to study everything from a logical positivist position." These two refrains often sustained me and other nurse researchers while developing and using purely qualitative research methods such as ethnonursing, ethnography, phenomenology, and others. At the same time, I was interested in what "scientific care" would mean and what kind of care this would constitute. The term *scientific* almost automatically led to the idea of care derived from the scientific method paradigm. I viewed nursing from both humanistic and scientific dimensions—to keep these lines of thinking open—until proven otherwise. They were used to guide my general thinking with these orientational definitions as I developed the theory (Leininger, 1978, 1981):

> Humanistic care (caring) *referred to understanding and knowing human beings in as natural or as human a way as possible, and to being with them in an assistive, helping, guiding or enabling way to help them achieve certain goals, improve, or ameliorate a human condition or lifeway, face disability, or to assist with dying. The goal of a humanistic care (caring) theory is to gain full understanding of human beings and their humanity, largely through inductive discoveries. In contrast, I viewed* scientific care (caring) *as referring to those precise, deductively predefined, logical, and measurable indicators identified to assist people using specifically controlled and manipulated variables to test rigorously overt care expressions.*

I believed these were two different approaches to care knowledge using different research paradigms. While both were important to nursing, I saw the urgent need for care knowledge to be derived inductively. I believed it was important to "tease out" covert humanistic care expressions of people for the epistemic and ontology of nursing knowledge. I believed *nursing science should be defined in a broad way as the creative study of nursing phenomena which reflects the systematization of knowledge using rigorous and explicit research methods within either the qualitative or quantitative paradigm in order to establish a new or to advance nursing's discipline knowledge.*

I envisioned the discovery of culture care knowledge as an evolutionary process largely from an inductive qualitative approach to obtain the people's viewpoints and experiences, and I did not see it as a revolutionary process in the Kuhnian (1970) sense. Hence, using theory and method together was important in care discoveries. I theorized that culturally based care undoubtedly existed a long time, but the findings had to be explicated and studied in-depth, primarily with qualitative methods to preserve and know the meanings and patterns of care. In the 1950s and 1960s, there was no other extant or competing theory like culture care, and so the world was open to the study of care phenomenon. Moreover, there was no competing or revolutionary Kuhnian "take over" approach for the theory in the sense of using a rapidly formulated deductive theory to arrive at urgent findings because of competing theories. The theory was born with little interest and no competition from other nurses in those days. It was the *first theory in nursing to focus systematically on the explication of human care from a transcultural perspective predicting that human care was the essence of nursing and a central, dominant, and unifying domain of nursing knowledge and practices.*

While pondering ideas for a theory of Culture Care, I soon recognized that the terms *care* and *caring* had been used interchangably or in different ways. Most importantly, care and caring had been used by nurses and lay persons with limited focus on their meanings and usages in different context. Care had been used as a noun such as "I gave care," "This patient needs care," "Care is needed with this patient." Here care often was used in rhetorical ways and as a cliche with limited meanings (Leininger, 1977, 1978, 1981). The term *caring*, as a gerund, also was being linguistically used in nursing as an *action* or *doing* component of nursing practices such as "I am caring for this patient," "This family has some urgent caring needs." It was clear that the meanings and usages of care and caring in nursing were ambiguous, covert, and needed to be studied in a systematic and rigorous way. Moreover, care meanings, attributes, characteristics, linguistic usages, and practice aspects in different nursing contexts and from a comparative transcultural perspective were urgently needed to advance nursing care knowledge. It also was clear that non-care, no care, or non-caring behaviors also were heard in nursing and needed to be examined for their meanings and uses, especially as related to beneficial or therapeutic caring.

I theorized that culture care undoubtedly had different linguistic uses, meanings, essences, patterns, expressions, functions, and structural features in different cultures that had to be explicated and studied in relation to health or well being by folk or lay carers and by professional nurses. I postulated that care or caring patterns included assistive, supportive, facilitative, and enabling acts, or attitudes that influenced the well being or the health status of individuals, families, groups, and institutions, as well as general human conditions, lifeways, and environmental context (Leininger, 1977, 1978, 1979, 1981, 1984a). It was imperative for nursing to discover these culture care dimensions in order to establish the epistemic and ontological substantive base of nursing's discipline knowledge. Without this knowledge, nursing could not become a caring profession or a legitimate nursing discipline. Culture care phenomena needed to be systematically discovered, studied, and interpreted within nursing's perspectives. Care had been too long the covert, unknown, and almost invisible aspect of nursing and health services. This meant studying actual or potential care and caring in different cultures and contexts.

Discovering culture care knowledge of different cultures from an *emic* or people-based perspective, and then studying care from nurses *etic* or professional perspectives was another unexplored area of much interest to the theorist. Identifying comparative perspectives of *emic* and *etic* care was predicted to provide new insights about differences and similarities between professional and generic (folk) or consumer-based care knowledge, attitudes, and practices. To study these dimensions of care worldwide or in all cultures was viewed as a long-term program of research in nursing that would cover several decades of work. Thus, from the beginning, the theory of Culture Care had been conceptualized from a worldwide perspective and as a longitudinal research program involving many nurses and people in order to establish comparative knowledge about what was universal and diverse about care (caring) phenomena in Western and non-Western cultures. I held, however, that as the findings were generated, they could be used in specific cultures studied for appropriate nursing decisions and actions in order to improve existing care practices. With most nurses doing only small scale hospital nursing activity studies or mini studies in the community, the global aspect of transcultural nursing theory was predicted to create conceptual difficulties and take time to discover. In fact, such a global program of research was held as very futuristic by my colleagues. The theory of Culture Care worldwide was viewed as imperative research for epistemic knowledge for the discipline of nursing in order to guide future nursing practices to meet some of the anticipated multicultural needs of clients in our rapidly changing world. Culturally congruent care, as the goal of the theory, is high in demand now and will be more so in the future.

THEORY DEFINITION AND SPECIFICS OF THE THEORY OF CULTURE CARE

As I developed the theory, I was confronted with definitions of theories that were constructed mainly from the logical positivist or the "received view" perspectives (Carter, 1985; Leininger, 1985a; Watson, 1985b). The idea of a theory being a set of interrelated concepts, definitions, propositions, or hypothesis with variables to be rigidly controlled and tested was not what I thought would be useful to explicate and understand largely covert culture care phenomena from a transcultural perspective. This traditional view of a theory and variants derived from the philosophy of logical positivist science could only lead to discrete, fragmented, and measurable bits and pieces of knowledge that would offer the researcher little chance to explain, understand, and predict human care from a holistic and integrated view. I wanted a theory that would help to discover both broad or common knowledge and specific care knowledge. As an anthropologist, I had learned how to do naturalistic or ethnographic and ethnologic inquiries to study unknown phenomena in the field, and how to use broad theoretical perspectives to discover tacit inductive and covert phenomena. I also had studied hypodeductive theories that tested a priori hypotheses and specific variables of interest to the researcher. I was concerned that the latter approach would greatly limit any in-depth discovery of meanings of humanistic cultural care within a culture and from many minorities or subcultural groups who feared such research approaches. I questioned the use of tightly or rigidly constructed hypotheses, specific variables, and use of "operational" definitions to study human behavior to get meaningful data. The researcher would have to establish an *a priori* hypothesis for which such ideas might have limited or no relevance to a culture. I also knew many cultures as unhappy in enduring manipulation control in their environments by researchers. The logical positivist or received view seemed inappropriate to study culture care phenomena transculturally.

The theory needed to be an open discovery, inductively derived approach to explicate, detail, and get meanings of culture care, patterns, expressions, and practices with *emic* people-based (inside culture) knowledge so that it would be credible or believable to the people being studied. Getting to the people's *emic* views was extremely important, more important than emphasizing the researcher's *etic* or externally derived presumed and pre-set specific ideas (Pike, 1954). The theory combined with the ethnonursing research method purported to discover how people cognitively knew, described, and interpreted care within their total culture lifeways, beliefs, and environment. The ethnonursing research method was developed to obtain such grounded people-based data (see Chapter 2). From 1959 to 1961, my mini ethnography and ethnonursing studies convinced me this was the extremely rich and meaningful research way to obtain full descriptive, accurate, and meaningful data from the people in their natural living environments (Leininger, 1965, 1985a,b,c, 1987a,b). Extremely important in obtaining credible, accurate, and reliable data was the close relationship between theory and research method being used. Not any available method or tool or triangulation of methods would be necessarily appropriate for this theory—a principle not fully understood in nursing to this day.

I defined *theory* as patterns or sets of interrelated concepts, expressions, meanings, and experiences that describe, explain, predict, and can account for some phenomena or domain of inquiry procured through an open creative and naturalistic discovery process (Leininger, 1978, 1985a, 1988c). This definition of theory provided a means for naturalistic discoveries within the theorist's broad hunches and tentative conceptualization of cultural care. I found Steven's (1979) theory provided for a general stance that a theory is effective if it allows discovery, explanation, interpretation, and prediction of certain phenomena. Watson's (1985a) later definition of a theory supported my general notion that "a theory is a statement that purports to account for or characterizes some phenomena" (p. 1). These later ideas about the nature and characteristics of a theory were helpful to reinforce and support my earlier thinking and research approach.

Therefore, it was quite acceptable for a theorist to have a broad theoretical framework to guide and stimulate his or her thinking and research, but it should not be so tight or rigid that it would not accommodate fresh data or new discoveries of phenomena being studied. For qualitative studies, broad theoretical frameworks with hunches, presuppositions, and theoretical assumptions were needed, as well as some predictions about the phenomena. The ethnonursing method with a broad culture care theoretical perspective would enable the researcher to learn from informants in their natural environmental contexts about their known or covert aspects of human care. Most importantly, the researcher needed to keep an open discovery posture to accommodate or to discover anew transcendental, spiritual, symbolic, metaphoric, and other people ideas related to human care and caring. Using the theory, the researcher must search for meanings and detailed descriptions with instances of culturally based care data. From several mini studies, however, I had discovered that culture care phenomena were largely embedded in the worldview, religious (or spiritual), kinship, and other areas of the social structure which were unfamiliar to nurse researchers. Documenting such meaning and importance to nursing would be a challenge.

In conceptualizing the theory of Culture Care, I held this central tenet: *Care is the essence of nursing and the central, dominant, and unifying focus of nursing.* I held that culture care would provide a distinctive feature by which to know, interpret, and explain nursing as a discipline and profession (Leininger, 1965, 1967, 1969a,b, 1976a,b,c, 1977, 1978, 1980, 1984a,b, 1988a,b,c, 1990a). I postulated further that *culture care* would provide the substantive knowledge to know, explain, interpret, predict, and legitimize nursing as a discipline and profession. Using the theory, then, could help to establish the nature, essence, meanings, expressions, and forms of human care or caring—a highly unique, credible, reliable, and meaningful body of knowledge for nursing. Understanding the why of cultural care differences and similarities among and between cultures would offer explanatory power to support nursing as an academic discipline and practice profession. Most importantly, the theory and ethnonursing research method could generate knowledge to help nurses care for people of diverse and similar cultures who needed to be understood, and helped in meaningful ways with our rapidly growing multicultural world (Leininger, 1970, 1977, 1978, 1989, 1990c).

I predicted that while there would be diverse culture care patterns, processes, meanings, attributes, functions, and structure of care worldwide, some *universals* also would exist. I postulated that human care practices existed in all human cultures since the beginning of *homo sapiens*, but their manifestations and uses remained undiscovered. I predicted that the worldwide knowledge and local culture knowledge gained from using the theory could radically transform nursing into a caring profession and discipline by virtue of new transcultural care substantive knowledge. It would constitute the substantive knowledge base to guide nurses' decisions and actions in assisting people under different human conditions or circumstances. Most importantly, I theorized that cultural care knowledge derived from the *people*, the *emic* culture knowledge, could provide the truest knowledge base for culturally congruent care so that people would benefit from and be satisfied with nursing care practices held to be healthy ways of serving them. The nurse's *etic*, or outsider knowledge, would have to be considered with the people's *emic*, or generic folk knowledge to discern areas of conflict or compatibility of ideas.

In my early studies of several cultures over time and in different ecologies, I could see the close and inextricable relationship between culture and nursing. This led me to see culture care as central to nursing, but also to predict that human caring was essential for human survival at birth, for human growth, to recover from illnesses, and to remain well. In the long evolution of *homo sapiens*, I predicted that cultural beliefs, values, norms, and patterns of caring had a powerful influence on human survival, growth, illness states, health, and well being. I viewed *culture* as the learned and transmitted values, beliefs, and practices that provided a critical means to establish culture care patterns from the people. Culture was seen to be dynamic but tenacious over time by the people who lived by and used culture care values. Culture was seen as the blueprint for living, remaining healthy, or for dying. Care was culturally defined and known to the people, and especially how they saw and knew care from their context. Culture care was conceptualized and predicted to provide some constancy, continuity, a familiarity, and credibility to the people. And since human beings are born, live, become ill, survive, experience life rituals, and die within a cultural care frame of reference, these life experiences have meanings and significance to them in any given culture or subculture. Moreover, these cultural care lived experiences were influenced by specific cultural values, worldview, social structure factors, language uses, ethnohistory, environmental context, and health care systems. These dimensions needed to be fully discovered over time periods to see their influence on human caring, well being, health, or illness, and to use this knowledge in people caring modes.

I theorized further that all cultures in the world had some kind of a *folk, indigenous, generic, or naturalistic lay care system*, and that some people (not all) had been exposed to *professional health care systems* with professional nurses and other personnel. The folk and professional health care systems were predicted to influence greatly the individual or groups access to and quality of care rendered to people in favorable or less favorable ways. These two major types of health systems were capable of providing human care that was healthy, satisfying, beneficial and congruent with the client's culture care values and needs. However, I also held that some professional nursing care practices might not always be congruent with the client's generic care, and so nurses would be challenged to recognize this and make appropriate changes in order to provide culturally congruent care. What was similar or different between the folk (or generic) care and the professional system was yet to be discovered. It was, indeed, a new area for nurses to discover care knowledge, and held great promise for transforming nursing practices as well as health care systems. From an anthropological perspective, the folk or indigenous care system was the oldest from a healing and curing view, whereas professional caring was recent in human history. Therefore, I conjectured that the favorable aspects of generic or folk care could be the epistemic and ontologic base of professional nursing knowledge, especially if brought together in meaningful ways. Combining generic and professional care could lead to people seeking health care services to receiving *culturally congruent* care. If this linkage of generic and professional care did not occur, culture conflicts, noncompliance behaviors, cultural stresses, imposition practices, and a host of other unfavorable nursing care problems already seen within nursing services would arise (Leininger, 1967,

1970, 1978, 1981, 1984a,b). I defined folk (or generic) and professional care as follows (Leininger, 1978, 1980, 1981):

Generic Care (caring): *refers to culturally learned and transmitted lay, indigenous (traditional) or folk (home care) knowledge and skills used to provide assistive, supportive, enabling, facilitative acts (or phenomena) toward or for another individual, group or institution with evident or anticipated needs to ameliorate or improve a human health condition (or well being), disability, lifeway, or to face death.*

Professional Nursing Care (caring): *refers to formal and cognitively learned professional care knowledge and practice skills obtained through educational institutions that are used to provide assistive, supportive, enabling or facilitative acts to or for another individual or group in order to improve a human health condition (or well being), disability, lifeway, or to work with dying clients.*

To provide culturally congruent care for individual or group well being or for cultural institutions was held as essential by discovering how generic and professional systems were alike or different.

My theoretical framework went further in that I predicted that the primacy of people relying on culture care, (generic or professional care expectations) was crucial to help people remain well, function, or survive each day. Human beings in any culture anticipated and experienced care or non-caring behaviors within their familiar cultural context. Culture care existed but was not consciously recognized as a pattern of functioning each day with groups, individuals, or in social institutions. Healthy culture care modalities were to help people stay well or to receive beneficial, satisfying, and effective care by health professionals, especially through nursing services. To fully understand and predict culture caring, the nurse would need to use care data as influenced by religion, kinship, language, technology, economics, education (formal and informal), cultural values and beliefs, and the physical (ecological) environment. An awareness of the people's (emic) knowledge was held to be imperative to accurately assess, know, and understand the world of the client(s) and to design and implement culturally congruent care that could lead to client wellness or health. I also postulated that care with caring modalities was so powerful and important to healing and curing, that curing could not occur without caring. The latter prediction is a profound idea still unexplored fully today.

The purpose of Culture Care theory was to discover human care diversities and universalities in relation to worldview, social structure, and other dimensions cited, and then to discover ways to provide culturally congruent care to people of different or similar cultures in order to maintain or regain their well being, health, or face death in a culturally appropriate way (Leininger, 1985c, 1988a,b,c). The goal of the theory is to improve and to provide culturally congruent care to people that is beneficial, will fit with, and be useful to the client, family, or culture group healthy lifeways. The nurse is challenged by the theory to discover transcultural human care knowledge that can guide provision of congruent care, such knowledge also contributing to the fundamental base of nursing knowledge. Nursing practices now and in the future would be culture specific due to heightened culture human rights and needs in a growing and legalistic multicultural world. The findings from the theory would be used toward providing care that blends with culture values, beliefs, and lifeways of people, and is assessed to be beneficial, satisfying, and meaningful to people of designated cultures.

Since I took the position that care *is* nursing and essential for human well being and health, I realized in the 1950s that I took a stance quite different from a later subgroup of nurses in the United States who, in the early 1980s, excluded care from their views of nursing (Fawcett, 1984, 1989). These nurses contend that *person, nursing, health,* and *environment* are central to the metaparadigm of nursing. It is difficult to believe that in the 1980s nurses would so patently omit human care. Did they fear studying human care because it could not be measured or fit the logical positivist theory development approach? Is it possible they had never seen clients experience care or seen nurses provide care? These few nurse leaders attempted to explain nursing with nursing, which preempted and violated the discovery of the phenomena of nursing by explaining the same thing with the same explanation—a philosophic contradiction to the discovery process. They also used *person* as central or distinctive to nursing. From both an anthropological and nursing perspective, the use of the term *person* has serious problems when used transculturally, as many non-Western cultures do not focus on or believe in the concept *person,* and often there is no linguistic term for person in a culture, family and institutions being more prominent. While *environment* is very important to nursing, I would contend it is certainly not unique to nursing, and there are very few nurses who have advanced formal study and are prepared to study a large number of different types of environments or ecological niches worldwide. These *a priori claimed* concepts had serious problems except for that of health. Again, as a concept health is not distinct to nursing although nursing plays a major role in health attainment and maintenance—many disciplines have studied health. Fortunately, many nurses are realizing the inadequacies of these metaparadigm concepts and have shifted to care as central to nursing. There is actually a groundswell of research interest by nurses since 1982 to study care, which gives further credence to care as the essence of nursing and of central interest to nurses.

In conceptualizing nursing from the 1940s onward, it had always seemed natural and self-evident from clinical and professional work to focus on what is and could be seen in practice as central to nurses patterned activities and modes of thinking, which was *caring for others.* *Caring for others* in need of assistance was historically a "calling," usually from religious interests, then a vocation, and later as essential professional knowledge and as an art and skill (Leininger, 1981, 1984a,b,c). The long-standing focus on care and caring phenomena was central to nursing and to my thinking, professional life experiences, and from public or societal expectations of nurses. The humanistic and scientific dimensions of care remained of theoretical and professional interest with the prediction that care, and especially culturally based care, would enable humans to attain wellness or maintain well being. In the early days and since, I firmly held to the following axioms that served as guides in developing the theory: "Care is nursing"; "Care is healing"; "Care is the nurse's way of being with and helping people"; "Care is the heart and soul of nursing"; "Care makes the difference in wellness or illness states"; and "Care can cure" (Leininger, 1977, 1980, 1981).

Grounded in anthropological insights and the nature of nursing, I believed that nursing was a transcultural care phenomenon and lived experience. As a result, I postulated that the nursing profession that claims to care for all people who seek nursing services, whether on a local, national, or worldwide basis, would be obligated to discover transcultural nursing care knowledge with a global comparative view.

Thus, the theory and Sunrise Model were conceptualized to be used in the discovery of all cultures over time. The nursing profession was challenged to pursue the study of care with all cultures in the world. For nursing to be recognized and function as a transcultural nursing discipline and profession, however, this global and longitudinal view of the theory required documentation and systematic study (Leininger, 1978, 1981, 1984b, 1989).

From the beginning, I was intrigued with the idea of transcultural care as central to nursing *worldwide* with a *comparative* focus. I theorized that if nurses had transcultural knowledge of many cultures, it would be possible to teach and provide care that was congruent with the people's lifeways, rather than use etic care imposition or culture-bound professional practices (Leininger, 1967). The study of human care transculturally, as pursued by nurses, would provide a comparative body of knowledge that would be formally taught in schools of nursing in the future as care principles, practices, policies, and perhaps laws. It would guide nurses who work with people of many different cultures to be knowledgeable, sensitive, competent, and effective in caring for and with culture strangers. Moreover, I held that this comparative discipline knowledge of culture care diversities and universalities would constitute knowledge essential to twenty-first century health care. When brought into teaching, curriculum, administration, clinical community practices, consultation, and nursing research, transcultural care knowledge would lead to near revolutionary changes. Although such thinking in the 1950s was "unreal" to most nurses, it seemed realistic for the future of nursing—a theory of nursing was needed to know and explain nursing worldwide. It was time to prevent cultural imposition practices, cultural care negligence, cultural care conflicts, and many other practice and education problems one could see then and by the end of this century. Interestingly, four decades later, nurses are now keenly feeling and demanding transcultural care knowledge to help them function in a tense multicultural world.

Finally, in conceptualizing the theory, I envisioned and predicted three major modalities to guide nursing judgments, decisions, or actions so as to provide *cultural congruent care* that is beneficial, satisfying, and meaningful to people nurses serve (Leininger, 1978, 1988b,c). The three modes are: (1) *cultural care preservation* and/or *maintenance;* (2) *cultural care accommodation* and/or *negotiation;* and (3) *cultural care repatterning* or *restructuring*. These diverse modes were derived from my direct experiences in using culture care knowledge to assist clients in several Western and non-Western cultures. The three predicted modes were care-centered and based on the use of generic (*emic*) care knowledge along with professional (*etic*) care knowledge obtained from research using the theory and depicted in the Sunrise Model (see Figure 1).

The nurse grounded in culture care knowledge would plan and make decisions with clients with respect to these three modes of action or decision which was predicted to be in accord with the care data obtained from findings in the upper part of the model. It also was theorized that sometimes only one dominant mode of action might be needed, such as using culture care preservation. For example, a Chinese-American client might express the need for herbal tea to ease a "nervous stomach," for this generic care practice has worked well in the past and is still held important today by many Chinese-American clients. It was predicted that there would be many instances of using *culture care accommodation or negotiation* between nurse and family when the later expected (or demanded) accommodation with their food, spiritual needs, family contacts, and in other areas. For example, Arab-Muslim families value total family participation when assisting a sick family member. For a sick Muslim child in the hospital, the mother is *obliged* and *responsible* to stay with him or her (Leininger, 1981-1989; Luna, 1990). In response, the nurse would need to plan and make accommodations for the mother and family to provide the most beneficial and satisfying care possible. There are many additional examples of cultural care accommodation involving culture food preferences, religious practices, kinship needs, child care, and treatment practices that are held to be imperative to provide beneficial (healthy) or satisfying care.

Cultural care repatterning and restructuring was another nursing care modality theorized as extremely important, but again would require nurses to have culture care knowledge to help repattern caring lifeways. As the nurse works with the client in a *coparticipant way*, the nurse theorizes ways to develop repatterning or restructuring of nursing care. This mode requires that the nurse possess an extensive culture knowledge base and make creative use of it. Repatterning or restructuring of care requires being very attentive or sensitive to the people's lifeways. It also involves assessing how nursing practices may

Figure 1
Leininger's Sunrise Model to Depict Theory of Cultural Care Diversity and Universality

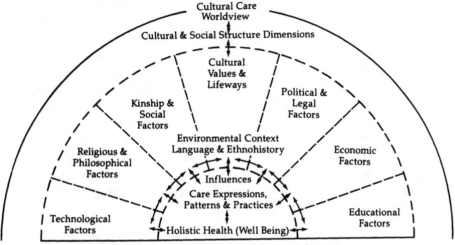

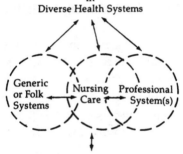

Individuals, Families, Groups, Communities, & Institutions in Diverse Health Systems

Nursing Care Decisions & Actions

Cultural Care Preservation / Maintenance
Cultural Care Accommodation / Negotiation
Cultural Care Repatterning / Restructuring

Culture Congruent Nursing Care

Code ←→ Influences

facilitate helping a client maintain wellness, and especially when he or she returns home. For example, nurses may repattern or restructure care related to eating, sleeping, and smoking lifeways found harmful to client(s) both by nurse and client. Together the nurse and client creatively design a new or different care lifestyle for the health or well being of the client. This mode requires the use of both generic and professional knowledge and ways to fit such diverse ideas into nursing care actions and goals. Care knowledge and skills should always be repatterned for the best interests of the clients. Likewise, care institutions need to restructure and repattern their ways to serve consumers. Thus, all care modalities require *coparticipation of nurse and clients (consumers) working together* to identify, plan, implement, and evaluate each caring mode for culturally congruent nursing care. These modes can stimulate nurses to design nursing care using new knowledge and culturally based ways to provide meaningful and satisfying holistic care to individuals, groups, or institutions.

ASSUMPTIVE PREMISES OF THE CULTURE CARE THEORY

In light of the above theoretical conceptualizations, philosophical position, beliefs, and predictive theoretical hunches, several assumptive premises had been formulated at the outset and refined through time to guide nurses in their discovery of Culture Care phenomena. These assumptive theoretical premises or tenets include (Leininger, 1966, 1970, 1973c, 1976a,b, 1978, 1980, 1981, 1984a, 1988a,b,c):

1. Care is the essence of nursing and a distinct, dominant, central, and unifying focus.

2. Care (caring) is essential for well being, health, healing, growth, survival, and to face handicaps or death.

3. Culture care is the broadest holistic means to know, explain, interpret, and predict nursing care phenomena to guide nursing care practices.

4. Nursing is a transcultural humanistic and scientific care discipline and profession with the central purpose to serve human beings worldwide.

5. Care (caring) is essential to curing and healing, for there can be no curing without caring.

6. Culture care concepts, meanings, expressions, patterns, pro-cesses, and structural forms of care are different (diversity) and similar (towards commonalties or universalities) among all cultures of the world.

7. Every human culture has generic (lay, folk, or indigenous) care knowledge and practices and usually professional care knowledge and practices which vary transculturally.

8. Culture care values, beliefs, and practices are influenced by and tend to be embedded in the worldview, language, religious (or spiritual), kinship (social), political (or legal), educational, economic, technological, ethnohistorical, and environmental context of a particular culture.

9. Beneficial, healthy, and satisfying culturally based nursing care contributes to the well being of individuals, families, groups, and communities within their environmental con-text.

10. Culturally congruent or beneficial nursing care can only oc-cur when the individual, group, family, community, or cul-ture care values, expressions, or patterns are known and used appropriately and in meaningful ways by the nurse with the people.

11. Culture care differences and similarities between professional caregiver(s) and client (generic) care-receiver(s) exists in any human culture worldwide.

12. Clients who experience nursing care that fails to be reason-ably congruent with the client's beliefs, values, and caring lifeways will show signs of cultural conflicts, noncompliance, stresses, ethical or moral concerns, and slow recovery.

13. The qualitative paradigm and criteria provide new ways of knowing and different ways to discover epistemic and ontological dimensions of human care transculturally.

These assumtive theoretical premises were used as guides to systematically study the theory and to discover if they prevailed with regard to culture care phenomena.

The following major tenets are used to examine systematically the theory with the ethnonursing method: 1) Culturally-based care has *diversities* (differences and variabilities) and some *universal* (common) features; 2) The worldview, socio-cultural factors, and other dimensions in the Sunrise Model *influence* care outcomes for congruent care; 3) Generic (emic) and professional beliefs and practices provide for valuable data for culture care practices; 4) The three predicted theoretical modes for nursing actions and decisions, namely a) *culture care preservation* and/or *maintenance*; b) *culture care accommodation* and/or *negotiation*, and c) *culture care repatterning* and/or *restructuring* provide credible data for congruent, safe, and beneficial care. Through co-participation of nurse and client on the decisions and actions, culturally congruent care can be realized.

ORIENTATIONAL DEFINITIONS

Since the major methods to study the theory of Culture Care have been within the qualitative paradigm using the ethnonursing method, orientational definitions are appropriate rather than the traditionally used operational definitions of quantitative paradigmatic studies. The definitions below are cited to provide only a broad orientational research focus in relation to the theory so as to permit new discoveries and to identify and explicate inductively phenomena from informants and situations of how people know, experience, and define these ideas or phenomena under study. Hence, the definitions are purposefully not tightly or rigidly formulated with *a priori* relational variables within each definition. These orientational definitions are used explicitly as guides to study the domain or areas related frequently to the theory (Leininger, 1981, 1985a,c, 1988a,c):

1. *Care* (noun) refers to abstract and concrete phenomena related to assisting, supporting, or enabling experiences or behaviors toward or for others with evident or anticipated needs to ameliorate or improve a human condition or lifeway.

2. *Caring* (gerund) refers to actions and activities directed toward assisting, supporting, or enabling another individual or group with evident or anticipated needs to ameliorate or improve a human condition or lifeway, or to face death.

3. *Culture* refers to the learned, shared, and transmitted values, beliefs, norms, and lifeways of a particular group that guides their thinking, decisions, and actions in patterned ways.

4. *Cultural care* refers to the subjectively and objectively learned and transmitted values, beliefs, and patterned lifeways that assist, support, facilitate, or enable another individual or group to maintain their well being, health, to improve their human condition and lifeway, or to deal with illness, handicaps, or death.

5. *Culture care diversity* refers to the variables and/or differences in meanings, patterns, values, lifeways, or symbols of care within or between collectivities that are related to assistive, supportive, or enabling human care expressions.

6. *Culture care universality* refers to the common, similar, or dominant uniform care meanings, patterns, values, lifeways or symbols that are manifest among many cultures and reflect assistive, supportive, facilitative, or enabling ways to help people. (The term *universality* is not used in an absolute way or as a significant statistical finding.)

7. *Nursing* refers to a learned humanistic and scientific profession and discipline which is focused on human care phenomena and activities in order to assist, support, facilitate, or enable individuals or groups to maintain or regain their well being (or health) in culturally meaningful and beneficial ways, or to help people face handicaps or death.

8. *Worldview* refers to the way people tend to look out on the world or their universe to form a picture or a value stance about their life or world around them.

9. *Cultural and social structure dimensions* refers to the dynamic patterns and features of interrelated structural and organizational factors of a particular culture (subculture or society) which includes religious, kinship (social), political (and legal), economic, educational, technologic, and cultural values, ethnohistorical factors, and how these factors may be interrelated and function to influence human behavior in different environmental contexts.

10. *Environmental context* refers to the totality of an event, situation, or particular experiences that give meaning to human expressions, interpretations, and social interactions in particular physical, ecological, sociopolitical and/or cultural settings.

11. *Ethnohistory* refers to those past facts, events, instances, experiences of individuals, groups, cultures, and institutions that are primarily people-centered (ethno) and which describe, explain, and interpret human lifeways within particular cultural contexts and over short or long periods of time.

12. *Generic (folk or lay) care system* refers to culturally learned and transmitted, indigenous (or traditional), folk (home based) knowledge and skills used to provide assistive, supportive, enabling, or facilitative acts toward or for another individual, group, or institution with evident or anticipated needs to ameliorate or improve a human lifeway, health condition (or wellbeing), or to deal with handicaps and death situations.

13. *Professional care system(s)* refers to formally taught, learned, and transmitted professional care, health, illness, wellness, and related knowledge and practice skills that prevail in professional institutions usually with multidisciplinary personnel to serve consumers.

14. *Health* refers to a state of well being that is culturally defined, valued, and practiced, and which reflects the ability of individuals (or groups) to perform their daily role activities in culturally expressed, beneficial, and patterned lifeways.

15. *Culture care preservation or maintenance* refers to those assistive, supporting, facilitative, or enabling professional actions and decisions that help people of a particular culture to retain and/or preserve relevant care values so that they can maintain their well being, recover from illness, or face handicaps and/or death.

16. *Culture care accommodation or negotiation* refers to those assistive, supporting, facilitative, or enabling creative professional actions and decisions that help people of a designated culture to adapt to, or to negotiate with, others for a beneficial or satisfying health outcome with professional careproviders.

17. *Culture care repatterning or restructuring* refers to those assistive, supporting, facilitative, or enabling professional actions and decisions that help a client(s) reorder, change, or greatly modify their lifeways for new, different, and beneficial health care pattern while respecting the client(s) cultural values and beliefs and still providing a beneficial or healthier lifeway than before the changes were coestablished with the client(s).

18. *Cultural congruent (nursing) care* refers to those cognitively based assistive, supportive, facilitative, or enabling acts or decisions that are tailor made to fit with individual, group, or institutional cultural values, beliefs, and lifeways in order to provide or support meaningful, beneficial, and satisfying health care, or well-being services.

The above major definitions are related to the theoretical framework and assumptive premises. The definitions of conceptual terms or phrases are stated to provide an open discovery perspective related to the goals of the theory and the theoretical framework.

SUNRISE ENABLER MODEL: CONCEPTUAL DIMENSIONS OF THE THEORY

With the theoretical framework, assumptive premises, and orientational concepts presented above, the Sunrise Model (see Figure 1) is presented to help the reader visualize different dimensions of the theory. The Sunrise Model is designed to depict a total view of the different but very closely related dimensions of the theory. The model is not a conceptual model *per se*, nor is it an abstract and general system of concepts and proportions as viewed by Fawcett (1989) and other theorists of similar interests. Instead, the model is used as in many social and physical sciences, as a cognitive map to orient and depict the influencing dimensions, components, facets, or major concepts of the theory with an integrated total view of these dimensions. It is important for the reader to know that I refer to this theoretical framework as both abstract and concrete aspects of a theory whose goal is to discover inductively and explain, interpret, and predict culture care knowledge and its influencers in order to understand and develop ways to provide culturally congruent nursing care. The reader, there-fore, becomes aware that there are different ways to conceptualize theories and that the theory is not the same as a conceptual model. In the strictest sense, models are known as image depictions, which re-flects the major purpose of the present model.

In using the Sunrise Model, the reader keeps in mind the total gestalt of diverse influencers to describe and explain care with health and well being outcomes. These dimensions or influencers of culture care are not to be viewed as isolated, fragmented, or unrelated parts. Instead, they are held to be inextricably and closely interrelated to each other, very much like a view of the total functioning of human beings, or the totality of one's cultural world. Like a culture, this model has wholeness and interrelatedness with the nature of the full connections to be studied in relation to human care. The Sunrise Model has been developed and refined over the past three decades to provide a gestaltic picture of these major dimensions or interrelated components of the theory. Interestingly, it has undergone approximately ten revisions in order to depict as fully and clearly as possible the conceptual dimen-sions of the theory and how they are generally perceived to be linked together so that one can see diverse care influencers or individuals, groups, families, communities, institutions, or whomever one is study-ing in relation to the major tenets as assumptions of the theory. Essen-tially, the model helps the researcher envision a cultural world of different life forces or influencers on human conditions which need to be considered to discover human care in its fullest ways. At no time is the model intended to depict casual, linear, or logical positivistic rela-tionships, or a rigid social structure system perspective. In keeping with the qualitative paradigm and the theory, the model guides the researcher to study and "tease out" the epistemics and ontological aspects of human care or caring within these diverse components so that a substantive base of culture care knowledge can be discovered for the discipline of nursing. The model keeps the researcher alert to different dimensions of potential or actual influencers on human care and health using the inductive qualitative ethnonursing method.

In using this model with the theoretical framework and the assump-tive premises, it is important to state that the researcher begins with his or her domain of interest or inquiry, so he or she may start the discov-ery process anywhere. Usually, however, the researcher begins with the worldview and works from the top to the bottom of the Sunrise Model. But it is possible that the nurse researcher may want to begin the exploration by focusing on care and nursing in the professional system (lower part of the model). The nurse, therefore, would study care of individuals or groups in the hospitals or homes, and gradually move the exploration to worldview, cultural, and social structural dimensions, and cover kinship, religion, and other areas depicted in the model. At the same time, the researcher remains focused on the domain of study and moves within a rough research plan influenced by how the research unfolds to obtain *emic* data from the informants and culture context. Frequently, the researcher starts at the top of the model with the worldview and social structure features and then gradually explores the professional and generic health care systems as well as possible modes of nursing actions and decisions. For example, the nurse may be interested in discovering the meaning, patterns, and practices of care and caring with a Mexican-American family. Here, the nurse centers on the family as the focal point (not the individual), and discusses with the family their ideas and practices about care in their family caring ways. The researcher continues to tease out how religion, family beliefs, and specific cultural values and practices tend to influence Mexican-American health or well being. The discovery process continues until all the remaining factors depicted in the model are studied to obtain a comprehensive picture including economic, education, political, environmental context, language, and worldview. Throughout the ethnonursing discovery, the researcher remains keenly aware of the ethnohistory environmental context, and the total situation or events that give meaning to what is being shared or observed with the Mexican-American family within or outside home life. The researcher may focus on specific family caring experiences and events that have influenced care, such as family values and their folk care or health system. If the Mexican-American family had experiences in a professional health system with personnel, their experiences would be explored at a time the informant wishes to talk about hospital care. After the researcher teases out information related to all components of the model and with attention to specific language terms about care, well being, illnesses, and related information, there usually emerges some meaningful patterns or themes about care meanings, experiences, and cultural taboos in relation to well being. Ideas about what the informants believe would be appropriate nursing decisions and actions are identified and considered to provide culturally congruent Mexican-American family care. With informants usually expressing many valuable ideas, the discovery of culturally congruent care becomes an exciting one. In addition, when considering the three modes of action or decisions, it is possible that *culture care preservation or maintenance mode* may be emphasized by the Mexican-American family. It also is possible that the family may want or expect several *culture care accommodations* to be made by the nurse for the family in order to regain their well being, and so this modality of care also may be used. There also may be data to support *cultural care repatterning or restructuring* with the family. For example, in childcare, *emic* information may show that the Mexican-American family needs to consider the grandmother as a caregiver because the young Mexican-American mother must work for family income and survival. Thus, the nurse and family work together on a repatterning plan with the grandmother to help care for the children while the mother and father work outside the home. The several daily life experiences that must be restructured so that the grandmother role can be realized often involve many other details as well. From this example, one can see how practical this model can be in examining the Culture Care theory in a concrete and practical way, as well as in discovering intriguing abstract phenomena in care patterns, such as the interaction of Mexican-American family with presumed "spiritual" forces, or with certain institutionalized beliefs.

The researcher, therefore, can use the model with flexibility and in creative ways as one studies and remains sensitive to the individual, group, family, culture (or subculture), or a community being studied. At all times, the researcher keeps in mind the domain of inquiry being explored with the general tenets of the theory. Moving with the natural situation and the informants' ideas related to care, health, and other aspects is always important. Studying culture, community, or institutions requires great skill and knowledge, for one must have some previous knowledge about the culture, community, or institution to help initiate and pursue the exploration. This "holding knowledge," however, must not get in the way of what the researcher is discovering anew. Often, the researcher may need to suspend consciously or hold in abeyance literature that may interfere with the research. Anthropological or transcultural ethnohistorical knowledge helps the researcher "cue into" rather quickly the meanings and ideas the informants may be expressing through special terms and uses in the culture. Some knowledge helps one to grasp accurately what one hears, sees, or experiences in the particular context being studied using confirmation with informants. This previous knowledge should never be imposed on informants, but should be used as a back-drop of ideas about the phenomena being studied. Courses in transcultural nursing, qualitative research, care seminars, and in cultural or social anthropology are most helpful to ensure a well-conducted qualitative ethnonursing study. In general, the better prepared in transcultural nursing, culture, and language, the easier it is to tease out and make sense of what is heard and seen. Throughout the study of the theory, the researcher seeks in-depth meanings, patterns, expressions, characteristics, and structures of care in relation to *emic* and *etic* knowledge. Documenting statements and confirming informant interpretations and observations are essential, including biopsychosociocultural factors.

It also is important to keep in mind while using the model and theoretical ideas that social structure factors are dynamic and tend to change over time in any culture in slow or moderate pace (seldom rapidly). The contemporary and past ethnohistory data provides rich and important information to examine factors influencing social structure and other aspects with any culture or representative of a culture. Some care expressions and patterns from informants may be culturally specific, while others may be covert, general, or perceived as universal for the culture. The Sunrise Model is used as a valuable cognitive map to guide researchers through different dimensions and to check on areas covered or not covered during the study.

The Sunrise Model often becomes like an imprinted cognitive map to help the researcher check on areas that need to be examined to obtain a full and accurate account of the people or informants' knowledge about culture care. The arrows on the model indicate *influencers*, but are not causal or linear relationships. The arrows flow in different areas and across major factors to depict the interrelatedness of factors and the fluidity of influencers. The dotted lines indicate an open world or an open system of living reflective of the natural world of most humans. The upper part of the model is extremely important but often more challenging to nurses because it often leads to discovery of embedded, backstage, or deeply valued and meaningful data about human care and well being. It requires that the researcher use not only nursing insights but also social science knowledge, liberal arts, and the humanities to tease out and understand areas of vital importance to a culture and caring ways. How social structure factors influence individuals, groups, and cultures in relation to care is often most revealing. Fortunately, because most nurses are prepared today in institutions of higher education, they have knowledge about these broad areas of knowledge and can draw on and use them in this discovery process.

The researcher will be encouraged to know that most culture informants are quite willing to share ideas about care when they feel trusted by the nurse researcher and when the researcher shows a real genuine interest in them and their perspectives. However, there will be some culture informants who feel threatened by being asked about their culture and care. Such informants tend to hold the public image that nurses are like physicians, studying only symptoms, diseases, treatments, and "using new drugs and surgery procedures." After a trusting relationship is established with informants, the researcher will find that informants often enjoy and express considerable pride, pleasure, and interest in having *their* ideas center focus, rather than any symptom or disease finding when they go to health personnel. Indeed, for many informants, it is refreshing to discuss meanings of care (including psychophysical and sociocultural) within their culture perspectives. While exploring culture care ideas with informants, the researcher, however, must guard against dichotomizing received ideas or overemphasizing mental and physical conditions. In regard to data from physical, emotional, spiritual, family, political, and other aspects, a holistic perspective must prevail. Such dichotomization leads to the "parts-whole" dichotomy of knowing people and is usually not congruent with how most cultures know and view care and health. Hence, such dichotomization is not depicted or used in the theory and the model.

When the researcher has obtained data from all dimensions of the model and has given full attention to the general theoretical framework of the theory with the intent of open discovery, the researcher will have obtained much rich, thick, dense, or saturated data with many important ideas about culture care and its linkage with health or well being. These data also will provide cues about nursing care decisions and actions that will give confidence to the researcher with respect to the three modes of nursing decisions and actions previously named: cultural care preservation or maintenance, cultural care accommodation or negotiation, and cultural care repatterning or restructuring—an important part of the theory to be studied.

From the examples given above and from those examples of culture care studies presented in this book, the reader will discover how the data are used in a culture-specific or more common universal way to provide culturally congruent care. At all times, the clients, clients' families, or cultural groups are actively involved in this discovery process as coparticipants. This is an important principle to maintain to get rich data and to help informants feel involved rather than researched out in an uncomfortable way. It helps to keep health maintenance and prevention of nursing care practices alive and important to participants. Since all the data collected is grounded or people-based data, the actions and decisions will have special meanings, and the informants will be more likely to carry out decisions or care plans over a long period of time, than if the informant(s) had no part in the research process *per se*. Most importantly, in the discovery process, informants will usually identify non-caring behaviors. The nurse researcher must be ready to listen to these informant ideas—they may refute or challenge what nurses ideally believe in or hold as professional truths belonging to nurses. When using the theory, the author and other researchers have found that non-caring meanings and patterns are usually shared later and become most valuable to understand the missing aspects of caring behavior, or to formulate ways to design congruent culture care from non-caring descriptors. With each caring (care) construct, often non-caring expressions and meanings will be shared if the informant feels it is safe to share ideas with the nurse researcher.

The reader will note that the author does not use the term *nursing intervention* in the theory nor in the model. This is purposeful, as it is a term that is often culture bound to Western professional nursing ideologies. Interventions tend to communicate to *some* cultural informants ideas of cultural interferences and imposition practices. All too often, some health practitioners do interfere with cultural lifeways and beliefs of cultures by their so-called interventions and lack of culture knowledge. Hence, the caring nurse generally wants to work with and be congruent with the norms and values of the culture. Likewise, the idea of "nursing problems" is not used by the theorist, as all too often the client may not have a problem, or the problem may not be seen as relevant to the people by the nurse. Indeed, nursing problems may not be the people's problems. It is always fascinating to find nursing problems formulated in advance for nursing research as quite different when seen through the lens of another culture. Thus, further support is provided for the use of qualitative ethnonursing research methods to pursue an open discovery and not a preconceived culture posture.

Using the theory with the Sunrise Model as a guide to discover new perspectives about human care, the researcher continuously searches for care differences and similarities with a culture, a group, or individual. Major contrasts with human care between Western and non-Western cultures also will appear by way of differing structural dimensions within the two societies. However, the researcher keeps an open discovery position in the systematic examination of the theory because of acculturation factors, sudden changes, and other conditions in a society that can make a difference about care practices and interpretations. Identifying care themes and constructs such as trust, acceptance, comfort, engrossment, stimulation, and many others are extremely important, for these constructs usually have very rich insights to document and understand. The theory is broad enough in scope to explore many aspects of care patterning with individual representations of a culture and over time. Of course, the use of the theory depends on the skill of the researcher in understanding and using the theory with the ethnonursing or another appropriate qualitative method. Focusing on care meanings and lived-through experiences (not unique to phenomenological methods) with a focus on culture care requires sensitive strategies to uncover such information. It also requires a good measure of patience, immersion in the data, and analytical abilities to periodically assess and synthesize data to be sure one has tapped the full fund of knowledge about care with the informants. A keen sense of ethical rights of informants and the culture is imperative for this kind of study. The research mentor is extremely valuable here in ensuring ethical rights of informants along with seminars on ethical aspects of qualitative research.

A FEW GLIMPSES OF FINDINGS
FROM THE THEORY

Although I and others have discovered and substantiated considerable culture care data using the theory over the past three decades, only a few culture care patterns will be shared here. Other specific findings related to culture care values and meanings will be shared in the subsequent chapters.

To date, 54 cultures in Western and non-Western worlds have been studied with the theory and 172 care constructs have been identified with specific meanings, usages, and interpretations (Leininger, 1960 to 1990). These care constructs are important dominant themes that provide ideas to guide nursing care practices as the *central fulcrum* for nursing care actions and decisions. The care constructs with dense social structure and other supported findings help nurses to focus on the primacy and power of care rather than medical symptoms, diseases, or tasks. Currently, *emic* culture care knowledge from Western and non-Western cultures shows greater *diversity* than similarities or commonalities in cultural values, usage, and meanings. The social structure and worldview of Western and non-Western cultures are strong influencers on care practices leading to health or well being. Recognition of such differences that have been embedded in the social structure and worldview are important for nurses to realize—often, they are little known and studied in nursing. Worldview and social structure data are usually packed with very rich knowledge about epistemic care, health, well being, and non-caring data of all cultures studied.

Findings also reveal some major differences between the client's cultural knowledge of care (*emic*) and that of professional nurses and other health personnel (*etic*) care viewpoints in hospital contexts. The greatest differences appear most frequently in hospital contexts rather than in home-care setting studies (Leininger, 1965, 1990). As a consequence of these culture care differences between the client and nurse (often identified as physicians by informants) in the hospital, cultural conflicts, stresses, noncompliance, slower client recovery, and questionable positive health benefits are experienced by clients. Other themes from my research and several graduate transcultural students reveal the following:

1. There are more signs of diversities than universalities among the 54 cultures, and especially between Western and non-Western cultures.

2. Culture care meanings and practices are difficult to tease out largely because they are embedded in the social structure, in non-Western cultures especially in kinship, religious beliefs,

and political factors; whereas in Western cultures care is viewed largely as high-tech tasks, cost factors, political decisions, and problems with language to understand clients' care needs.

3. The cultural context and care values make a major difference in how care is expressed and how care takes on meanings to clients and especially families or cultures.

4. Care meanings and their uses often require knowledge of the culture and local language.

5. High technology nursing practices in Western cultures tends to increase the distance between the client and the nurse (or professional staff), and especially within hospital or clinic institutionalized settings which frequently use high-technology nursing practices.

6. While generic (lay or folk) practices of a culture provide valuable care knowledge to guide professional nursing practices, generic care is still very little understood and valued by nurses and other health professionals.

7. Clients who have been involved as key or general informants with nurse researchers using Culture Care theory with the ethnonursing research method generally have expressed highly positive feelings, pride, and hope that more nurses will "get close to clients" and enter their broader life worldview.

8. Clients see that "their cultural ideas, beliefs, and lifeways must be fully considered by professional health personnel to help them appropriately."

CONSIDERATIONS TO EVALUATE AND ANALYZE THE THEORY

As students and scholars of nursing continue to expand their knowledge and analysis theory development, they soon will realize that, among theorists, there is considerable diversity in ways to analyze, evaluate, or "test" a theory. With many new methods for nurses to use (16–20) within the qualitative paradigm, there is an urgent need to reconsider how theories are evaluated. Otherwise, nursing theories will be incorrectly evaluated or improperly assessed. During the past decade, there has been a tendency for nurses to standardize or prescribe what constitutes a theory and what constitutes a theoretical or conceptual framework model, and what should be included or excluded in a nursing theory as well as concepts for nursing's metaparadigm and how to analyze a theory (Fawcett, 1983, 1989; Meleis, 1985; Walker & Avant, 1988). Theory and research scholars in most disciplines realize there usually are many different ways to test or evaluate a theory. Most importantly, it is essential to maintain communication with colleagues and an open discovery posture when evaluating a theory. Relying on conventional analyses or evaluation processes as defined by logical positivism can lead to false conclusions and restrictive perspectives.

Theory construction or development is a creative process. When deciding on the most appropriate way to evaluate the theory, however, evaluative criteria must be *congruent* to or *fit* with the theory. It is especially important not to standardize or rapidly proclaim what should be included or excluded in theory evaluations or to state what constitutes a theory by a few interested persons from a debatable paradigm. Such assumed "rectitude" often leads to noncreative scholars and followers. It is especially a questionable practice in a relatively young field or discipline to standardize testing or evaluations of theories as it often preempts some of the most creative and productive ideas available. Often, such premature standardization closes the doors to the discipline's real potential or actual scholars.

Today, the four proclaimed concepts of *health, nursing, person,* and *environment* (as discussed earlier) seem no longer acceptable to many nurses who value and believe in human care. There also are questions about Donaldson and Crowley's (1977) three theoretical statements as the focus of the discipline of nursing. Hence, there are important debates and queries about the central concepts and focus of nursing's discipline, as well as how theories are developed and analyzed. Currently, most nursing theories are developed and analyzed with criteria related to the quantitative paradigm, which is of concern to qualitative theorists (Leininger, 1985a; Munhall, 1982). In fact, this is a serious matter, leading as it does to quite different theories, because the purposes and goals of qualitative research are very different from those developed in the quantitative paradigm. Nurse theorists and users of the theories need to evaluate qualitatively constructed theories with qualitative criteria. In general, while the qualitative paradigm is a different approach to theory development, this fact is still little acknowledged today.

A number of quantitative-oriented nurse theorists or users of a theory based on experimental or quasi-experimental methods "test" their theories with the goal of producing *measurable* and objective results with generalizations. Such theories tested within the quantitative paradigm are tightly constructed and controlled to obtain definitive quantifiable results. Today, more nurse theorists are developing theories within the qualitative paradigm and their goal is not to "test" theories for measurable outcomes or for wide population generalizations. The qualitative theorist develops the theory inductively with the goal of establishing meanings, understandings, patterns, processes, characteristics, and attributes of some phenomenon under study. The theorist uses qualitative criteria to "*systematically evaluate*" or "*establish credibility*" of the theory. Qualitative theorists and researchers find it inappropriate to use quantitative criteria, such as validity and reliability, to appraise qualitative theories. Hence, theory developers and users must be aware of the important differences in the uses, goals, and outcomes of the two paradigms with the theories (Leininger, 1985a,b, 1990a).

In general, it is imperative that theories which are developed within the qualitative paradigm use qualitative criteria, rather than quantitative criteria, as the two paradigms have very different purposes and goals (Leininger, 1985a, 1990a; Lincoln & Guba, 1985; Reason & Rowan, 1983). Empirical (five senses), logical, experimental evaluations of a theory with operational definitions, hypotheses, and measurement scales are *not* congruent or appropriate to use with qualitative constructed theories. Indeed, objectivity and logical deductions under controlled circumstances may severely limit knowing and understanding qualitative phenomenon. A nurse studying a theory focused on abstract phenomena, transcendentalism, supernaturalism, mythical ideas, illusionary experiences, and concrete phenomenon will find that testing and measuring these phenomena is virtually impossible, unrealistic, and highly inappropriate with quantitative criteria. Hence, when reading nursing theory books today with their evaluations, questions, and modes of analysis, keep in mind that they are written almost completely within the quantitative paradigm when used to evaluate a nursing theory

(Fawcett, 1983, 1989; Walker & Avant, 1983; Chinn, 1983). Moreover, the steps in theory construction, analysis, and evaluation are usually made explicit in logical positivist theory for quantitative theory findings.

Today and in the future, we will see more qualitative paradigm theories in nursing. During the past three decades as a leader in this movement, I have identified criteria to evaluate qualitative theories which are presented in Chapter 2. Some important *questions* to help evaluate a qualitative theory in order to preserve the philosophy and purposes of the qualitative paradigm include the following (see also Chapter 2) (Leininger, 1985; Lincoln & Guba, 1985):

1. Do the findings from the study provide sufficient *credible and "thick data"* from the informants and other sources to support the domain and tenets of the theory?

2. Do the findings from the study give evidence to *confirm* findings of the theory in relation to the domain of inquiry and/or research questions and theory tenets?

3. Do the findings from the study reflect *saturation* of ideas with thick and full accounts about the meanings, expressions, and other qualitative indicators to support the theoretical tenets under study?

4. Do the findings show a *pattern of recurrency* to substantiate the theoretical tenets, questions, or general domain of inquiry?

5. Do the findings give evidence of sufficient data to support *meaning-in-context* in relation to the theoretical ideas under study?

6. Do the findings show evidence of *transferability to similar contexts* in relation to the theory?

7. Do the findings reflect *accurately* the ideas, experiences, or beliefs as known to the key and general informants and the researcher's observations and participatory experiences over time?

Reflecting on current and traditional ways of evaluating or testing nursing theories, the following brief comments can be offered:

1. *Origins of the theory*—this criterion is of much interest, but not essential to establish the credibility of a qualitative theory.

2. *Logical adequacy* of a theory is usually *not* of great importance in qualitative studies, and can be detrimental to exploring largely unknown, *illogical*, subjective, and transcendental data offered by informants. One must remember that a theory which has *logical structure* and its *own concepts*, definitions, and rigid formulations may be quite inappropriate for the culture or social setting being studied. Logic may reside in the researcher's world, but may not be known or understandable in the informants' conceptual and lived world.

3. *Usefulness* of a theory focuses on how practical or helpful the theory is to the discipline. Culture Care theory, for example, does have practical features but there also may be some impractical features because of new ideas that may take some time before they become "useful" to nursing with current norms and practices. The theory, however, may be very useful to establish what potentially may be needed now and in the future. For example, the use of folk care practices may make the theory look useless, impractical, or irrelevant to nursing, and yet generic folk care may be extremely useful in advancing nursing and in working with clients.

4. *Generalizability of the theory* refers essentially to wide use and statistical support for the theory to be used with groups, populations, etc. In qualitative theoretical research, however, as Lincoln and Guba (1985) state, *generalizations are not the goal.* Instead, the goal is to obtain findings that are meaningful to particularized individuals or groups. A theory can be extremely valuable even though it is *not generalizable* to many people and populations. Such findings can provide in-depth knowledge of a particular culture, individual, family, or group.

5. The concept of *parsimony* used to evaluate most nursing theories is problematic in that some theories are comprehensive, complex, and open to wide discovery of multiple factors, and are not constructed to be restrictive and tight with few variables, hypotheses, and other quantitative features. A qualitative theory constructed to seek in-depth study of undiscovered or unknown phenomenon can seldom be stated or presented in a parsimonious way nor should it be. The use of a few

equations, explanations, or a specific mathematical equation are often inappropriate as these features support quantitative studies and tend to reduce understanding of phenomena.

6. *Usefulness* of the theory refers to the above as the practical, concrete, and helpful ways that the theory and the findings can be used by the discipline. Indeed, there may be both impractical and non-useful outcomes from qualitative theories and concomitant research findings. Sometimes qualitative data from a theory may not be meaningful or fit the context or present situation; yet such findings are often valued as knowledge discovered even though it cannot be applied instantly or used in all applied or clinical situations.

In sum, nurse theorists and users of theories are beginning to realize there are different ways to develop, analyze, and evaluate nursing theories. To limit theory development and testing to quantitative paradigmatic thinking greatly curtails discovering nursing's covert and elusive phenomena today and in the future. A new generation of nurse theorists are now developing and analyzing theories within the qualitative paradigm and they will be expected to use qualitative criteria. Indeed, the "turning point" as discussed by Capra (1983) for physical sciences, and by the author since the 1950s, is now being realized by more nurses today. Consequently, new knowledge in nursing is being discovered by different theories, methods, and with appropriate criteria within the two major types of qualitative or quantitative paradigmatic perspectives. The theory of Culture Care is one such theory providing new knowledge with specific and broad perspectives to advance nursing knowledge.

NOTES

[1] In keeping with qualitative research methods and writing, the first person will be used as a direct and personalized way to the reader's experience and ideas.

[2] The term *construct* was used in the theory to refer to several concepts or ideas that are embedded in and used to know fully the term or a domain of inquiry. Construct is a much broader and more inclusive term than concept, for it has many implicit and explicit meanings that have to be teased out in research processing.

REFERENCES

Ashley, J. (1976). *Hospital paternalism and the role of the nurse.* New York: Teacher's College Press.

Benner, P., & Wrubel, J. (1989). *The primacy of caring: Stress and coping in health and illness.* Menlo Park, CA: Addison-Wesley.

Bevis, E. O. (1981). Caring: A life force. In M. M. Leininger (Ed.), *Caring: An essential human need.* Detroit: Wayne State University Press, 49–59.

Bevis, E. O., & Murray, J. (1979). *Caring curriculum and teaching process.* Unpublished paper. National Research Care Conference, Salt Lake City, UT.

Brunner, J. (1962). *On knowing.* Cambridge: Belnap Press.

Capra, F. (1983). *The turning point.* New York: Bantam.

Carter, M. (1985). The philosophic dimensions of qualitative nursing science research. In M. M. Leininger (Ed.), *Qualitative research methods in nursing.* Orlando, FL: Grune & Stratton, 27–32.

Chinn, P. L. (1983). *Advances in nursing theory development.* Rockville, MD: Aspen.

Donaldson, S. K., & Crowley, D. M. (1977). Disciplining of nursing: Structure and relationship to practice. In M. V. Batey (Ed.), *Optimizing environments for health. Nursing's unique perspective. Communicating Nursing Research* Vol. 10 (pp. 1–22). Boulder, CO: WICHE.

Fawcett, J. (1983). Hallmark of success in nursing theory development. In P. L. Chinn (Ed.), *Advances in nursing theory development.* Rockville, MD: Aspen.

Fawcett, J. (1984). The metaparadigm in nursing: Present status and future refinements. *Image: The Journal of Nursing Scholarship, 16*(3), 84–87.

Fawcett, J. (1989). *Analysis and evaluation of conceptual models of nursing,* (Second edition), Philadelphia: F. A. Davis.

Gaut, D. (1981). Conceptual analysis of caring. In M. M. Leininger (Ed.), *Caring: An essential human need.* Detroit: Wayne State University, 17–24.

Gaut, D. (1984). A theoretic description of caring as action. In M. M. Leininger (Ed.), *Caring: The essence of nursing and health.* Thorofare, NJ: Slack, 17–24.

Gaut, D. & Leininger, M. M. (1991). *Care: The compassionate healer.* New York: National League for Nursing.

Henderson, V. (1966). *The nature of nursing,* New York: Macmillan.

Hofling, C., & Leininger, M. M. (1960). *Basic psychiatric concepts in nursing.* Philadelphia: J. B. Lippincott.

Johnson, D. (1959). The nature of science of nursing. *Nursing Outlook, 7*(5), 291–294.

Kalisch P., & Kalisch, B. (1987). *The changing image of the nurse.* Menlo Park, CA: Addison-Wesley.

Kuhn, T. S. (1970). *The structure of scientific revolutions (2nd ed.).* Chicago: University of Chicago Press.

Larson, P. (1987). Comparison of cancer patients' and professional nurses' perceptions of important nurse caring behaviors. *Heart and Lung, 16,* 187-193.

Leininger, M. M. (1965). *Culture care as a central theoretical concept in the discipline and profession of nursing.* Unpublished paper. Denver: University of Colorado.

Leininger, M. M. (1966). *Convergence and divergence of human behavior: An ethnopsychological comparative study of two Gadsup villages in the Eastern Highlands of New Guinea.* Unpublished doctoral dissertation. Seattle: University of Washington.

Leininger, M. M. (1967). The culture concept and its relevance to nursing, *Journal of Nursing Education, 6*(2), 27-39.

Leininger, M. M. (1969a). Ethnoscience: A promising research approach to improve nursing practice. *Image: The Journal of Nursing Scholarship, 3,* 22-28.

Leininger, M. M. (1969b). Nature of science in nursing. Conference on the nature of science in nursing. *Nursing Research, 18*(5), 388-389.

Leininger, M. M. (1970). The culture concept and American culture values in nursing. In *Nursing and anthropology: Two worlds to blend.* New York: John Wiley & Sons, 45-52.

Leininger, M. M. (1972). *Using cultural styles in the helping process and in relation to the subculture of nursing.* Nursing papers at the Illinois Psychiatric Institute, May 13-14, Chicago, IL, 1971. Illinois Psychiatric Institute, 43-61.

Leininger, M. M. (1973a). *Becoming aware of types of health practitioners and cultural imposition.* In American Nurses Association 48th Convention paper. Kansas City: American Nurses Association, 9-15.

Leininger, M. M. (1973b). *Contemporary issues in mental health nursing.* Boston: Little, Brown & Co.

Leininger, M. M. (1973c). Towards conceptualization of transcultural health care systems. *Health Care Issues.* Philadelphia: F. A. Davis, 3-22.

Leininger, M. M. (1976). Doctoral programs for nurses. Trends, questions, and projected plans. *Nursing Research, 25*(210), 210.

Leininger, M. M. (1976a). Caring: The essence and central focus of nursing. American Nurses Foundation. *Nursing Research Report, 12*(1), 2, 14.

Leininger, M. M. (1976b). Towards conceptualization of transcultural health care system: Concepts and a model. In M. M. Leininger (Ed.), *Transcultural health care issues and conditions.* Philadelphia: F. A. Davis, 3-22.

Leininger, M. M. (1976c). *Transcultural health care issues and conditions:* Philadelphia: F. A. Davis.

Leininger, M. M. (1977). The phenomenon of caring: Caring the essence and central focus of nursing. American Nurses' Foundation. *Nursing Research Report*, 12(1), 2-14.

Leininger, M. M. (1978). *Transcultural nursing: Concepts, theories, and practices*. New York: John Wiley & Sons.

Leininger, M. M. (1979). *Transcultural nursing*. New York: Mason.

Leininger, M. M. (1980). Care: A central focus of nursing and health care services. *Nurses and Health Care*, 1(3), 135-143.

Leininger, M. M. (1981). *Care: An essential human need*. Thorofare, NJ: Slack.

Leininger, M. M. (1981-89). *Ethnocare and ethnohealth of ten cultures in urban environmental contexts*. Unpublished manuscript. Detroit: Wayne State University Press.

Leininger, M. M. (1983). Cultural care: An essential goal for nursing and health care. *The American Association of Nephrology Nurses and Technicians*, 10(5), 11-17.

Leininger, M. M. (1984a). *Care: The essence of nursing and health*. Detroit: Wayne State University Press. Reprinted in 1988.

Leininger, M. M. (1984b). Transcultural nursing: An essential knowledge and practice field for today. *The Canadian Nurse*, 41-45.

Leininger, M. M. (1984c). Southern rural black and white American lifeways with focus on care and health phenomenon. In *Care: The essence of nursing and health*. Detroit: Wayne State University Press. Reprinted in 1988.

Leininger, M. M. (1985a). *Qualitative research methods in nursing*. Orlando, FL: Grune and Stratton.

Leininger, M. M. (1985b). Ethnography and ethnonursing: Models and modes of qualitative data analysis. In *Qualitative research methods in nursing*. Orlando, FL: Grune & Stratton, 33-72.

Leininger, M. M. (1985c). Transcultural care diversity and universality: A theory of nursing. *Nursing and Health Care*, 6(4), 209-212.

Leininger, M. M. (1986). Care facilitation and resistance factors. In Z. Wolf (Ed.), *Clinical care in nursing*. Rockville, MD: Aspen, 1-24.

Leininger, M. M. (1987a). Importance and uses of ethnomethods: Ethnography and ethnonursing research. In M. Cahoon (Ed.), *Recent advances in nursing*. London: Churchill Livingston, 17, 23-25.

Leininger, M. M. (1987b). *Care: Discovery and uses in clinical and community nursing*. Detroit: Wayne State University Press, 1-30.

Leininger, M. M. (1988a). *Care: The essence of nursing and health*. Detroit: Wayne State University Press.

Leininger, M. M. (1988b). *Care: An essential human need*. Detroit: Wayne State University Press.

Leininger, M. M. (1988c). Leininger's theory of nursing: Cultural care diversity and universality. *Nursing Science Quarterly*. Baltimore: Williams & Wilkins Press, 2(4), 11–20.

Leininger, M. M. (1989). Transcultural Nursing: A worldwide necessity to advance nursing knowledge and practice. In J. McCloskey & H. Grace (Eds.), *Nursing issues*. Boston: Little, Brown & Co.

Leininger, M. M. (1990a). Ethnomethods: The philosophic and epistemic basis to explicate transcultural nursing knowledge. *Journal of Transcultural Nursing*, 1(2), 40–51.

Leininger, M. M. (1990b). *Leininger-Templin-Thompson ethnoscript qualitative software program: User's Handbook*. Detroit: Wayne State University Press.

Leininger, M. M. (1990c). Historic and epistemologic dimensions of care and caring with future directions. In J. Stevenson (Ed.), *American academy of nursing*. Kansas City, MO: American Nurses Association Press, 19–31.

Leininger, M. M., & Watson, J. (1990d). *The caring imperative in nursing education*. New York: National League for Nursing.

Lincoln, Y., & Guba, G. (1985). *Naturalistic inquiry*. Beverly Hills: Sage.

Luna, L. (1989). Transcultural nursing care of Arab Muslims. *Journal of Transcultural Nursing*, 1(1), 22–27.

Meleis, A. (1985). *Theoretical nursing: Development and progress*. Philadelphia.

McGlothlin, W. (1960). *Patterns of professional education*. New York: G. P. Putnam & Sons.

Munhall, P. L. (1982). Nursing philosophy and nursing research: In apposition or opposition? *Nursing Research*, 31, 176–177, 181.

Nightingale, F. (1859). *Notes on nursing: What it is and what it is not*. London: Harrison and Sons.

Orem, D. (1980). *Nursing: Concepts of practice*. McGraw-Hill.

Orlando, I. J. (1961). *The dynamic nurse-patient relationship*. New York: G. P. Putnam & Sons.

Parson, T. (1939). *The professors and social structure: Social forces*. The College Book Company.

Peplau, H. (1952). *Transcultural health care issues and conditions*. Philadelphia: F. A. Davis.

Pike, K. (1954). *Language in relation to a unified theory of the structure of human behavior*. Glendale, CA: Summer Institute of Linguistics.

Ray, M. (1981). Philosophical analysis of caring. In M. M. Leininger (Ed.), *Caring: An essential human need*. Thorofare, NJ: Slack, 25–36.

Ray, M. (1987). Technological caring: A new model in critical care. *Dimensions in Critical Care Nursing*, 6, 166–173.

Reason, P., & Rowan, J. (1981). *Human Inquiry: A source book of new paradigm*. New York: John Wiley & Sons.

Reilly, D. E. (1975). Why a conceptual framework? *Nursing Outlook, 23,* 566–569.

Rieman, D. (1986). The essential structure of a caring interaction: Doing phenomenology. In P. Munhall & C. Oiler (Eds.), *Nursing research: A qualitative perspective.* Norwalk, CT: Appleton-Century-Crofts.

Roach, S. (1984). *Caring: The human mode of being, implications for nursing.* Toronto: Faculty of Nursing, University of Toronto. (Perspectives in Caring Monograph 1.)

Roach, S. (1987). *The human act of caring.* Ottawa: Canadian Hospital Association.

Rogers, M. E. (1970). *An introduction to the theoretical basis of nursing.* Philadelphia: F. A. Davis.

Spradley, J. (1979). *Ethnographic interview.* New York: Holt, Rinehart and Winston.

Spradley, J. (1980). *Participant observation.* New York: Holt, Rinehart and Winston.

Stevens, B. J. (1979). *Nursing theory: Analysis, application, evaluation.* Boston: Little, Brown & Co.

Walker, L., & Avant, K. (1983). *Strategies for theory construction in nursing.* Norwalk, CT: Appleton & Lange.

Watson, J. (1979). *Nursing: The philosophy of science care.* Boston: Little, Brown & Co.

Watson, J. (1985a). *Nursing: Human science and human care: A theory of nursing.* Norwalk, CT: Appleton-Century-Crofts.

Watson, J. (1985b). Reflections on different methodologies for the future of nursing. In M. M. Leininger (Ed.), *Qualitative research method in nursing.* Orlando, FL: Grune & Stratton, 27–32.

Some Key Updated References

Leininger, M. (1995) *Transcultural Nursing: Concepts, Theories, Research and Practices* (Second Edition) Columbus, OH. McGraw Hill College Custom Series.

Leininger, M. (1997) Overview and Reflection of the theory of Culture Care and the ethnonursing research method. *Journal of Transcultural Nursing,* 8(2) pp. 32–51.

Leininger, M. and M. McFarland. *Transcultural Nursing, Concepts, Theories, Research, and Practices* (Third Edition) New York: McGraw Hill Co.

Part

II

ETHNONURSING RESEARCH STUDIES TO REFLECT USES OF CULTURE CARE THEORY

In this section, ethnonursing research is presented as a method specifically designed to study Leininger's theory of Culture Care Diversity and Universality. This method was the first nursing research method conceived and designed in the early 1960s to study a nursing theory and related nursing phenomena. Included here are the philosophy, rationale, and major features of the ethnonursing method along with research guidelines, principles, "enablers," and qualitative criteria to evaluate the theory within the qualitative paradigm.

This first chapter serves as a general methodological framework for the subsequent chapters that follow, and shows the close relationship of the ethnonursing method with the use of Culture Care theory. Each research study focuses on different cultures or subcultures with specific domains of inquiry conceptualized within Leininger's Culture Care theory. The use of the method with the theory reveals the importance of the ethnonursing research method to study specific nursing phenomena with a theoretical perspective to generate new nursing knowledge or different nursing perspectives.

2

Ethnonursing: A Research Method with Enablers to Study the Theory of Culture Care

Madeleine M. Leininger

The ultimate goal of a professional nurse scientist and humanist is to discover, know, and creatively use culturally based care knowledge with its fullest meanings, expressions, symbols, and functions for healing, and to promote or maintain well being (or health) with people of diverse cultures in the world.

Leininger

In the past history of nursing, nurse theorists and researchers have borrowed and depended on research methods from other disciplines to study or test nursing phenomena. The idea of nurses developing their own nursing research methods to study nursing phenomena and specifically nursing theories has not been a dominant practice until recently. Today there are a few nurse researchers who are beginning to realize that nurses may need to develop their own research methods and strategies to study particular nursing domains, problems, or questions. This awareness has occurred largely because of the inadequacy of borrowed methods to study highly complex, covert, and embedded nursing phenomena such as human care and well being.

When considering past norms of nurse researchers, it is clear that nurses rely strongly on established research methods in order to adhere to the tenets of logical positivism or the "received view" of empirical scientists (Carter, 1985; Leininger, 1985a). To develop new research methods to study nursing phenomena was untenable because nurses felt compelled to use the scientific method to obtain reliable and valid data and to have their research recognized by other "hard core" logical positivists. Moreover, the culture of nursing reflected largely "other-directed" (Leininger, 1970) decisions and practices until recent years, and so most nurses would not consider that they could be self-directed and have sufficient confidence to develop their own research methods. Indeed, nurses have been quick to use ready-made methods and standardized instruments already in use and validated by largely non-nursing methodologists. Thus, the idea to develop nursing research methods to study nursing phenomena was a radical and bold new step which this author took in the early 1960s. It was still a more courageous step to develop a research method to study a specific nursing theory such as cultural care. These and related trends set the context for discussing the ethnonursing research method as an essential nursing method to study a nursing theory.

In this chapter, the author presents the purpose, rationale, and philosophy for the ethnonursing research method. Specific features of the method are given along with the research process and principles, research enablers, and other aspects of the method. The chapter serves as background framework for several research studies that follow and demonstrates the use of the method with the Culture Care theory. The research philosophy, process, and enabling tools are an integral and important part of the ethnonursing research method.

PURPOSE AND RATIONALE FOR ETHNONURSING METHOD

The central purpose of the ethnonursing research method was to establish a naturalistic and largely *emic* open inquiry discovery method to explicate and study nursing phenomena especially related to the theory of Culture Care Diversity and Universality. This research method was designed to tease out complex, elusive, and largely unknown nursing dimensions from the people's local viewpoints such as human care, well being, and health and environmental influencers. In the 1950s and 1960s, there were no appropriate nursing research methods to explicate and to know and understand the nature, essence, and characteristics of human care, and of actual or perceived nursing phenomena. The use of borrowed research methods was quite inadequate to study in-depth human caring and from a transcultural perspective. In those days, I had already identified human care as central to nursing, but there was a critical need to know the meanings, expressions, patterns, functions, and structure of human care and caring. Without such knowledge, nursing could not support or justify its existence as a profession or a discipline. As a nurse leader eager to make nursing a legitimate, scholarly, and well-grounded discipline, I held that nurses needed research methods to establish the scientific, humanistic, epistemic, and ontologic bases for nursing's unique discipline perspectives especially focused on human care (Leininger, 1969). How people knew and experienced human care was essential for nurses to describe, document, and explain so that this knowledge could ultimately guide nursing practices. An open discovery and naturalistic people-centered research method was needed that would permit people to share their ideas about care in a spontaneous and informative way with nurse researchers.

From my continuing clinical nursing studies, I realized that care was an ambiguous and often elusive phenomena that was extremely difficult to study (Leininger, 1976, 1980, 1981). From an anthropological perspective, I realized that care was extremely difficult to identify as it was embedded in the worldview, social structure, and cultural values of a particular culture. Revealing embedded and undiscovered care phenomena required an inductive and open inquiry method that was familiar to human groups. Nursing needed a research method that would help nurses discover and fully know the many elusive and unknown ideas about human care, and especially while working with people of different cultures.

Prior to the decade of the 1960s, as a nurse leader and researcher, I was cognizant that care had not been systematically explicated in nursing and different health care and cultural settings. If human care was to become the essential and distinctly claimed feature of nursing, such systematic explication was necessary. The idea of an ethnonursing research method which was people- or client-centered rather than researcher-centered also seemed necessary to know human care and its influence on the health and well being of people from different cultures in the world. Most assuredly, quantitative research methods (e.g., the experimental method) seemed questionable at best and inappropriate at worst to study human caring. Care meanings, perceptions, patterns, and experiences hardly could be studied at a distance, or manipulated, tightly controlled, and measured by quantitative methods. To lead people to credible and meaningful insights about humanistic care based on accurate findings so as to establish an epistemics of care knowledge required another method. Indeed, researchers that treated people as objects or non-humans could only lead to non-humanistic care data and debatable results. Clearly, such an approach was not congruent with the nature of nursing and human care practices, or to discover care knowledge essential for the profession. As caregivers, nurses are expected to get close to people and to establish and maintain intimate caring relationships. Research methods that relied on creating distance and controlling informants, as previously discussed, would limit the discovery of and learning about care meanings, structure, and processes. Thus, the then current quantitative methods in use by the scientific community were inappropriate to study human care and nursing care practices.

To study care phenomena required an openness to examining subjective, intersubjective, spiritual, or supernatural experiences as well as those experiences lived through human care. In addition, a research method was needed to discover, document, preserve, and accurately interpret care meanings and experiences of different cultural groups. This necessitated a perspective on methodology that was quite different from that prevailing in experimental and other types of quantitative methods used by nurses. The ethnonursing inductive and naturalistic research method was needed to discover the nature, essence, and distinguishing features of human care in different life contexts.

Another major reason to establish the ethnonursing research method was interest in discovering differences between *generic* or *native folk (naturalistic) care* (informally learned indigenous knowledge) and *professional nursing care* (learned through formal educational systems in nursing) among different cultures. I had speculated about differences between generic and professional care, but a research method was needed to tease out the subtle and elusive aspects of these sources of care. As a nurse anthropologist, I was aware that folk practices (and undoubtedly folk care) had been practiced by cultural groups for hundreds of years, and that "modern" professional nursing was a recent development in human history. Discovering generic or naturalistic care was held essential to know and to use in developing professional nursing care practices (Leininger, 1976, 1981). In the early 1960s, during my field study with the Gadsup of the Eastern Highlands of New Guinea (Leininger, 1966), I had come to realize that generic care was essential to know and understand in order to provide meaningful, congruent, and acceptable care—the goal of Culture Care theory. However, generic care was unknown and had not been considered for systematic discovery in professional nursing prior to the 1960s. Therefore, I predicted that generic care would be quite different from professional nursing (Leininger, 1970, 1978, 1981).

In the late 1950s, I learned by chance about Pike's (1954) use of the terms *emic* and *etic* in linguistic studies and thought that they would be most helpful to explicate and understand human care transculturally. At that time, although *emic* and *etic* were unknown in nursing, and had not been used in anthropological field research, I could see their usefulness as part of the ethnonursing research method to study care and other nursing phenomena. According to Pike, *emic* referred to the local informants or inside views of people whereas *etic* referred to the outsider's views of a culture. While studying the Gadsup of New Guinea, I had used these concepts (*emic* and *etic*) and found they greatly helped to reveal the meanings of ideas regarding the values, beliefs, norms, rituals, and symbols of care, health, and illness (Leininger, 1966, 1970). *Emic* ideas about Gadsup spiritual or ancestral beliefs became known to me with an *emic* focus on traditional ideas and experiences of the people. It is clear that the *emic* view also was needed to discover human care with other cultures regarding their history, social structure, environment, biological, ecological, and many other factors. *Etic* knowledge about professional nursing views also was needed to obtain a full understanding about human caring or care.

Most importantly, the ethnonursing method was conceived and developed to overcome the limitations and philosophical tenets of logical positivism, the use of the prevailing "scientific method," and other conventional features and goals of the quantitative paradigm to study nursing phenomena. Nursing was different from many established disciplines and its researchers needed better ways to discover its distinctive body of knowledge. As such, the conceived new and different ethnonursing method was viewed as the answer to discover the true essence, nature, patterns, and expressions of human care so as to advance nursing care knowledge (Leininger, 1969, 1978, 1981, 1984).

ETHNONURSING: ITS MAJOR FEATURES

Since the ethnonursing research method was the first of its kind developed to study nursing phenomena, it was conceptualized and developed from a nursing perspective (Leininger, 1978, 1985b, 1987, 1990a). The prefix, *ethno*, was chosen to refer to people, or a particular culture, with a focus on their worldview, ideas, and cultural practices related to nursing phenomena. Ethnonursing was developed as a research method to help nurses systematically document and gain greater understanding and meaning of the people's daily life experiences related to human care, health, and well being in different or similar environmental contexts (Leininger, 1980, 1985b, 1987, 1990a). My anthropological experiences with ethnography, ethnoscience, and ethnology in the early 1960s provided some rich insights of ways to study people and as a basis to develop the ethnonursing method. People-centered research with an *emic* focus required a friendly naturalistic approach that permitted people to share their ideas, beliefs, and experiences with research strangers or investigators unknown to the people being studied. It also was clear that the goals, purposes, and phenomena of anthropological research were different from those of nursing. As a result, the ethnonursing method was oriented to discover nursing's central interests or phenomena within the scope of human caring.

Discovery of *actual* or *potential* people-centered care, well being, and health phenomena as well as non-caring practices predicted to lead to illness, disability, or death was the primary purpose for developing the ethnonursing method. New insights from diverse cultures obtained from a holistic care perspective (biophysical and psychocultural) were needed to establish professional nursing within a discipline perspective both humanistic and scientific. I defined *ethnonursing* as a qualitative research method using naturalistic, open discovery, and largely inductively derived *emic* modes and processes with diverse strategies, techniques, and enabling tools to document, describe, understand, and interpret the people's meanings, experiences, symbols, and other related aspects bearing on actual or potential nursing phenomena (Leininger, 1978, 1985a, 1990a).

Establishing the ethnonursing research method required an approach radically different from the traditional quantitative paradigm (Leininger, 1985a). In the early 1960s, while the qualitative and quantitative paradigms and their features were largely unknown to nurses, their attributes were becoming identifiable. The ethnonursing method was designed to discover how things really were and the way people knew and lived in their world. The method focused on *learning from the people through their eyes, ears, and experiences* and how they made sense out of situations and lifeways that were familiar to them. The method required direct naturalistic observations, participant experiences, reflections, and checking back with the people to understand what one observed, heard, or experienced. It required that the ethnonurse researcher enter into a largely unknown world, remaining with the people of concern for an extended time, to learn first-hand meaningful constructions specific to the natural context or lived environment at hand. It meant that the realities of individuals, groups, or collectives were developed over time by enculturation or socialization processes and influenced by a variety of cultural and environmental factors. The use of *a priori* judgments, scientific hypotheses, and the testing of the researcher's interests or variables was not congruent with the ethnonursing method. Instead, with the ethnonursing method, the researcher had to suspend or withhold fixed judgments and predetermined truths to let the people's ideas come forth and be documented (Leininger, 1985b, 1987). Exploring the informants' world to discover vaguely known or unknown ideas about human care and other nursing phenomena was a dominant focus. The researcher had to be sensitive and responsive to the people's ideas and to interpret ideas that gave meaning to the informants' views and cultural lifeways about human care or non-caring along with the factors influencing the phenomena discovered.

Since the mid 1950s, I had perceived care as the essence of nursing, and what distinguished nursing from other health professionals (Leininger, 1967, 1970, 1976, 1980, 1984). However, I realized that human care required systematic investigation with a method appropriate to discover the full subjective and objective human meanings, patterns, and values of care in different cultures. This research goal was essential to establish the epistemics or roots of nursing knowledge for the discipline and profession of nursing. Because nurses claimed to care for all people, a research method was needed to discover what was universal or diverse about human care transculturally. Generic or people-based care could only be fully known by studying care from the people in their natural contexts such as the home, workplace, or wherever people lived and functioned each day and night, and in different cultures. Thus, the ethnonursing method functioned as a means to obtain new foundational or substantive nursing knowledge to establish human care as the discipline's knowledge base. While this goal was yet to be recognized by nurse researchers and scholars, it remained for me a preeminent guide to differentiated nursing care decisions and actions in professional practices.

As a nurse and anthropologist, I pondered why human care had not been systematically studied and why it remained a largely unexplored area in the 1950s. I also wondered why human care transculturally had not been studied by anthropologists. I soon realized that care and its relationship to well being was awaiting discovery by nurses. But, again, to study the ambiguous and invisible phenomenon of human care from a transcultural perspective (Leininger, 1978, 1980) required a uniquely focused research method that included transcultural human care phenomena as well as other largely unknown dimensions of nursing such as *health*, *well being*, and *environmental contexts* in their historical, religious, kinship, language, technologic, environmental, biocultural, and other aspects. To obtain care knowledge from such broad dimensions of social structure and other factors required an inductive ethnonursing approach to grasp the totality of cultural care and to establish ultimately holistic nursing care practices over practices derived from the fragmented, predetermined, disease and symptom medical model then in use.

From my perspective, nursing was far too narrowly oriented and ethnocentric to discover holistic care in cultural and social contexts and to discover transcultural human care. Cultural care within the tenets of the theory provided the broadest and most comprehensive holistic means to discover care and related nursing knowledge. Most importantly, my anthropology field experiences had led me to realize that care, well being, health, illness, and other related aspects of nursing were largely embedded in worldview and complex social structure factors related to kinship, cultural values, religion, environmental, worldview, biological, and language expressions, and so these dimensions had to be explicated and fully known in nursing.

While developing and refining the ethnonursing method in the early 1960s, I found myself quite alone in the study of human care from a transcultural nursing perspective. I also realized there were no research mentors or professional nurses available or interested in examining my new ethnonursing method. As a result, I developed and refined the method largely from my ongoing ethnonursing research experiences and with graduate students whom I encouraged to study care from a transcultural nursing viewpoint. These realities required that I spend considerable time establishing the method and educating students, which delayed the sharing of ideas with other nurses. However, the method was developed, refined, and did attract many nurse researchers whose feedback was helpful. Unquestionably, nurse researchers who were firmly entrenched within logical positivism and the quantitative scientific methods in the 1950s and 1960s regarded the ethnonursing qualitative method as "too soft." It did not have measurable and statistical outcomes as required by the "received view" of the logical positivists (Carter, 1985; Leininger, 1985b, 1987, 1990a; Watson, 1985). Moreover, the idea of nursing developing its *own* method to study nursing phenomena was not acceptable in those early days. Nursing, we must remember, was then trying to become "scientific" by joining the league of other "hard-core" quantitative scientists and emulating their ways.

It is of historical interest that before going to the Eastern Highlands of New Guinea, I conceptualized the ethnonursing method and developed some enabling guides such as the *Stranger-Friend Model* (Figure 1)

Figure 1
Leininger's Stranger to Trusted Friend Enabler Guide*

The purpose of this enabler is to facilitate the researcher (or it can be used by a clinician) to move from mainly a distrusted stranger to a trusted friend in order to obtain authentic, credible, and dependable data (or establish favorable relationships as a clinician). The user assesses him or herself by reflecting on the indicators as he/she moves from stranger to friend.

Indicators of Stranger (Largely etic or outsider's views) Informant(s) or people are:	Date Noted	Indicators as a Trusted Friend (Largely emic or insider's views) Informant(s) or people are:	Date Noted
1. Active to protect self and others. They are "gate keepers" and guard against outside intrusions. Suspicious and questioning.		1. Less active to protect self. More trusting of researchers (their "gate keeping is down or less"). Less suspicious and less questioning of researcher.	
2. Actively watch and are attentive to what researcher does and says. Limited signs of trusting the researcher or stranger.		2. Less watching the researcher's words and actions. More signs of trusting and accepting a new friend.	
3. Skeptical about the researcher's motives and work. May question how findings will be used by the researcher or stranger.		3. Less questioning of the researcher's motives, work and behavior. Signs of working with and helping the researcher as a friend.	
4. Reluctant to share cultural secrets and views as private knowledge. Protective of local lifeways, values and beliefs. Dislikes probing by the researcher or stranger.		4. Willing to share cultural secrets and private world information and experiences. Offers most local views, values and interpretations spontaneously or without probes.	
5. Uncomfortable to become a friend or to confide in stranger. May come late, be absent and withdraw at times from researcher.		5. Signs of being comfortable and enjoying friends and a sharing relationship. Gives presence, on time, and gives evidence of being a "genuine friend".	
6. Tends to offer inaccurate data. Modifies "truths" to protect self, family, community, and cultural lifeways. *Emic* values, beliefs, and practices are not shared spontaneously.		6. Wants research "truths" to be accurate regarding beliefs, people, values and lifeways. Explains and interprets *emic* ideas so researcher has accurate data.	

* Developed and used since 1959: Leininger.

82

Figure 2
Leininger's Ethnonursing Enabler
Observation-Participation-Reflection Phases

Phases: 1 ⟶ 2 ⟶ 3 ⟶ 4

Primary	Primary	Primary	Primary
Observation &	*Observation*	*Participation*	*Reflection &*
Active Listening	with limited	with continued	*Reconfirmation*
(no active	participation	observations	of findings
participation)			with informants

and the *Observation-Participation-Reflection Model* (Figure 2). These enablers helped guide me in entering and remaining with the people to study their lifeways in relation to nursing care phenomena in a systematic and reflective way. The *Stranger-Friend Model* became an important part of the ethnonursing method and has been an essential guide for the researcher to obtain accurate and credible data. It was a fascinating and rewarding research experience to discover rich and meaningful data by entering the people's world as a coparticipant. I soon realized that the ethnonursing method was important to discover nursing caring ways of feeding infants, dealing with pain and anxiety, supporting people in lifecycle events and crises, finding different ways to help people, and instructing people to maintain their well being. Explication of such caring aspects of nursing and the full epistemics of care phenomena required the ethnonursing method. Specific techniques, strategies, and the use of several enabling guides were valuable to tease out the elusive, complex, and ambiguous aspects of care (as a noun) and caring (as an action) with individuals, families, and groups of different or similar cultural care systems.

EPISTEMIC AND PHILOSOPHICAL VALUES TO SUPPORT THE ETHNONURSING METHOD

Philosophically, the term *ethnonursing* was purposefully coined for this research method because *ethno* comes from the Greek word, *ethos*, and refers to "the people" or culture with their lifeways. The suffix *nursing* was essential to focus the research on nursing's phenomena concerned primarily with the humanistic and scientific aspects of human care, well being, and health in different environmental and cultural contexts (Leininger, 1978, 1980, 1984, 1985b, 1988). Therefore, the ethnonursing research method was designed to discover how people knew and experienced these major but insufficiently explored areas of nursing phenomena from a transcultural context and perspective in relation to the theory of Culture Care Diversity and Universality. Discovering such a potentially large base of nursing knowledge would provide the epistemic, historic, and ontological "roots" as well as contemporary sources of nursing's discipline knowledge (Leininger, 1980, 1984, 1990a).

Philosophically and epistemologically, the sources of ethnonursing knowledge were held to be *grounded with the people* as the *knowers* about human care and other nursing knowledge. It was the ethnonurse researcher's task as the *knowee* to learn from the people nursing phenomena and the factors influencing care and health from the local knowers' viewpoints and daily and nightly lived experiences. The knowers were seen as teachers who would share their experiences, insights, and other knowledge of interest with the researcher. Obtaining such grounded data was essential to establish the epistemics and ontological nature and features of human care. Grounded data discoveries had long been part of ethnographic method as a way of knowing and generating theoretical data since the early, creative work of Bronislaw Malinkowski (1922) with the Trobrianders in the mid-nineteenth century and with Franz Boas (1924) and his detailed work with the North American Indians. These pioneers set the idea of grounded, detailed, and epistemic sources of knowledge from "the people" long before the work of Glaser and Strauss (1967) and other later qualitative methodologists. While I valued grounded discovery with the ethnonursing method to obtain full, rich data directly from people about human care and related nursing phenomena, I used both the *emic* (local) with *etic* (non-local) method to obtain a more complete understanding of the phenomena of interest to nursing. This philosophical posture, that indigenous or local people were able to cognitively describe, know, explain, interpret, and even predict human care patterns, was an entirely new perspective to nurses in the 1960s and is still so today with some nurses. Indeed, some nurses question this philosophical posture believing that professionals are the "knowers" of care and "medical truths" and that their mission is to "instruct or teach" clients who are "non-knowers" of what is best for them. Granted, nurses have professional knowledge, but it may not reflect culturally based knowledge that largely guides human decisions and actions.

The ethnonursing method, therefore, was a way of discovering, knowing, and confirming people's knowledge about care, and ways to keep well, or how they can become ill or disabled. For the ethnonurse researcher, the challenge is to be an interested friend of the people and to participate with them in discovering their past and current cultural beliefs, values, and ideas about human care, health, well being, and other nursing dimensions. The ethnonurse researcher develops skill in teasing out or explicating the people's ideas about human care meanings, expressions, forms, patterns, and general care experiences as lived. This required the use of relaxed, open-ended inquiry modes done in nonaggressive or nonconfrontive ways. It also required a genuinely interested mode of listening to and confirming informants' ideas. This approach was held essential for informants to become the primary sharers and definers of ideas in discussion with the researcher, which could ensure accurate and meaningful interpretation of those ideas. Being a humble and open learner is as vital to this research method as it is a reversal of roles from the conventional scientific method which assumes, at least here, that the researcher holds, by logical inferences, other research studies, or from previously learned professional expertise, superior knowledge. Keeping an "open mind" and suspending personal beliefs, past professional experiences, and research experiences were essential attributes of the method and philosophy.

More specifically, as launched in the early 1960s, this ethnonursing research method had several general philosophical and research features to study ideas related to Culture Care Diversity and Universality (Leininger, 1966, 1970, 1978, 1985b, 1987, 1990a). First, the method required the researcher to move into familiar and naturalistic people settings to study human care and related nursing phenomena. The use of contrived, artificially controlled settings or being manipulative was not acceptable to obtain credible and accurate people-based data. Likewise, a tightly or rigidly controlled research design was not desired as the nurse researcher was expected to "move with the local people or situation" as the people told their past or present story, events, or lived experiences. The researcher was challenged to enter the *emic* or local world and to gradually become an active and genuinely interested learner. An ethnonursing research design could be used as rough schema (or sometimes with a very limited schema) to guide the research process. But whatever design or guide was used, it had to accommodate or *move with* the people or local informants' lifeways and their patterns of knowing and sharing ideas bearing on human caring within their local environmental context, human ecology, or framework.

Second, by necessity, the ethnonursing method reflected detailed observations, reflections, descriptions, participant experiences, and data derived from largely unstructured open-ended inquiries, or from enabler strategies. Open statements such as, "I would like to learn about your views, ideas or experiences about caring for others or self, in this setting or culture," are used (Leininger, 1985b, 1987, 1990a). Open-ended frames such as, "I would appreciate it if you would tell me more about _____" [whatever is being shared], or on a special event also are used. In addition, *emic*, local folktales, stories, or spontaneous narratives are elicited as well as *etic* ones to show any contrasts and similarities. Many additional examples of inquiry modes are given in other works (Leininger, 1984, 1985b; Wenger, 1985). Some suggestions from Spradley's (1979) ethnographic interviews are helpful, but his participant-observation research method is not the same as the ethnonursing method. In addition, learning to enter into a strange world requires some willingness to risk uncertainties and to become comfortable with strangers. It means developing skills to be an astute observer, listener, reflector, and accurate interpreter by taking a learner's role in the most naturally possible way. Being able to tolerate highly ambiguous, uncertain, subjective, or vaguely known complex sets of ideas requires patience, time, and genuine interest in others, an essential feature of the ethnonursing method. Some of these attributes can be found with people-sensitive nurses who have perfected these skills in their clinical practices and in teaching.

Third, the ethnonursing method requires that the researcher's biases, prejudices, opinions, and preprofessional interpretations be withheld, suspended, or controlled so that informants can present *their emic ideas and interpretations* rather than those of the researcher. Learning to value and respect the people's views and experiences when well, sick, disabled, oppressed, dying, or whatever human condition they are experiencing is an important skill with the method. Being cognizant of the researcher's views and any prejudices requires centering on the informant, active listening, and self-reflection often with a research mentor. The philosophical position that the individuals and cultural groups "can make sense out of their world" is often difficult for any professional nurse because of past dominant emphases on "knowing all about people being ill or having a specific diseased condition." However, informants can share ideas that make sense to them and are important to them whether ill or well. Avoiding a reinterpretation of the informant's ideas to fit professional knowledge and expectations is important. As such, research mentors prepared in the method are extremely valuable for the conduct of this method. Experienced ethnonurse researchers who have lived through and used the method can deal with the novice researcher's tendencies related to ethnocentrism, biases, prejudice, and reinterpretation tendencies. The mentor can help the researcher remain sensitive to research proclivities in order to obtain accurate and credible ethnonursing knowledge. Through reflection and clarification with the researcher, the research mentor can reduce ethnocentric tendencies and arrive at informant-based meanings and interpretations. These mentors also are challenged to help the novice nurse researcher who has been strongly enculturated in the use of quantitative research ideologies, techniques, precise measuring of data, and other tendencies that can seriously limit the full and accurate discovery of qualitative ethnocare phenomena. Mentors experienced in the ethnonursing method are also extremely important to assess ethical and moral issues related to informant "secrets," confidentiality, obtaining process consent, and recordings of detailed people data. They are especially useful in "teasing out" *generic* and *professional* care findings from large volumes of qualitative data and in analyzing all data collected. Having external nurse panelists who are not prepared in the method or in the culture are of limited use and may impose their ideas onto rich and new findings from an ethnonursing study.

Fourth, the ethnonursing method requires that the researcher focus on the *cultural context* of whatever phenomena are being studied. The cultural context refers to the totality of the situation or lifeway at hand (Leininger, 1970, 1987, 1990a). To discover and fully understand cultural context, often there are both contemporary and ethnohistorical underpinnings to consider as well. Since the 1960s, and in order to interpret cultural research findings accurately, I have held the idea of cultural context as an extremely important focus of my thinking and research. Grasping the full meaning of cultural context means examining historical, biosocial, cultural values, language expressions, technology, material, and symbolic referents of the people's environment being studied. Any removal of cultural contextual data, or "surgical pruning," can markedly reduce the credibility, accuracy, and meaning of what was seen, heard, or experienced. I have used the qualitative criterion of *meaning-in-context* in all of my field research emphasizing the importance of describing and detailing diverse factors impinging on the meanings of human care, health, or well being of the cultures. Inclusion of cultural context remains an essential aspect of ethnonursing research. Contextual data also provides thick descriptions to establish the study's credibility. Thick descriptions about human care with multiple external or internal cultural factors, symbols, and beliefs will help the researcher identify embedded "truths" about human care, well being, and the lifeways of the people. However, teasing out contextual data from the social structure and worldview takes time, patience, and cultural sensitivity.

Allowing the people themselves to come forth "to take control" of their knowledge and experiences to share their *emic* cultural viewpoints, values, and lifeways are important. The inductive *emic* approach helps to prevent researchers from using preconceived judgments or *a priori* views of modifying informants ideas. In general, obtaining full, thick, and detailed accounts of cultural care situations, events, or happenings through direct observations, participation, and interviews over time is critical to confirm and establish meaningful patterns of culture care. The ethnonurse researcher remains a coparticipant with informants to discover these detailed accounts and to see how the people practice human care in their daily and nightly lives.

With ethnonursing research, it is important to obtain in-depth particularistic or diverse accounts while searching for commonalities (Leininger, 1988, 1989). Ideographic or particularized patterns and situations are usually considered more important than broad-sweeping nomothetic generalizations with qualitative studies (Lincoln & Guba, 1985; Reason & Rowan, 1981). Arriving at generalizations to be applied to large numbers of people or population groups is not the goal of qualitative or ethnonursing research, and is, therefore, very different from quantitative research goals (Lincoln & Guba, 1985; Leininger, 1985b, 1990a). Instead, the goal of ethnonursing research is to know as fully as possible actual or potential nursing phenomena such as the meanings and expressions of human caring in different or similar contexts.

By focusing on some phenomena, the researcher often discovers new insights and ways people interpret and explain their world of knowing. For example, I discovered that there were gender differences between the adult Gadsup males and women regarding protective and surveillant care. Gadsup men had different ways to provide public protective care that contributed to the well being of the extended clan members, and felt a responsibility to provide protective care. The women also provided some protective care, but they were skilled in providing nurturant and surveillant domestic care activities, and not public care (Leininger, 1970, 1978). I also discovered that the Gadsup do not follow Erikson's (1963) stipulated stages of growth and development. Instead, the Gadsup had several phases of human development that were part Gadsup caring and nurturance and surveillance through the lifecycle. These comparative emic and etic differences have provided refreshing new lifecycle insights that care expressions, meanings, and interpretations were different from those in our Western culture. Such ideographic or particularistic findings have provided some entirely new perspectives to transcultural nursing knowledge. I also realized that many New Guinea findings were not generalizable to other cultures, but were more culture specific or relativistic as to Gadsups due largely to enculturation, social structure, and ethnohistorical factors. Such findings of a particular culture provide in-depth quality data, rather than generalized data about thousands of unknown "subjects" which limits understanding of the people.

Still characteristic in the use of the ethnonursing method is to give attention to the sequence of events or the ethnohistory of how care lifeways and patterns developed over time. Discovering how human care was traditionally viewed and how it may have changed with individuals and groups often provides fresh insights about cultural changes and variabilities in the culture. The use of ethnohistorical data from anthropologists or social science historians can be useful as background information to show how changes have occurred over time and under different circumstances. It is the task of the nurse researcher, however, to focus specifically on nursing phenomena in relation to ethnohistorical data. For example, human care practices often change drastically due to certain cultural events: major wars, feuds, coups, or major migrations to a new culture. The people's interpretations or explanation of these changes can provide meaningful explanations of the dynamic aspects of the culture. Such historical change practices contrast sharply with quantitative studies where historical data are viewed as threats to validity and reliability of a study and must be avoided or controlled (Polit & Hungler, 1983).

In conducting an ethnonursing study, the researcher uses a broad theoretical framework to guide the study such as the theory of Culture Care. However, theoretical frameworks should be broad enough to accommodate local or particular cultural care factors and serve as a general guide to inquiry. The researcher remains active to identify if the data supports or refutes the general or specific theoretical premises, and remains alert to the theoretical assumptions or presuppositions as guiding study parameters. Although ethnonurse researchers usually have a general theoretical framework in mind with a domain of inquiry, it is yet possible to conduct the study without any theory, and generate the theory in the process of conducting the study (Leininger, 1985b). The theory of Culture Care Diversity and Universality provides a broad schema about cultural care to help the researcher reflect on the theoretical tenets as well as the assumptions and major components of the theory such as worldview, social structure, cultural care values and beliefs, environment, and other dimensions held to influence human care. The theoretical framework also serves as an important guide to search for holistic and particular cultural factors about human care and caring, and to guide the analysis of data by covering all ethnonursing findings. Accordingly, a specific method of data analysis was developed as part of the ethnonursing method to provide systematic data analysis in relation to theoretical assumptions. Enablers were developed to explicate or tease out data related to the social structure and other components of the theory.

RESEARCH ENABLERS TO DISCOVER HUMAN CARE AND RELATED NURSING PHENOMENA

In accord with any method, the methodologist develops not only the major features of the method, but also techniques, strategies, and tools that can be used with the method to attain envisioned purposes. It is the methodological features with specific techniques and tools that differentiate one research method from others. In the late 1950s and before conducting my first ethnonursing and ethnography, I conceived of the idea "enablers" as ways to explicate, probe, or discover in-depth phenomena that seemed as complex, elusive, and ambiguous as human care. I disliked the term *instrument* as it was too impersonal, mechanistic, and fit with objectification, experimentation, and other methods and logical features of the quantitative paradigm. I also disliked the idea of the researcher being "the instrument" as it, too, harked of a cold, detached, and impersonal investigator. The idea of enablers and friendly researcher communicated a participatory and cooperative way to obtain ideas that were often difficult to know immediately or without gentle probing of informants willing to share their ideas. Enablers were congruent with the qualitative paradigm and as a means to explicate cultural care. In this section, some major enablers will be discussed briefly as I developed them and as part of the ethnonursing research method. Although I have developed several unique enablers during the past three decades, I will present only those of major importance that are frequently used by ethnonurse researchers to study comparative cultural care. The several ethnonursing research studies that follow this chapter have used these common enablers, and some researchers have developed their own specific enablers for a particular focus of their study.

Leininger's Stranger-Friend Enabler

I developed this model, the first enabler, before conducting my first ethnonursing and ethnography field study in the Eastern Highlands of New Guinea in the early 1960s (see Figure 1) (Leininger, 1985b). Although some aspects of the model were stimulated from reading Berreman's (1962) paper *Behind Many Masks*, it was reconceptualized with new practical indicators to help ethnonurse researchers move from a stranger to friend role when studying people with any nursing phenomena. The model was designed with the philosophical belief that the researcher should always assess and gauge the researcher's relationships with the people being studied in order to enter or get close to the people or situation under study. It was anticipated that the researcher needed to move from a stranger or distrusted person to a trusted and friendly person during the ethnonursing research process to obtain accurate, sensitive, meaningful, and credible data. Based on my extensive field work, I held that researchers, usually as *etic* strangers (outsiders), needed to be trusted *before* they would be able to obtain any accurate, reliable, or credible data. Initially, most cultural groups or informants find the researcher an outsider or a distrusted stranger until proven otherwise and someone to watch in regard to actions, motives, and behaviors. While a distrusted stranger, the people are generally quite reluctant to share their ideas with the researcher. On repeated occasions, and while a distrusted stranger, I have found that initial research data are often superficial, inaccurate, and incomplete (Leininger, 1970, 1978, 1985a). This is understandable—culture informants must protect themselves, their people, and their ideas until the informants know the researcher(s). This was further evident with psychological "standardized" tests, such as Holtzman, Thematic Apperception Test (TAT), and Rorchach, which I tried with the Gadsup and received non-truths in the stranger phase.

The pattern of moving from stranger to trusted friend can be identified in all research studies that I have mentored over the past three decades with 15–20 cultures (Leininger, 1970, 1978, 1985a,b). The purpose, therefore, of the Stranger-Friend Model is to serve as an assessment or reflection guide for the researcher to become consciously aware of own behaviors, feelings, and responses, and as one moves into and works to collect data for confirmation of cultural "truths" (Leininger, 1985b). Each of the indicators or characteristics for the stranger or friend in Figure 1 are used and studied over time to identify patterned behaviors and expectations of people-centered studies. They have been established as credible and reliable indicators with approximately 30 cultures (Leininger, 1985a,b).

The Stranger-Friend Model also serves as a gauge for the researcher's progress with some researchers remaining in the distrusted role longer than others. In using the model, the goal is to move from stranger to friend in order to help ensure a credible, meaningful, and accurate study. The model can be used by the researcher in hospital settings, in community contexts, and in many other places where nurses study nursing phenomena. Becoming aware of self-behavior as a researcher as well as observing those being studied is a major task for the researcher while actively participating with the people. This Stranger-Friend enabler is especially useful as nurse's study nurse-client, nurse–group, nurse–family relationships in the hospital or home. The model keeps the researcher alert to different indicators identified in the model, and the researcher learns to appraise the progress of the study by remaining sensitive to verbal feedback or responses from the people. This enabler is essential to all people-centered investigations, and, therefore, has been used by many researchers besides nurses involved in qualitative investigations. It is an enabler that can be used for all humanistic qualitative studies to facilitate the research process, get close to people, and obtain accurate data in a sensitive and skilled manner within different life contexts.

Observation-Participation-Reflection Enabler (O-P-R)

I developed the Observation-Participation-Reflection Model in the early 1960s, and have refined and used it for three decades along with many graduate students. The model was derived from the traditional participant-observation approach used in anthropology, but was modified in several ways and with the added focus of reflections to fit the philosophy, purposes, and goals of ethnonursing method (see Figure 2). The model also is different from the conventional anthropological "participant-observation" approach in that the process was reversed. With the O-P-R Model, the researcher is expected to devote a period of time making observation *before* becoming an active participant. This resequenced role serves the important function of allowing the nurse researcher to become fully cognizant of the situation or context before becoming a full participant or "doer." In addition, the reflection phase has been added to provide important and essential confirmatory data from the people studied. Reflection is done throughout the research process, but especially during the last phase of research. Thus, there are four phases rather than two phases found with the traditional participant-observation phases of anthropology. These phases were especially conceptualized and developed to fit with the people-centered nursing ways that professional nurses are expected to work within their daily experiences.

To perfect the O-P-R Model for ethnonursing studies, I, with many graduate students, have refined it several times during the past three decades (Leininger, 1978, 1985b, 1990a). The users find that the model provides a most helpful and systematic way to enter into, remain with, and conclude an ethnonursing study with individuals, groups, communities, and cultures related to human caring and nursing. This model helps the researcher get close to the people, study the total context, and obtain accurate data from the people. The most difficult phase for most nurse researchers is the first phase of observation because most nurses find it difficult to remain in a focused observer role before becoming a participant. Nurses who are active doers and who have not learned to do sustained observing before acting find that this model helps them learn about the importance of observing for a period of time before becoming an active participant and centering on context.

Reflection is an integral part of the ethnonursing method. Reflection on the phenomena observed or ideas heard helps the nurse to reflect on all contextual aspects of the research before proclaiming or interpreting an idea or experience. At the conclusion of the study, the researcher reflects back on all findings to recheck and confirm them primarily with key informants. Reflection on small and large segments of the data is essential at every phase of the research process as it helps one to study meanings-in-context and other aspects of the data. The O-P-R phases are a critical and important feature of the ethnonursing research method to ensure accurate observations and interpretations of findings. This enabler has been described in other sources (Leininger, 1985b, 1987; Wenger, 1985a), and by researchers who have used the ethnonursing method in this book.

Leininger's Phases of Ethnonursing Data Analysis Guide as An Enabler

A major concern of qualitative researchers has been to find ways to systematically analyze large amounts of field data. To meet this challenge, I developed and refined the Phases of Ethnonursing Data Analysis Guide (see Figure 3) as another enabler to facilitate the research process. This guide was developed and refined during the past several decades as a part of the ethnonursing method to provide rigorous, in-depth, and systematic analysis of qualitative ethnonursing research data, and especially research findings bearing on the theory of Cultural Care (Leininger, 1987). This enabler has been used by many nurses and by other researchers to analyze qualitative data, and

Figure 3
Leininger's Phases of Ethnonursing Analysis for Qualitative Data*

Fourth Phase

Major Themes, Research Findings, Theoretical Formulations, and Recommendations

This is the highest phase of data analysis, synthesis, and interpretation. It requires synthesis of thinking, configuration analysis, interpreting findings, and creative formulation from data of the previous phases. The researcher's task is to abstract and present major themes, research findings, recommendations, and sometimes theoretical formulations.

Third Phase

Pattern and Contextual Analysis

Data are scrutinized to discover saturation ideas and recurrent patterns of similar or different meanings, expressions, structural forms, interpretations, or explanations of data related to the domain of inquiry. Data are also examined to show patterning with respect to meanings-in-context and along with further credibility and confirmation of findings.

Second Phase

Identification and Categorization of Descriptors and Components

Data are coded and classified as related to the domain or inquiry and sometimes the questions under study. *Emic* or *etic* descriptors are studied within context and for similarities and differences. Recurrent components are studied for their meanings.

First Phase

Collecting, Describing, and Documenting Raw Data (Use of Field Journal and Computer)

The researcher collects, describes, records, and begins to analyze data related to the purposes, domain of inquiry, or questions under study. This phase includes: recording interview data from *key* and *general* informants; making observations, and having participatory experiences; identifying contextual meanings; making preliminary interpretations; identifying symbols; and recording data related to the phenomenon under study, mainly from an *emic* focus, but attentive to *etic* ideas. Field data from the condensed and full field journal is processed directly into the computer and coded.

* Leininger, M. M., (1987, 1990, and current revisions in 1991).

remains an important systematic data analysis method for qualitative studies. Currently, this method is replacing qualitative data analysis that is vague, ambiguous, or questionable such as doing a "content analysis" in which *all* data are analyzed in nonsystematic ways.

The Data Analysis Guide offers four sequenced phases of analysis. The researcher begins data analysis on the first day of research and continues with regular data coding, processing, and analysis of all data until all data are collected. The researcher uses the four levels of data analysis as seen in Figure 3. The data are continuously processed and reflected on by the researcher at each phase (originally, the model had six phases in 1965, but the tool has been refined and perfected to four phases).

As one examines the four phases in Figure 3, the major characteristics of each phase are presented (Leininger, 1987). In Phase I, the researcher analyzes grounded and detailed raw data before moving to Phase II. In Phase II, the researcher identifies the *descriptors, indicators,* and *categories* from the raw data in Phase I. In Phase III, the researcher identifies the *recurrent patterns* from the data as derived from Phase I and II. In Phase IV, *themes* of behavior and other *summative research findings* are presented and abstracted from the data as derived from the three previous phases. At all times, research findings from the data analysis can be traced back to each phase and to the grounded data in Phase I. This interphase check is essential to preserve *emic* data and to confirm findings by checking back on the findings at each phase. The systematic data analysis process is extremely detailed and is essential to understand the data and to trail back on the findings or conclusions. This process of data analysis is detailed and rigorous but essential to meet the criteria of qualitative data showing how the researcher met the criteria of credibility, recurrent patterning, confirmability, meaning-in-context, and other criteria of a qualitative study.

Data from ethnonursing interviews and the enablers such as the Observation-Participant-Reflection Model, Stranger-Friend Model, Health Care Life History Model, and others are incorporated in the total ethnonursing mode of data collection and analyses. The culminating abstraction and identification of themes in Phase IV constitute the highest level of data analysis. This phase also is the most difficult level of analysis as it requires critical analysis of all data and keen intellectual abilities to synthesize data and abstract meanings from the four phases so that conclusions are credible and understandable.

Phase IV of data analysis also requires skill to synthesize findings related to contextual findings, cultural interpretations, language analysis, social structure, and other influencers of human care and well being. To conduct an accurate synthesis, the researcher must be fully immersed in the data and know the data well. The researcher must carefully preserve relevant verbal statements, meanings, and interpretations from informants in a meaningful way and not reduce data to spurious or questionable themes. Attention is given to special linguistic terms and verbatim statements, subjective and experiential data of *emic* and *etic* content. In addition, the key informant's interpretations of diverse themes and commonalities are identified. Ethnohistorical facts, artistic expressions, worldviews, material cultural items, values and beliefs, and many other aspects influencing cultural care and health are presented. Actually each phase of analysis builds on and supports previous phases of analysis so that confident, accurate, and meaningful findings are evident. When the data analysis is completed in a systematic way, the researcher feels strongly and convincingly that the analysis is credible and fully reflects the domain of inquiry with research questions related to the theory.

A caveat should be noted with research assistants and nurses who have had no preparation with the ethnonursing method and this data analysis—they will have difficulty unless prepared by a teacher experienced with the method. Questionable findings can be identified using research assistants and analyzers who have not had experience and who have not studied the method. For those prepared in the method, it offers a highly rewarding process to make sense out of large or small volumes of ethnonursing qualitative data. Luna's (1989) study of American Lebanese Arab-Muslims and other studies in this book provide examples of detailed and rigorous analyses of data using the four phases of Leininger's data analysis. These studies provided new knowledge and insights about culture care transculturally.

Leininger-Templin-Thompson Ethnoscript
Qualitative Software (LTT)

To facilitate the above systematic mode of data collection, processing, and analysis, the Leininger-Templin-Thompson Ethnoscript Qualitative Software (LTT) was developed around 1985 (Leininger, 1990b).

The LTT Software was designed as a tailor-made means to process large amounts of ethnonursing data for the Culture Care theory (Leininger, 1987). This software is used with ethnonursing data analysis in that the researcher can directly process large amounts of detailed qualitative data by use of microcomputers. Data focusing on the worldview, social structure, cultural values, language, environmental context, historical facts, folk, and professional health care systems, specific caring modes, and other data are computer coded and processed (Leininger, 1990b). Currently other software are being explored to preserve all key and general informant data, and other field data collected from the enablers. Researchers can process field data directly to their laptops or desktop computers. The LTT software is user-friendly and provides a complete and comprehensive account of data generated in relation to Culture Care theory. While the LTT software is a major facilitator in processing the large amounts of data generated for the Culture Care theory, it can be used with other qualitative nursing theories as well, where naturalistic detailed data need to be processed systematically. LTT software has been used since 1985, and several of the studies presented in this book reflect its use. With new and different types of data processing software being developed everyday, researchers are constantly exploring them for use in Culture Care theory data analysis and other purposes.

Acculturation Enabler Guide

An Acculturation Enabler Guide was created by the author to help assess the extent of acculturation of an individual or group with respect to a particular culture or subculture (see Figure 4). This enabler was developed as part of the ethnonursing research method to assess the extent to which individuals or groups of a particular culture are more traditionally or nontraditionally oriented, and to identify cultural variability or universality features (Leininger, 1978, 1991). The acculturation enabler was developed with thought to the components of the Culture Care theory in order to assess cultural variabilities of

Figure 4
Leininger's Acculturation Health Care Assessment Enabler for Cultural Patterns in Traditional and Nontraditional Lifeways*

Name of Assessor _____ Date: _____

Informants or Code No. _____ Sex: _____ Age: _____

Place or Context of Assessment: _____

Directions: This enabler provides a general qualitative profile or assessment of traditional or nontraditional orientation of informants of their patterned lifeways. Health care influencers are assessed with respect to worldview, language, cultural values, kinship, religion, politics, technology, education, environment, and related areas. This profile is primarily focused on *emic* (local) information to assess and guide health personnel in working with individuals and groups. The *etic* (or more universal view) also may be evident. In Part I, the user observes, records, and rates behavior on the scale below from 1 to 5 with respect to traditional or nontraditionally oriented lifeways. Numbers are plotted on the summary Part II to obtain a qualitative profile to guide decisions and actions. The user's brief notations on each criterion should be used to support ratings and reliable profile. This enabler was *not* designed for quantitative measurements, but rather as a qualitative enabler to explicate data from informants.

Part I: Rating of Criteria to Assess Traditional and Nontraditional Patterned Cultural Lifeways or Orientations

Rating Indicators:	Mainly Traditional 1	Moderate 2	Average 3	Moderate 4	Mainly Nontraditional 5	Rater Value No.
Cultural Dimensions to Assess Traditional or Nontraditional Orientations						
1. Language, Communication & Gestures (Native or Non-native). Notations: _____						___
2. General Environmental Living Context (Symbols, material & non-material signs). Specify: _____						___
3. Wearing Apparel & Physical Appearance. Notations: _____						___

Rating Indicators:	Mainly Traditional 1	Moderate 2	Average 3	Moderate 4	Mainly Nontraditional 5	Rater Value No.
4. Technology Being Used in Living Environment. Notations: _____						_____
5. World View (How person looks out upon the world). Notations: _____						_____
6. Family Lifeways (Values, beliefs and norms). Notations: _____						_____
7. General Social Interactions and Kinship Ties. Notations: _____						_____
8. Patterned Daily Activities. Notations: _____						_____
9. Religious (or Spiritual) Beliefs and Values. Notations: _____						_____
10. Economic Factors (Rough cost of living estimates and income). Notations: _____						_____
11. Educational Values or Belief Factors. Notations: _____						_____
12. Political or Legal Influencers. Notations: _____						_____
13. Food Uses and Nutritional Values, Beliefs, & Taboos. Specify: _____						_____

Rating Indicators:	Mainly Traditional 1	Moderate 2	Average 3	Moderate 4	Mainly Nontraditional 5	Rater Value No.
14. *Folk* (Generic or Indigenous) *Health Care* (*-Cure*) Values, Beliefs & Practices. Specify: _____						
15. *Professional Health Care* (*-Cure*) Values, Beliefs & Practices. Specify: _____						
16. Care Concepts or Patterns that guide actions i.e. concern for, support, presence, etc.: _____						
17. Caring Patterns or Expressions: _____						
18. Views of Ways to: a) Prevent illnesses: _____ b) Preserve or maintain wellness or health: _____ c) Care for self or others: _____						
19. Other Indicators to support more traditional or nontraditional lifeways:						

Part II: Acculturation Profile from Assessment Factors

Directions: Plot an X with the value numbers rated on this profile to discover the orientation or acculturation gradient of the informant. The clustering of numbers will give information of traditional or nontraditional patterns with respect to the criteria assessed.

Criteria	1 Mainly Traditional	2 Moderate	3 Average	4 Moderate	5 Mainly Nontraditional
1. Language & Communication Modes					
2. Physical Environment					

Criteria	1 Mainly Traditional	2 Moderate	3 Average	4 Moderate	5 Mainly Nontraditional
3. Physical Apparel & Appearance					
4. Technology					
5. World View					
6. Family Lifeways					
7. Social Interaction & Kinship					
8. Daily Lifeways					
9. Religious Orientation					
10. Economic Factors					
11. Educational Factors					
12. Political & Legal Factors					
13. Food Uses					
14. Folk (Generic) Care-Cure					
15. Professional Care-Cure Expressions					
16. Caring Patterns					
17. Curing Patterns					
18. Prevention/Maintenance Factors					
19. Other Indicators					

* Note: This enabler has been developed, refined, and used for three decades (since the early 1960s) by Dr. Madeleine Leininger. It has been frequently in demand by anthropologists, transcultural nurses, and others. It has been useful to obtain informant's *orientation* to traditional or nontraditional lifeways. It provides qualitative indicators to meet credibility, confirmability, recurrency and reliability for qualitative studies. This copyright enabler may be used if the *full title* of the enabler, recognition of *source* (M. Leininger), and *publication outlet* (*Journal of Transcultural Nursing, 1991*) is cited. The author would also appreciate a letter to know who has used it with focus and summary outcomes.

Note: The assessor may total numbers to get a summary orientation profile. Use of these ratings with written notations provide a wholistic qualitative profile. More detailed notations are important to substantiate the ratings.

individuals and groups of a particular culture along major lines of differentiating cultural experience.

During the past three decades, this enabler has been used, modified, confirmed, and perfected with many informants and contexts so that several dimensions of the theory could be assessed in relation to acculturation factors such as social structure, worldview, and human care factors. With this enabler, the researcher can obtain a profile of the extent and areas of acculturation with respect to traditional or nontraditional cultural orientations. Data from the tool are analyzed and reported in the findings in different creative ways such as pictorial graphs, bar graphs, narratives, or informant or group profiles. There is provision for written narrative statements to support the cultural assessments in each area. The researcher may want to use percentages or simple numerical data to show the directions or a degree of acculturation which is in keeping with qualitative analysis. To date the acculturation enabler has high credibility, reliability, and confirmability as it has been used with many cultures over the past three decades to identify specific characteristics or patterns of a culture bearing on cultural aspects, care, and related nursing phenomena. It is one of the few major acculturation enablers available in nursing, anthropology, and the social sciences.

Life History Health Care Enabler

Previously published and discussed in *Qualitative Research and Nursing* (Leininger, 1985c, 119–133), the reader is referred to this publication for a full account of the enabler's purposes and uses in ethnonursing and related qualitative research studies. The Life History Health Care enabler is a guide to obtain longitudinal data from selected informants of their "lived through life span experiences," and with focus on care and caring (or related nursing aspects). Life histories have long been of value in anthropology. Today nurses are learning how to use full life histories to study nursing and health care practices. Ideas for this enabler were derived from several authors' experiences and from anthropological life histories.

It is of interest that clients and families often enjoy talking about their life history accounts, and especially with the middlescent and elderly adults. Hence, this enabler was designed to obtain a full and systematic account from informants about their caring healthy, or less healthy, lifeways and how care beliefs and practices influenced their well being. Enormously rich and detailed data have been obtained from the use of this enabler especially with respect to human caring and health values, expressions, and meanings (Leininger, 1985c). Nurse researchers using the ethnonursing method are encouraged to use this enabler to tease out historic insights about health care values and practices, especially related to generic and professional care patterns and practices. The life history guide has been useful in obtaining longitudinal narratives about the informants' special experiences in folk and professional health systems in homes and institutions. It can be used as a reliable and credible method in its own right with five to ten full health care histories with key informants and as part of the ethnonursing method.

Other Enablers: Options for the Researcher

Over time, I have developed other enablers such as those focused on: (1) Cultural Care Values and Meanings; (2) Culturalogical Care Assessment Guide; (3) Audio-Visual Guide; and (4) Generic and Professional Care Enabler Guide (Leininger, 1985a, 1988). Due to space limitations, these enablers will not be presented here. It is important to note, however, that the researcher who uses the ethnonursing method to study Cultural Care theory can develop different kinds of enablers to study in depth different domains of inquiry related to Cultural Care theory and as noted by several research accounts in this book.

ETHNONURSING RESEARCH PROCESS

With the above philosophy, rationale, and enablers in mind, the ethnonursing research process is presented. Nurse researchers need to envision the general research process of conducting an ethnonursing study. Figure 5 is presented as a visual guide to the general sequence of an ethnonursing researcher process. While this sequence offers general guidelines, the researcher may modify the process to fit with the

Figure 5
Leininger's Phases of Ethnonursing Research

1. Identify the general intent or purpose(s) of your study with focus on the domain(s) of inquiry phenomenon under study, area of inquiry, or research questions being addressed.
2. Identify the potential significance of the study to advance nursing knowledge and practices.
3. Review available literature on the domain or phenomena being studied.
4. Conceptualize a research plan from beginning to the end with the following general phases or sequence factors in mind.
   a) Consider the research site, community, and people to study the phenomena.
   b) Deal with the informed consent expectations.
   c) Explore and gradually gain entry (with essential permissions) to the community, hospital or country wherever the study is being done.
   d) Anticipate potential barriers and facilitators related to: gatekeepers expectations, language, political leaders, location, and other factors.
   e) Select and appropriately use the ethnonursing enabling tools with the research process, e.g. Leininger's *Stranger-Friend Guide* and *Observation-Participation-Reflection Guide* and others. The researcher may also develop enabling tools or guides for their study.
   f) Chose key and general informants.
   g) Maintain trusting and favorable relationships with the people conferring with ethnonurse research expert(s) to prevent unfavorable developments.
   h) Collect and confirm data with observations, interviews, participant experiences, and other data. (This is a continuous process from the beginning to the end and requires the use of qualitative research criteria to confirm findings and credibility factors).
   i) Maintain continuous data processing on computers and with field journals reflecting active analysis and reflections, and with discussions with research mentor(s). Computer processing with Leininger/Templin/Thompsons's software is a helpful means to handle large amounts of qualitative data.
   j) Frequently present and reconfirm findings with the people studied to check credibility and confirmability of findings.
   k) Make plans to leave the field site, community, and informants in advance.
5. Do final analysis and writing of the research findings soon after completing the study.
6. Prepare published findings in appropriate journals.
7. Help implement the findings with nurses interested in findings.
8. Plan future studies related to this domain or other new ones.

research setting or context. Most importantly, the ethnonursing process needs to remain flexible so that the researcher can *move with the people* and in accord with the naturalistic developments and human research conditions. As the researcher moves from a stranger to a friend to collect and process data, flexibility and modifications in the research plan often are needed. Nonetheless, the ethnonursing research process as depicted in Figure 5 helps the researcher to perceive him or herself when entering, remaining in, or leaving informants as part of the research sequence whether in the hospital, community agency, urban street clinic, rural communities, or many other places. Careful use of the ethnonursing research process also helps the researcher to ensure a complete and comprehensive study by being attentive to areas that must be considered to systematically and fully study a theory such as Culture Care. Any credible research method contains desired ways to carry out a sound method of investigation for a complete, credible study, and this process is offered to help the researcher attain this goal.

Although the particular phases of the Ethnonursing Research Process are not discussed here, they have been identified and discussed in other publications, and readers are encouraged to study these sources (Leininger, 1985a, 1985b, 1987, 1989, 1990a). Derived underpinnings and general philosophical premises to support the ethnonursing process also are discussed in the works of Guba (1990), Lincoln and Guba (1985), Reason and Rowan (1985), Heron (1981), and Spradley (1979).

GENERAL ETHNONURSING PRINCIPLES TO SUPPORT THE RESEARCH METHOD

In light of the philosophical, epistemic, and ontological bases and the purposes for the ethnonursing method, some general summative principles can be stated to guide the nurse researcher in using the method. The first principle the ethnonursing researcher requires is *to maintain an open discovery, active listening, and a genuine learning attitude in working with informants in the total context in which the study is conducted.* The researcher's attitude and willingness to be an active learner and to discover as much as possible from the informants and the culture is extremely important for a sound ethnonursing study. The researcher remains an active learner about the people's or client's world by becoming involved in and showing a willingness *to learn from the people*. Discovering and learning about the meanings, expressions, values, beliefs, and patterns of human care also requires active listening, suspending judgments, and reflecting about informant ideas. Informants usually are willing to respond to an active listener who is genuinely interested in them, their lifeways, and viewpoints. Learning from the knowers (informants) may be difficult for some nurse researchers who are skilled clinicians, administrators, or in other roles where subject matter expertise prevails. An awareness of ethnocentric biases or if nurses act like they know and can explain everything, can greatly hinder learning from others. The nurse researcher, therefore, needs to be aware of ethnocentric views and biases. Being a humble learner also is not always easy if female nurses are eager to assert their rights and knowledge especially to patriarchal informants. Learning from strangers and respecting what strangers shared with you and without moral (right or wrong) judgments is important as well as respecting cultural secrets.

The second principle the ethnonurse researcher requires is to *maintain an active and curious posture about the "why" of whatever is seen, heard, or experienced, and with appreciation of whatever informants share with you*. Being an active participant and reflector about phenomena means becoming sensitive to the local *emic* viewpoints and reflecting on *etic* professional ideas. Searching for the "why" means remaining interested in the informant's different or similar views to that of the nurse. It means a willingness to explore new or different ideas about human caring from folk (generic) and professional viewpoints. Explanations and interpretations of informant cultural care are views that need to be respected and not demeaned because they are different from professional nursing ideas. Observing and pondering about the "why" of care expressions and action modes from both indigenous and professional care givers often provides new insights about unknown aspects of care. Exploring caring behaviors related to care constructs such as touch, assisting others, protection, support, comfort, and other largely undiscovered culture-specific care concepts necessitates time, patience, and teasing out of vague ideas to get to the epistemics or knowledge sources. The ethnonurse becomes an unrelenting researcher to obtain specific meanings, functions, and expressions of care with their relationships to well being, health, illness, death, or to any human condition.

The third ethnonursing principle is to *record whatever is shared by informants in a careful and conscientious way for full meanings, explanations, or interpretations to preserve informant ideas.* This means that the nurse researcher needs to value whatever is shared and try to grasp the diverse and common linkages about human caring. It also means that informants and others in the culture usually are able to interpret and make sense out of their beliefs, experiences (subjective and real), and decision modes if permitted to do so by the researcher. Sometimes it is difficult for the researcher to make sense out of cultural data of what one sees and hears, but the more one trusts local informants the more one can learn about cultural care and health patterns or experiences. Patience and a willingness to listen and reflect on informant ideas are essential to comprehend and fully understand care and related phenomena. For example, the researcher often records deviant, ambiguous, or questionable ideas with interpretations suspended or withheld until their meanings become understandable with help from informants' diverse expressions. Such diverse expressions must be preserved as well. Not only do they provide significant help in the understanding of informant ideas, often they are indicators of cultural changes, areas of conflicts, or special modes of expressing cultural care practices.

The fourth ethnonursing principle is to *seek a mentor who has experience with the ethnonursing research method to act as a guide.* An experienced mentor who has conducted ethnonursing studies can be most helpful in examining the research process at hand. He or she also can help to reduce biases, prejudices, prejudgments, and questionable interpretations that do not support grounded data. An experienced research mentor provides an opportunity for the researcher to reflect on the findings and to make meaningful linkages with diverse and similar findings. Moreover, an experienced qualitative mentor can help process large amounts of qualitative data when the research feels overwhelmed and not able to move or "get hold of the data." Often, when strange cultural linkages may be difficult to make, the researcher mentor can reflect on the ideas in a way that facilitates the researcher's analysis. Finally, the research mentor can be very helpful to present and publish ethnonursing research findings which are often presented in long, detailed reports.

A fifth ethnonursing principle is to *clarify the purposes of additional qualitative research methods if they are combined with the ethnonursing method such as combining life histories, ethnography, phenomenology, or ethnoscience.* Such combinations are possible, but the *reasons* and *purposes* for combining several methods must be made clear at the outset and with the domain of inquiry as well as with the theory and the research purposes. Actually, the nurse researchers do not need to use additional research methods unless absolutely necessary, and if another method is used it should fit the paradigm and study purposes. Nurses who have not been well prepared in qualitative research methods may fail to realize that the qualitative and quantitative paradigms have very different goals and purposes (Leininger, 1985a; Lincoln & Guba, 1985) and ethnomethods and paradigms should not be mixed. As I have stated in other publications (Leininger, 1987, 1990a), *one can mix methods within a paradigm, but not mix methods of different paradigms as it violates the purposes and integrity of each paradigm.* If methods are used from different paradigms, then the researcher does not fully understand the purposes and philosophy of each paradigm. Currently, there are a host of serious problems with nurses using "triangulation," mixing both qualitative and quantitative methods and paradigms with limited to no rationale stated except "more methods seem better than less." As a consequence, much confusion prevails and such study results are very questionable and have limited credibility. It is possible, however, to do sequential qualitative or quantitative studies (or the reverse), but not simultaneously or by merging methods and paradigms. For further guidance on the rationale and focus of the two paradigms and mixing methods, the reader is encouraged to read reliable and substantive articles on ethnomethods (Leininger, 1990a, 40–51), and other writings by other qualitative experts (Guba, 1990; Lincoln & Guba, 1985; Reason & Rowan, 1981).

INFORMANTS: KEY AND GENERAL

Key and general informants are important in any ethnonursing research study. The ethnonurse researcher, however, does not have "samples," "objects," "subjects," "cases," and "populations" (Leininger,

1985b), but does work with key and general informants such as individuals, families, and groups of people in diverse contexts, institutions, or communities. Key and general informants become a major source for nurse researchers to learn about people and their cultural care, well being, health, and general lifeways as influenced by a variety of factors. *Key informants* are persons who have been thoughtfully and purposefully selected (often by people in the culture or subculture) to be most knowledgeable about the domain of inquiry of interest to nurse researchers. Key informants are held to reflect the norms, values, beliefs, and general lifeways of the culture, and are usually interested in and willing to participate in the study. In contrast, *general informants* usually are not as fully knowledgeable about the domain of inquiry, but do have general ideas about the domain, and are willing to share their ideas. After the researcher has involved key informants in several sessions, general informants are used to reflect on how similar or different their ideas are from key informants. Such information from key and general informants helps to identify the diversity or universality of ideas about human care and other nursing phenomenon.

During the past three decades of ethnonursing research, I have discovered that it requires from three to five informant sessions of approximately one to two hours to obtain in-depth insights, full meanings, interpretations, and other data that are often embedded in diverse social structure factors and in different human care experiences (Leininger, 1989, 1990a). Since general informants provide reflective information and are not key informants, less time is given to them. Ethnonursing studies in which the researcher spends limited time or only one or two sessions with key informants can result in unreliable and inaccurate data. As a result, the researcher does not get to "backstage" or to the "cultural secrets" of informants, and the findings may be questionable. Key informants are the main source to check and recheck data collected as to its internal (emic) and external (etic) relevance, meanings, accuracy, and dependability because they are the in-depth source of information along with direct observations and participant experiences.

When conducting a *maxi* or *macro ethnonursing* study, *12 to 15 key* informants are needed or approximately *twice* the number of *key informants to general informants.* If a *mini* or *macro ethnonursing* study is being conducted (or one smaller in scope), the researcher needs 6 to 8 *key* and *12 to 16 general* informants. A ration of 1:2 is the general rule to follow for key to general informants with three to five sessions with the former and one session with the latter. These numbers of key and general informants have been established through three decades of research and in accord with other nurse researchers. We must remember, however, that large numbers of informants alone are not the rule; instead, the focus is on obtaining in-depth knowledge to understand fully the phenomena under study (Leininger, 1985a, 1987; Lincoln & Guba, 1985). The use of large "samples" for qualitative studies generally leads to superficial knowledge, less credibility on interpretations and explanations, and limited insights about the "why" and "how" of particular care phenomena.

The ethnonursing method also requires that the nurse have appropriate language skills to communicate with people in the culture and to interpret ideas and written documents. The researcher must be able to "cue-in" to what informants are talking about relative to the topic under discussion. This may require nurses to learn the language of a culture to study cultural care phenomena as language and culture are closely linked. Language becomes the means to understand meanings, patterns, and other *emic* or *etic* expressions and interpretations so critical to ethnonursing studies. Many different meanings of kinds and patterns of care are often found in special language expressions that must be carefully written with detailed interpretations. Ethnohistorical data about care, health, well being, or illnesses also are expressed in special language statements over different timespans that the researcher must know how to explore with informants in written and spoken language. Most importantly, the nurse researcher needs to be aware of not imposing professional or personal language ideas on the data, or to interpret the data from the researcher's linguistic expressions, viewpoints, or phrases. When this occurs, one can anticipate less accurate knowledge of cultural care meanings from the people. In general, language skills with attention to the informants' ways of expressing are essential to conduct a successful, accurate, and credible ethnonursing study.

Keeping a field journal with *condensed* and *expanded* notes with focus on the theory and the Sunrise components is essential to a comprehensive ethnonursing study (Leininger, 1985a, b, 1990a). The field (or clinical) journal offers the researcher the means to record data directly from the people in both condensed and expanded forms. The Sunrise Model serves as a cognitive map that covers the major components of the theory while collecting and analyzing the findings. The Sunrise Model also serves as a comprehensive guide to the ethnonurse researcher while recording grounded or raw field data and when checking on areas still not fully explored. The field journal covers data related to the worldview, social structure, ethnohistorical, environmental factors, folk, and professional features as areas to be explored as potential influencers of human care. The field journal remains the primary data source along with computer data processing of all field data. As discussed earlier, ethnonursing data are collected and processed with the use of the Leininger-Templin-Thompson Ethnoscript Qualitative Software, or with other available computer software. However, the LTT was designed especially to code, classify, and process data bearing on Culture Care theory.

QUALITATIVE CRITERIA TO ETHNONURSING RESEARCH STUDIES

Since qualitative and quantitative paradigms have very different purposes, goals, and predicted outcomes, the nurse researcher must be knowledgeable about and use qualitative criteria for ethnonursing studies. Since the purpose of ethnonursing research studies is to discover the nature, essence, attributes, meanings, characteristics, and understandings of particular phenomena under study, use of qualitative criteria is imperative. The researcher is challenged to discover diversities and universalities in relation to the theory and the qualitative paradigm (Leininger, 1987, 1990a; Guba, 1990; Lincoln & Guba, 1985; Reason & Rowan, 1981). During the past 30 years, I have developed and used specific criteria for qualitative paradigmatic investigations as presented below (Leininger, 1970, 1978, 1989, 1990a). In recent years, Lincoln and Guba and a few other methodologists have added their support to use similar criteria and these developments support these criteria.

1. *Credibility*—refers to the "truth," accuracy, or believability of findings that have been mutually established between the

researcher and the informants as accurate, believable, and credible of their experiences and knowledge of phenomena. These truths, beliefs, and values (largely from *emic* findings) have been substantiated through the researcher's observations and with documentation of meanings-in-contexts, specific situations, or events. In addition, direct experiences of the researcher with the people over time and the people's interpretations or explanations are used to substantiate this criterion.

2. *Confirmability*—refers to the repeated direct and documented evidence from largely observed and primary informant source data, and with repeated explanations or interpretive data from informants about certain phenomena. Confirmability means reaffirming what the researcher has heard, seen, or experienced with respect to the phenomena under study. It reflects evidence of the informants restating or reaffirming ideas or instances that have occurred over time in familiar and natural living contexts. "Audit trails" (Lincoln & Guba, 1985) or "confirmed informant" checks (Leininger, 1990a) with direct people feedback are ways to establish confirmability.

3. *Meaning-in-context*—refers to data that has become understandable with relevant referents or meaning's to the informants or people studied in different or similar environments. Situations, instances, settings, and life events or experiences with meanings known to the people are evident. This criterion focuses on the significance of interpretations and understanding of the actions, symbols, events, communication, and other human activities within specific or total contexts in which something occurred or happened.

4. *Recurrent Patterning*—refers to repeated instances, sequence of events, experiences, or lifeways that tend to reoccur over a period of time in designated ways and contexts. Repeated experiences, expressions, events, or activities that reflect identifiable sequenced patterns of behavior over time are used to substantiate this criterion.

5. *Saturation*—refers to the "taking in" of occurrences or meanings in a very full, comprehensive, and exhaustible way

of all information that could generally be known or understood about certain phenomena under study. Saturation means that the researcher has conducted an exhaustive exploration of whatever is being studied, and there is no further data or insights coming forth from informants or observed situations. There is a redundance of information in which the researcher gets the same (or similar) information, and the informants contend "there is no more to offer as they have said or shared everything." Data reveals redundancies and duplication of content with similar ideas, meanings, experiences, descriptions, and other expressions from the informants or from repeated observations of some phenomena.

6. *Transferability*—refers to whether particular findings from a qualitative study can be transferred to another *similar context or situation* and still preserve the particularized meanings, interpretations, and inferences of the completed study. While the goal of qualitative research is not intended to produce generalizations, but to obtain in-depth knowledge of a particular study, this criterion looks for any general similarities of findings under *similar* environmental conditions, contexts, or circumstances that one might make from the findings. It is the researcher's responsibility to establish if this criterion can be met in a new research context.

Currently, these six qualitative criteria can be studied more fully in other publications (Leininger, 1990a; Lincoln & Guba, 1985) but also in other nurse research studies now available in this book and others. It is of interest that Lincoln and Guba (pp. 290–338) used the criteria of transferability, credibility, dependability, confirmability, but fail to identify the importance of meaning-in-context, saturation, and recurrent patterning. These later criteria are held to be extremely important to establish the soundness of most qualitative studies. It should be noted that the use of internal and external validity or reliability measurements are not appropriate, nor can they be used meaningfully with qualitative studies as the purposes and goals of the qualitative and quantitative paradigms are very different.

In this chapter, I have provided an overview of the ethnonursing research method within the qualitative paradigm to show how this method can be used to systematically study Culture Care theory. While it is possible that Culture Care theory can be studied with other qualitative or quantitative methods, I believe that the latter greatly limits obtaining in-depth, complex, and embedded care phenomena. Instead, the ethnonursing method has been designed to achieve this goal and to explicate largely unknown and elusive aspects of human care from transcultural perspectives. Nursing phenomena such as care, well being, healing, health, environmental contexts, and other undiscovered or vaguely discovered nursing phenomena remain a challenge to document fully in regard to their epistemic, ontological, and culturally relevant forms. Over the past three decades, I have made several revisions and refinements with the ethnonursing method, the Sunrise Model, and the theory to perfect it so as to explicate human care and related nursing phenomena. As a result, a new and different way of discovering, knowing, and interpreting humanistic and scientific care is available. Humanistic and scientific dimensions of care are being established with research findings largely with the use of the ethnonursing research method and other methods within the qualitative paradigm. Unquestionably, the ethnonursing method has become one of the most rigorous and relevant ways to discover human care and many other untapped nursing phenomena. As the only known research method to link nursing theory with the nursing research method, it also is important to use with care findings to improve people care transculturally. It is the method that is helping to establish the epistemic and ontologic of nursing knowledge for the discipline and profession of nursing.

REFERENCES

Berreman, G. (1962). *Behind many masks*. Society for Applied Anthropology. Ithaca, NY: New York.

Boas, F. (1924). The methods of ethnology. *American Anthropologist*, (22), 311–321.

Carter, M. (1985). The philosophical dimensions of qualitative nursing science research. In M. M. Leininger (Ed.), *Qualitative research methods in nursing*. Orlando, FL: Grune & Stratton, 27–32.

Erikson, E. (1963). *Childhood and society* (2nd ed.). Toronto: W.W. Norton.

Glaser, B. G., & Strauss, A. L. (1967). *The discovery of grounded theories: Strategies for qualitative research.* Chicago: Aldine.

Guba, E. (1990). *The paradigm dialog.* Newbury Park, CA: Sage.

Heron, J. (1981). Philosophical basis for a new paradigm. In Reason & Rowan, (Eds.), *Human inquiry: A sourcebook of new paradigm research.* New York: John Wiley & Sons.

Leininger, M. M. (1966). *Convergence and divergence of human behavior: An ethnopsychological comparative study of two Gadsup villages in the Eastern Highlands of New Guinea.* Unpublished doctoral dissertation. Seattle: University of Washington.

Leininger, M. M. (1967). The Culture concept and its relevance to nursing. *Journal of Nursing Education, 6*(2), 27–39.

Leininger, M. M. (1968). The significance of cultural concepts in nursing. *Minnesota League for Nursing Bulletin, 16*(2), 5–9.

Leininger, M. M. (1969). Nature of science in nursing. Conference on the nature of science in nursing. *Nursing Research, 18*(5), 388–389.

Leininger, M. M. (1970). *Nursing and anthropology: Two worlds to blend.* New York: John Wiley & Sons.

Leininger, M. M. (1976). Caring: The essence and central focus of nursing. American Nurses Foundation, *Nursing Research Report, 12*(1), 2, 14.

Leininger, M. M. (1978). *Transcultural nursing: Concepts, theories, and practices.* New York: John Wiley & Sons.

Leininger, M. M. (1980). Care: A central focus of nursing and health care services. *Nursing and Health Care,* 135–143.

Leininger, M. M. (1981). *Care: An essential human need.* Detroit: Wayne State University Press.

Leininger, M. M. (1984). *Care: The essence of nursing and health.* Detroit: Wayne State University Press.

Leininger, M. M. (1985a). *Qualitative research methods in nursing.* Orlando, FL: Grune & Stratton.

Leininger, M. M. (1985b). Ethnography and ethnonursing: Models and modes of qualitative data analysis. In *Qualitative research methods in nursing.* Orlando, FL: Grune & Stratton, 33–72.

Leininger, M. M. (1985c). Life health care history: Purposes, methods and techniques in *Qualitative research methods in nursing.* Orlando, FL: Grune & Stratton, 119–132.

Leininger, M. M. (1987). Importance and uses of ethnomethods: Ethnography and ethnonursing research. In M. Cahoon (Ed.), *Recent advances in nursing.* London: Churchill Livingston, 17, 23–25.

Leininger, M. M. (1988). *Care: Discovery and uses in clinical and community nursing.* Detroit: Wayne State University Press.

Leininger, M. M. (1989). Ethnonursing: A research method to generate nursing knowledge. Unpublished Paper of the *Proceedings of Qualitative Summer Research Conferences*. Detroit: Wayne State University.

Leininger, M. M. (1990a). Ethnomethods: The philosophic and epistemic basis to explicate transcultural nursing knowledge. *Journal of Transcultural Nursing, 1*(2), 40–51.

Leininger, M. M. (1990b). *Leininger-Templin-Thompson ethnoscript qualitative software program: User's Handbook*. Detroit: Wayne State University.

Leininger, M. M. (1991, Winter). Leininger's acculturation health care assessment tool for cultural patterns in traditional and non-traditional lifeways. *Journal of Transcultural Nursing, 2*(2).

Lincoln, Y. & Guba, G. (1985). *Naturalistic inquiry*. Beverly Hills: Sage.

Luna, L. (1989). *Care and cultural context of Lebanese Muslims in an urban community: An ethnographic and ethnonursing study conceptualized within Leininger's theory*. Unpublished Dissertation. Detroit: Wayne State University.

Malinowski, B. (1922). *Argonauts of the western pacific*. New York: E.P. Dutton.

Pike, K. (1954). *Language in relation to a unified theory of the structure of human behavior*. Glendale, CA: Summer Institute of Linguistics.

Polit, D., & Hungler, B. (1983). *Nursing research: Principles and methods*. Philadelphia: J.B. Lippincott.

Reason, P., & Rowan, J. (1981). *Human Inquiry: A sourcebook of new paradigm research*. New York: John Wiley & Sons.

Strauss, A., & Corbin, J. (1990). *Basics of qualitative research*. Beverly Hills: Sage.

Spradley, J. (1979). *Ethnographic interview*. New York: Holt, Rinehart and Winston.

Spradley, J. (1980). *Participant observation*. New York: Holt, Rinehart and Winston.

Watson, J. (1985). Reflections on different methodologies for the future of nursing. In M. M. Leininger (Ed.), *Qualitative research methods in nursing*. Orlando, FL: Grune & Stratton, 343–351.

Wenger, A.F., (1985). Learning to do a mini ethnonursing research study: A doctoral student's experience. In M. M. Leininger (Ed.) *Qualitative research methods in nursing*. Orlando, FL: Grune & Stratton, 283–316.

Some Key Updated References

Leininger, M. (1995) *Transcultural Nursing: Concepts, Theories, Research and Practices* (Second Edition) Columbus, OH. McGraw Hill College Custom Series.

Leininger, M. (1997) Overview and Reflection of the theory of Culture Care and the ethnonursing research method. *Journal of Transcultural Nursing, 8*(2) pp. 32–51.

Leininger, M. and M. McFarland. *Transcultural Nursing, Concepts, Theories, Research, and Practices* (Third Edition) New York: McGraw Hill Co.

3

Culture Care of Philippine and Anglo-American Nurses in a Hospital Context

Zenaida Spangler

Transcultural nursing, an area of study and practice with human care focus as originated by Leininger (1970), has led to the development of new nursing knowledge and skills as well as improving client care. Conceived in the 1950s, the theory did not take a firm hold until the mid-1970s, when nursing scholars and clinicians gave more attention to culture as an important influence on nursing. Since then, numerous concepts, with several explicitly focused on culture care, have been studied and examined from different perspectives and with different cultures (Aamodt, 1972; Byerly, Molgaard, & Snow, 1979; Horn, 1978; Kendall, 1979; Leininger, 1970, 1976, 1977, 1978, 1979, 1980, 1981, 1984, 1988; Luna, 1989; Rosenbaum, 1990; Tripp-Reimer, 1982; Wenger, 1988). These studies have focused mainly on transcultural conceptions of care, health, and illness among care recipients, and have revealed unique and diverse expressions, patterns, and practices of care among cultures. They also have confirmed specific transcultural care concepts and practices that have in turn generated further studies and interest in nursing theory development, research, and practice (Leininger, 1978, 1980, 1981, 1984, 1988; Luna, 1989; Rosenbaum, 1990; Wenger, 1988). There is no doubt that these studies have contributed substantially to transcultural nursing knowledge and to the dissemination of this knowledge in education and practice.

While research, theory, and education were a dominant focus of transcultural nursing in the 1960s, 1970s, and 1980s, especially related to diverse cultures, research into the significance of caregivers from different cultures lagged behind. To date, there have been only few studies that have focused on different kinds of care given by nurses from different cultures. Recently, however, this void has been recognized, especially in the United States, where a nursing shortage has led to increased recruitment of nurses from different countries in the world (Pilette, 1989).

American institutions tend to recruit nurses from other countries without giving serious consideration to the nurses' cultural background, values, and adjustment needs (Maroun & Serota, 1988; Curran, 1989). As a result, such nurses express problems related to failing grades on state board licensing exams, difficulties in adjusting to high technologies in hospitals and clinics, and a host of miscommunications and misinterpretations (Aguino, Trent, & Deutsch, 1982; Arbeiter, 1988; Beyers, 1979; Maroun & Serota, 1988; Miraflor, 1976). These problems lead to disappointments, interpersonal conflicts, and other concerns. While some literature does examine cultural values, lifeways, and suggestions to facilitate adjustment for foreign nurses, these articles are few and tend to gloss over individual cultural differences and nursing care practices (Pilette, 1989). Likewise, there has been limited discussion about how nurses are prepared to move into a culture different from their own and provide quality care practices.

With an increasing number of nurses from other cultures coming to the United States, there is a need to explicate, analyze, and understand foreign nurses' beliefs and values, but especially their professional and folk (generic) cultural care beliefs, values, and practices. Undoubtedly, the nurses' care beliefs, values, and practices affect the care they give to patients and have a major influence on quality based nursing care. Differences in culture care beliefs, values, and practices could lead to major misunderstandings, conflicts, and inappropriate care. As such, the same interest and energy which are given to discover clients' psychophysiological and cultural care needs also should be given to study the cultural care dimensions and differences among nurses of different cultures. It is the so-called foreign nurses' "cultural care values" that have been little addressed, especially when used in another country.

PURPOSE AND RESEARCH QUESTIONS

This study will identify and analyze the similarities and differences in the nursing care values and caregiving practices of Anglo-American and Philippine nurses as revealed in practice in an American hospital context. The domains of inquiry were the nursing care values and caregiving practices of Anglo-American and Philippine nurses. The five research questions that guided this ethnonursing study follow:

1. What are the nursing care values and caregiving practices of Anglo-American and Philippine nurses practicing in an American hospital context?

2. What are the influences of culture on the nursing care values and caregiving practices of Anglo-American and Philippine nurses?

3. What are the similarities and differences in the nursing care values and caregiving practices of Anglo-American and Philippine nurses?

4. How do the similarities and differences between the Anglo-American and Philippine nurses influence nurse-to-nurse cultural care congruence?

5. What explains the differences in nursing care values and caregiving practices of Anglo-American and Philippine nurses?

CONCEPTUAL FRAMEWORK

As conceptualized within Leininger's theory of Culture Care (1978, 1981, 1988), the present study focused on care, its meaning, its interpretation, its symbolism, and its practices. Most importantly, however, the study focused on the ways each cultural group saw, experienced, and understood care within their culture as well as in the other nurses' culture. The identification and elucidation of cultural care meanings and experiences from the perspective of each culture required an understanding of each group's worldview, cultural values and beliefs, and social structure dimensions. These factors were predicted by Leininger to influence care expressions and behavior, and in turn the well being or health of individuals, groups, and institutions. Also predicted by Leininger was that language, which is closely linked to worldview and environment, would influence care and in turn the health status of clients. Indeed, the environmental context was an important area to study in this investigation. The Anglo-American and Philippine nurses practiced in an American hospital which, as a subsystem of the American culture, reflects and represents the various elements of the cultural and social structure dimensions specific to American cultural values in technology, economy, education, lifeways, and other aspects.

Of special interest was the discovery of cultural care congruence from the perspectives of caregivers who came from different cultures. Since the goal of Leininger's theory is to provide culturally congruent care, its conceptualization emphasizes the caregiver and care-recipient relationship in establishing cultural care congruence. Cultural care congruence provides an appropriate focus on the meaningful fit between the values, norms, and lifeways of caregivers and care-recipients which lead to beneficial and satisfying care outcomes. In this study, nurse-to-nurse cultural care congruence was conceptualized as a meaningful fit between the care values and caregiving practices of nurses from diverse cultures. The researcher predicted that nurse-to-nurse cultural care congruence would exist between nurses if they responded to their care values, beliefs, and practice differences or similarities with acts of "care preservation," "care accommodation," or "care repatterning." Also of particular interest were the culture care values within different cultural contexts of the hospital environment.

REVIEW OF THE LITERATURE

The literature review focused on two domains of inquiry: nursing care values and caregiving practices of nurses of different cultures. Unfortunately no studies were found which focused primarily on culture care differences and similarities between nurses of different cultures using Leininger's theory and qualitative ethnonursing method. As a result, only a few care papers relevant to this study will be reviewed. Rather than providing focus on culture care differences among nurses, these papers include selected scholarly discourse and research about care.

Visintainer (1986), in analyzing the characteristics of nursing theories and constructs as applied in practice, concurred with Leininger and other nursing scholars that care is the proper jurisdiction of nursing. To her, the goal of nursing is to improve a person's condition through the application of caring behaviors. Like Leininger, Visintainer suggested that nursing give a second look to theories of care and take advantage of their flexibility and amorphousness, for theories are not truths but tools with which to understand and alter the world.

Benner and Wrubel's (1989) work focused mainly on the role of caring in stress and coping, and not on cultural care factors among nurses of different cultures. The authors asserted that caring is extremely important because it sets up what matters to people, it defines what counts as stressful, and it determines what options are available for coping. Their premise was that caring is primary, it is an essential requisite for all coping, and it is the base of concern and connection with other people. From Benner and Wrubel's viewpoint, care is weakened by extreme individualism, autonomy, and high regard for technology.

Ray's (1984) research dealt with care in a large general hospital. The results provided new and interesting insights into the different meanings and practices of care within the hospital as a cultural institution. Using an ethnographic and participant-observation approach, Ray outlined an institutional care classification system with four major themes: psychologic, practical, interactional, and philosophic. Ray reported that although psychologic caring was valued, caring was greatly influenced by the culture, organizational features, and practical concerns of the institution. Practical caring was linked to economy and cost effectiveness and ranked second to organizational care values. Ray identified a shift in values from humanistic concerns to more practical material and technological values.

Thompson (1990) conducted an ethnonursing and ethnographic study of care to describe and to explain the meanings and experiences of care in the specialty of rehabilitation nursing. Led by Leininger's Culture Care theory, Thompson identified three themes which depicted the characteristic nature of care in rehabilitation nursing: care as enculturation, teamcare, and independence and conformity. Enculturation described the phenomenon of "clicking-in" to the rehabilitation process, an outcome which started with different expectations and knowledge between nurse and patient. This study reaffirmed the significance and relevance of elucidating and making explicit the meanings of care in institutional settings and in specialty areas.

Drew (1986) coined the term *exclusion* to represent non-caring and *confirmation* to mean caring. In her phenomenological study of patients' experiences with caregivers, Drew abstracted from patients' responses both exclusion and confirming actions of nurses. The experience of exclusion as described by patients included caregivers who "lacked emotional warmth," "starchy," "cold," "stiff," "mechanical," "insensitive," "dismissive," "lacked eye contact," and others. The experience of confirmation included positive descriptions such as "having a sense of energy," "wanting to be there," "caring what happens," "liking their work," and "having personality." Patients also reported negative consequences related to their experience of exclusion and beneficial effects from their experience with confirmation. This study supports Leininger's premise that care is essential for human health and survival as well as differential patterns of care expressions.

As mentioned, the review of literature on cultural care congruence between nurses of different cultures disclosed no major study in this area, and no study at all concerning Anglo-American and Philippine nurses. Nurse care scholars are, however, studying the philosophical, clinical, and institutional dimensions of care. This study appears as the first in-depth qualitative study of its kind to focus on culture care differences and similarities between caregivers of diverse cultures in a hospital context over time.

ETHNOHISTORY OF ANGLO-AMERICAN AND PHILIPPINE NURSES

In ethnonursing method, the available cultural history is presented to grasp the meaning of the culture and to derive possible meanings in context. In this section, a brief account of the cultural and ethnohistorical background of the Anglo-American and Philippine nurses follows.

Anglo-American Culture: Ethnographic Background

The term *Anglo* refers to Angles, one of the three Teutonic tribes (the other two being the Jutes and the Saxons) which invaded England in 500 A.D., displacing the Celts. According to Baugh (1957), the Celts called their conquerors *Saxons*, but later the terms *Angli* or *Anglia* emerged together with Saxon to refer to the Teutons in general. In time, *Anglia* became the root or source of the word "*England*" (literally, the land of the Angles), referring to the nation of the Teutons, and to the word *English*, which referred to the Teutons and the language they spoke. When colonists from England came to North America in the early 1600s, they brought with them their language and culture. The Anglos in the United States formed the mainstream of American culture and dominated this country's political, legal, economic, educational, religious, and artistic institutions. The dominant cultural group in the United States is comprised of white Anglo-Saxon Protestants, or "WASPs." However, in this country with diverse cultural, religious, and economic groups, middle-class whites have come to be regarded as Anglo-Americans (Arensberg & Neihoff, 1975; Hsu, 1955; Kluckhohn, 1949).

Kluckhohn (1949) sketched an explicit characterization of white middle-class Americans or Anglo-Americans. He noted that although significant regional, religious, and economic class differences exist, certain cultural traits transcend these differences, and Americans share some common life goals and some basic attitudes. Kluckhohn also called American culture a "culture of paradoxes" (p. 230) because he found complexities and inherent contradictions in its values. In describing a person to represent the American national character, he sketched a youth-oriented, individualistic, self-reliant, high-achieving, benevolent optimist who believes in equality and freedom. Kluckhohn characterized American individualism as the dramatization of the individual as activities, achievements, and their consequences become personalized. Individualism is intimately related to competition, success, and personal responsibility.

Du Bois (1955) characterized the values of the dominant American culture as based on persons' cognitive views of the universe, their relations to the universe, and their relationships with each other. She proposed that the American middle-class conceives the universe as mechanical, that individuals master nature, that people are equal, and that people are perfectible.

Social scientists who studied American culture and social structure noted the importance of the family in value formation (Mason, 1955; Slater, 1976; Veroff, Douvan, & Kulka, 1981). The basic unit of the American kinship system is the nuclear family, which is made up of father, mother, and children. Relatives by blood and marriage are recognized on both sides, however, kinship ties outside the nuclear family are weak. Mason described the American family as informal with the father in a dominant role as breadwinner and decision maker. Veroff, Douvan, and Kulka described the changing American family structure from 1957 to 1976, and chronicled changes in family roles particularly in the late 1960s and 1970s. According to these authors, the social upheavals that started in the late 1960s have changed some traditional roles of males and females in American family and society, and have brought about increased emphasis on relationships and parenting issues with males more willing than before to accept caring and nurturing responsibilities for children. Nevertheless, latter day parents stress the same value for individualism and self-reliance as earlier parents.

Leininger's (1970, 1978) characterization of American culture is related to nursing, and focused on the cultural values of optimal health, democracy, individualism, materialism and technology, achieving and doing, cleanliness, time, and automation. She noted that individualism places emphasis on the person as singularly special. The marked emphasis on the single person highlights the attention given to the rights, welfare, and privilege of the individual rather than the group. Leininger added that, although the ideal of democracy pervades American culture, gaps do exist between democratic beliefs and practices. The democratic ideal is reflected in the belief that all people regardless of race, creed, or gender should be treated equally.

Rokeach and Ball-Rokeach (1989) discussed stability and changes in American values found in four national surveys conducted in 1968, 1971, 1974, and 1981. They reported an increase in emphasis on equality between 1968 and 1971, a dramatic decrease between 1971 and 1974, and no change between 1974 and 1981. The authors noted a correlation between equality and anti-racist and liberal attitudes. They explained that the increase in emphasis on equality in 1971 may have been related to the civil rights movement and to Vietnam war protests occurring in that period. The dramatic decrease in the value placed on equality between 1971 and 1981 was accompanied by increases in the importance of "personal values emphasizing a comfortable life, sense of accomplishment, and excitement" (p. 779). These findings are consistent with the "me generation," the "yuppie" phenomenon, and increased racial tensions during the 1980s.

Philippine Culture and Ethnohistorical Dimensions

The Philippines is a group of approximately 7,107 islands, including three major islands: Luzon, Visayas, and Mindanao. Approximately 87 linguistic groups are present, and the language and dialects are important identifying features of the different Philippine ethnic groups (Asperilla, 1986; Pascacio, 1971). Pilipino, based on Tagalog, is the national language, although it is the native language of only one-sixth of the population (Yraola-Westfall, 1986). In many parts of the Philippines, Tagalog and English are learned as second and third languages, and it is common to hear people conduct business in English, Tagalog, or a combination of both (Casino, 1982; de la Costa, 1965; Karnow, 1989). While Tagalog or Pilipino is the national language, English is the language used in formal discourse, as in school instruction, science, political campaign oratory, and regional and international cooperation and diplomacy (Karnow, 1989; Pascacio, 1971).

The Philippine people are essentially Asian with strong Malayan influence characterized by the complex culture of the Indonesian Madjapahit Empire (de la Costa, 1965). Beyond these origins, trade with neighboring Asian countries, 300 years of Spanish colonization, and 50 years of American occupation have left indelible imprints on Philippine values, culture, and worldview. The contemporary Philippine culture reflects the complex and diverse heritage of its Malayan and colonial experience.

Hunt et al. (1963), a group of American and Philippine social scientists, have depicted traditional Philippine values. They noted that despite the wide acceptance of many Western values and technologies, the "bayanihan" type of social organization still prevails. *Bayanihan* is a Tagalog term derived from the word, *bayani*, translated literally in English as "hero." However, the term means a form of interpersonal relationship that stresses personal, face to face, and neighborly relationships. Inherent in this relationship is commitment and an obligation to help one's own people or "sariling tao." Hunt et al. described the "bayanihan" society as traditional, authoritarian, group-oriented, particularistic, in harmony with nature, and oriented to shame rather than guilt.

Landa-Jocano (1972), a Philippine anthropologist, characterized the Philippine value system within the context of Philippine social structure. He noted that kinship system and the family, the basic elements of Philippine social structure, define and order authority, rights, obligations, and modes of interaction in society. Within the Philippine family, seniority accords certain rights and obligations. For example, the older siblings assume the role of second parents. Respect for one's elders is a basic value expressed in kinship terms of respect such as "kuya," for older brother, "ati," for older sister, "na," for aunts or older women, and "ta," for uncles or older men. Respect is shown in deferential behaviors such as avoidance of open disagreement, remaining quiet or not answering back, and avoidance of extreme familiarity.

Several social scientists who studied Philippine society and culture (Barnett, 1966; Carroll, 1972; Eggan, 1971; Guthrie, 1971; Landa-Jocano, 1966; Lynch, 1964) noted that the systems of social interaction revolved around "obligation" systems which are sanctioned by the use of "amor propio," (personal esteem and honor) and "hiya" (shame). Within the obligation system, when one person helps another, the recipient of help is morally bound to repay the helper. This is referred to as "utang na loob." The same group of social scientists observed that interpersonal and social life operate by indirection aimed at maintaining a smooth interpersonal relationship. Lynch (1970) was the first to coin the phrase "smooth interpersonal relationship" as an English equivalent of "pakikisama," which he suggested was a Philippine value for getting along.

Landa-Jocano (1966) questioned the validity of "pakikisama" as a Philippine value. He suggested that "pakikisama," which was identified by Lynch (1964), was an artifact of comparing rural people from the Bicol region with Americans in the Philippines. He argued that the Americans in the Philippines were mostly missionaries, students, university professors, or peace corps volunteers, and were thus socially and educationally different from the rural Bicolanos.

Enriquez (1986), a Philippine anthropologist, also criticized Western accounts of Philippine values as superficial and the result of an insufficient understanding of the Philippine language. He was particularly critical of "pakikisama," or smooth interpersonal relationship, as a core Philippine value. Enriquez proposed that "pakikipagkapwa" is the superordinate Philippine value because it is the one that strikes at the core of the Philippine worldview. "Kapwa," associated with the English "others," designates the recognition of a shared identity between self and others. To Enriquez, "pakikipagkapwa" stresses the similarity of the other's dignity and being to one's own. He saw "kapwa" as defining a close tie between man and nature and as an openness to one's fellow being.

RESEARCH METHOD

Ethnonursing is primarily a qualitative and inductive nursing research method developed by Leininger and used in this study to explicate care, health, and illness phenomena. Since this method is more fully explained in other chapters, only those major features relevant to this study will be discussed.

This study was conducted in a 200-bed acute care hospital located in the Northeast. There were 9 key Anglo-American informants, 10 key Philippine informants, 13 general Anglo-American informants, and 16 general Philippine informants. The key and general informants were chosen for their specific and general knowledge about the domain of interest (Leininger, 1985; Spradley, 1979). While key and general informants were bearers of cultural knowledge, key informants possessed more in-depth knowledge about care practices and nurses' relationships. General informants possessed more commonplace knowledge and were not consistently involved in the observation-participation process to gain in-depth insights. Key informants worked full time and had worked in the hospital for a year or more. General informants worked part time and had worked in the hospital for less than a year. In keeping with the ethnonursing method, key informants were the focus of intense observation and interviews, while general informants were interviewed only once and were not observed when providing patient care.

Leininger's (1990) Observation-Participation-Reflection (O-P-R) Model was used as a conceptual field guide for systematic and rigorous data collection. The four sequenced phased—(1) primarily observation, (2) primarily observation with some participation, (3) primarily participation with some observation, and (4) reflective observation— were used with ethnonursing interviews and cultural assessments to identify nursing care values and caregiving practices of Anglo-American and Philippine nurses. These ethnonursing enabling tools were important to obtain ethnodemographic data, cultural information, and detailed cultural care congruence.

The study was analyzed using Leininger's Ethnonursing Phases of Qualitative Data Analysis, a method that provides highly systematic and rigorous analysis of raw data and at different levels of analysis. The researcher took notes and then extrapolated categories and tentative patterns from the thick, rich, textured events, experiences, and field interviews. As raw data were gathered, preliminary categories, patterns, and themes were identified, studied intensely and comparatively, verified with informants, and refined through rigorous analytic and critical thinking processes. The Leininger-Templin-Thompson Ethnoscript software was used as a valuable means to handle large volumes of qualitative data (Leininger, 1990). Data meanings and interpretations were derived and analyzed within the framework of Leininger's theory which included full consideration of the environmental and cultural caregiving contexts.

Throughout the research experience, the researcher relied on the characteristics and assumptions of qualitative research paradigm and the purposes of the ethnonursing research method to study the theory. The themes and other findings were evaluated by using Leininger's (1990) six criteria for evaluating qualitative research: credibility, confirmability, meaning-in-context, recurrent patterning, saturation, and transferability.

RESEARCH FINDINGS

Four diversity and two universal care themes were discovered. Diversity themes were based on the recurrent, observed, and expressed differences between Anglo-American and Philippine nurses, while universal themes were based on the recurrent, observed, and expressed similarities or commonalities between the two cultural groups.

Themes Related to Care and Cultural Diversities Between Anglo-American and Philippine Nurses

Four major themes comprised the care and cultural diversities discovered in the comparative analysis of data from Anglo-American and Philippine nurses.

Diversity theme one: Anglo-American nurses' care is characterized by promotion of autonomous care based on informed decision making and control of situations. Data from Anglo-American nurse informants supported the theme of care characterized by autonomous care and control of situations. This theme was supported by patterns derived from recurrent ethnonursing findings, such as promotion of independence or self-care, patient education, expectation that patients comply or conform to prescribed health regimen, and control of situations and conditions.

Anglo-American nurses expressed a stronger regard for promoting optimal independence and self-care than Philippine nurses. Statements from Anglo-American nurses pointed to the value of optimal caring for self as a major goal. For example, one Anglo-American nurse stated, "I think nurses must deal with patients. They must try to make a difference so patients don't end up coming back to the hospital for the same situation only because they neglected to care for themselves. You try to make a difference until they realize what is going on." The Anglo-American nurses' support and promotion of independence is consistent with the American value for self-reliance. As a result, Anglo-American nurses indicated that their major nursing goal was to help patients gain independence and attain ability to care for self.

To accomplish the goal of autonomous care, Anglo-American nurses stressed patient education. Nineteen of the 22 or 86 percent of the Anglo-American nurses in this study mentioned the value of patient teaching or education as the means to autonomous care. Others saw patient teaching as the ultimate in the nursing role as exemplified in the following statement, "The doctors leave the orders or what is supposed to be done. But the nurse has to act or tell the patient exactly how to put nursing care into it to get the patient to do what he has to do to get better. Basically, patient education, the teaching role of the nurses, is very important."

Patient education was valued more by Anglo-American nurses with baccalaureate degrees and to a lesser extent by nurses from associate and diploma programs. Anglo-American nurses who graduated during or prior to the 1960s tended to be somewhat less aggressive in pursuing patient education than more recent graduates.

Philippine nurses discussed patient education much less than Anglo-American nurses. In fact, only 30 percent of the Philippine nurses mentioned patient teaching as part of their nursing care. The hospital director of nursing education observed that the Philippine nurses were not strong in patient education. In her words, "Filipino nurses are good nurses but we have to coach them to do patient teaching. Those who have been here a while are better at it." Thus, it appeared that patient education is a value more profoundly held by Anglo-American than by Philippine nurses.

The Anglo-American nurses' high regard for autonomous care, which was encouraged through patient education, was, however, also linked to these nurses' demand that patients comply or conform to prescribed health care regimens. Anglo-American nurses expressed frustration when they thought patients' actions or behaviors "did not make sense" or did not conform to what they considered rational decisions. Anglo-American nurses showed frustration when they perceived their patients as "noncompliant." Although they wanted patients to care for themselves and to make choices and decisions, they wanted the patients' decisions and choices to be consistent with what they believed made sense or at least were in line with the accepted beliefs of health professionals.

Concepts of autonomous care and adherence to health regimen were not entirely alien to Philippine nurses. However, Philippine nurses included family members in their invocation of responsibility. Additionally, they used the term *cooperation* more often than *compliance* in reference to adherence to health care regimen. One Philippine nurse explained her reason for using the term *cooperation*. "In our culture, we get people to do something by persuading them, understanding their point of view, coaxing them, or even use of 'lambing' [indirect and gentle persuasion]." Thus it appeared that while the Anglo-American nurses appealed to reason and rationality, the Philippine nurses appealed to maintaining congenial and empathetic relationships.

The Anglo-American nurses' demand for control was reflected in their desire "to be on top of things." Anglo-American nurses, especially nurses in the Intensive Care Unit (ICU), were very cognizant of the precarious and ever changing conditions of their patients. They expressed value for keeping their patients' conditions stable. Stating that they "anticipate changes and prepare for them," these nurses accomplished this through vigilant assessment, frequent monitoring of vital signs, and knowing laboratory values. One Anglo-American nurse stated, "My priorities? I assess patients constantly. It is important to watch even the minute changes. I like to be on top of things." The Anglo-American nurses' acts of assessment and examination of laboratory values are professional acts which they acquired in their nursing education. However, the underlying value for control is very much consistent with the American value for "mastery of nature" or mastery of events. The Anglo-American nurses were aware that changes in patients' conditions will occur, and for some of these changes they had no direct control. Nevertheless, they exercised control by anticipating changes and preparing for them. In essence, the Anglo-American nurses maintained control by shaping and influencing existing situations, by acts involving vigilant assessment, anticipatory problem solving, and utilization of rational knowledge.

Diversity theme two: Philippine nurses' care is characterized by "obligation to care" based on the care values of physical comfort, respect, and patience. This theme epitomized the care values and caregiving practices of Philippine nurses and was supported by patterns of seriousness and dedication to work, provision of physical comfort, and respect and patience.

Philippine nurses claimed a sense of "duty," "conscience," and a "vocation-like" commitment to work, expressed in the following statements: "We have conscience. If we do not do our job, we feel guilty." "As a nurse and as a professional, you make a commitment—it is like a commitment on your part." The Philippine nurses' view of nursing care as a duty or obligation reflected some elements of self-effacement reminiscent of the earlier traditions of nursing education. Philippine nurses related that nursing as a duty, demanding a vocation-like commitment, was part of their nursing enculturation in Philippine schools of nursing. But the Philippine nurses' emphasis on duty and service was undoubtedly also influenced by their culture's hierarchical and authoritarian social structure that emphasized respect for authority, social acceptance, and group orientation where the common good outweighs individual desires and rights.

The Philippine nurses' newness to the United States also may have contributed to their emphasis on obligation or duty. Being new to the United States, they felt that they had fewer rights to make demands. Seventy percent of Philippine informants were in the United States under a working or H-1 visa which allowed them to stay for five years. Those who wanted to stay requested the institution to formally "sponsor" them. This arrangement placed them in a suppliant and dependent relationship with the institution. Unlike Anglo-American nurses who had choices and were free to seek employment anywhere, Philippine nurses were more constrained.

One aspect of the Philippine nurses' nursing care was their attention to patients' physical comfort. The majority of Philippine nurses stressed the importance of promoting physical comfort as illustrated by recurrent statements and patterned behavior modes. Statements made by Philippine nurses were: "The making of the bed—it is not the most glorified task in the ICU, but when you make the smoothest, most comfortable bed for your patients, you are showing your care." "To me, it is very important that patients are physically comfortable. I clean them up. I make sure their linens are smooth and they are positioned comfortably. I encourage them to talk while I attend to their physical needs. With our busy schedule, this is the best time to get to know the patient." To the Philippine nurses, the provision of physical comfort was also a way of developing relationships.

The Philippine nurses' attention to physical comfort, as a means to establish rapport, seemed even more prominent when compared to Anglo-American nurses who declared that making beds and baths were not a priority for them. The Philippine nurses' attention to patients' physical comfort to establish relationship was consistent with the self-giving cultural value of the theme "obligation to care." Nurses' work involving the body was considered menial manual work with low symbolic prestige. Philippine nurses were aware of the low status attributed by Anglo-American nurses to physical care. Nevertheless, the Philippine nurses' beliefs and values in the beneficial effects of physical comfort persuaded them to provide the care.

Philippine nurses cited the cultural values of respect and patience as those they had learned early in life and which prevailed in their care of patients. All Philippine informants described how their families inculcated the value of respect when they were growing up. They reported that respect was taught as an important element of caring which must be accorded to all human beings especially older persons such as parents, older brothers and sisters, older relatives, and persons in positions of authority.

Patience was another cultural care expression of respect. Philippine nurses equated patience with respect. One Philippine nurse stated: "If you respect a person, you do not rush him, you take your time, you listen to his point of view, and you do not insist on doing what you want." Philippine nurses claimed that they were patient by nature, and that this characteristic influenced their relationship with others and their care of patients, especially demanding patients. A Philippine nurse related, "We are very patient people so I think that is reflected in our work. We tolerate demanding patients a bit more. Some Americans tell us, how can you tolerate that patient? I would have told him off long time ago."

The patterns described above contributed to the care theme "obligation to care." This care theme was heavily influenced by Philippine worldview and cultural values and beliefs which emphasized duty, respect (especially hierarchical respect), patience, and relationships with others. Philippine nurses learned these cultural ways of caring in the structure of their immediate family and society. Although the Philippine nurses' acquiescent and self-effacing demeanor cast a shadow of weakness on their nursing care values and caregiving practices, their sensitivity, respect, patience, and attention to physical comfort and relationships had salutary effects on patient care.

Diversity theme three: Cultural differences between Anglo-American and Philippine nurses generated nurse-to-nurse conflicts. Cultural value differences between Anglo-American and Philippine nurses were significant enough to contribute to cultural misunderstandings and tensions. Both cultural groups, however, attempted to soften their differences by not discussing them openly or by attributing their intercultural conflicts to a myriad of reasons other than cultural. The nurses' reluctance to attribute their conflicts to cultural differences may in part be due to an inadequate understanding of the concept of culture. For example, one Anglo-American nurse stated, "Oh gee! I do not know if it is culture or just the way they were raised." It seems that the concept of culture was not cognitively known and integrated in the practice of nurses. Perhaps the nurses' refusal to attribute their conflicts to cultural differences also may have allowed them to interpret their differences as minor irritations with no real bearing on the way they provided nursing care. In fact, cultural differences between the two cultural groups did not seem to have affected patient care. Nievaard (1987), who investigated the relationship between nurses' communication and patient care, also reported that communication climate on nursing units did not affect nurses' attitude toward patients.

Despite denial that cultural differences led to conflicts, both Anglo-American and Philippine nurses were most aware and cognizant of their cultural differences. The areas of cultural differences recognized by the Anglo-American and Philippine nurses were: (1) language differences, (2) interaction and relational style differences, and (3) lifestyle differences. The conflicts which arose from these differences constituted the recurrent patterns which defined theme three.

Language was essential for intercultural communication to understand cultural thoughts, ideas, and gestures. Language differences between the Anglo-American and Philippine nurses constituted a major source of conflict between the two groups. Anglo-American nurses complained that Philippine nurses were cliquish, isolated others by speaking in Pilipino or Tagalog, and had difficulty expressing themselves in English. Philippine nurses were sensitive about the charge that they were isolating others by speaking Tagalog. They stated that they did not want to exclude or offend others when they spoke Tagalog, however, they indicated that they had difficulty expressing themselves fluently in English. They expressed a need to speak in their native language among themselves in order to articulate their feelings, ideas, and even jokes. One Philippine nurse stated, "It is hard to talk in English. When I get angry and speak in English, I stop and try to figure out what words to use. In Tagalog, my words come together with my feelings."

The differences in interaction and relational styles were closely related to language and were deeply embedded in the values and beliefs of the people within their cultural traditions. The Anglo-American and Philippine nurses held disparate values about their relational styles which were often misunderstood by both sides. Anglo-American nurses saw Philippine nurses as quiet, observant, tactful, patient, and slow-to-respond, and called them unassertive. In contrast, Philippine nurses saw the Anglo-American nurses as outspoken, impatient, bold, and fast-moving, and they viewed them as crass and insensitive. Some examples are offered to confirm this finding. One Anglo-American nurse observed, "I see most of our evening staff are Filipinos. I see that they are much quieter than the American nurses. They never complain, or very rarely. If they do, they complain for two minutes and apologize for three minutes." The Philippine nurses agreed with the Anglo-American nurses' assessment and explained, "Maybe it is the personality of Filipinos not to be assertive. Filipinos do not speak up. We were brought up—we do not tell our parents what we feel, what we want to do. Maybe, it also has to do with language." Related to the Philippine nurses' putative lack of assertiveness was the cultural value for understanding others or "kapwa tao" and maintaining smooth interpersonal relationship or "pakikisama." The Philippine nurses expressed the importance of seeing the other person's point of view, of not hurting other people's feelings, of avoiding confrontation, and use of "lambing" (use of playful coaxing or cajoling) when requesting something.

The Philippine nurses expressed perplexity over some aspects of the American ways of life. On the other hand, Anglo-American nurses also stated that they could not understand some things that Philippine nurses did. These areas of lifestyle differences related to many subjects including family relationships, religiosity, male–female relationships, legal issues, food, social gatherings, and others. For example, some Philippine nurses wondered why many elderly Americans are placed in nursing homes, because in their homeland this practice does not prevail. Anglo-American nurses wondered why Philippine nurses leave husbands and young children in the Philippines to work in the United States. The Philippine nurses who had been in the United States less than five years expressed the greatest conflict with the host culture. Thus, major cultural diversities were observed and confirmed in daily Anglo-American and Philippine nurses' relationships.

Diversity theme four: Philippine nurses worked to achieve care congruence with Anglo-American nurses through cultural care preservation, accommodation, and repatterning. In considering Leininger's predicted three modes of actions or decisions to achieve culture care congruence, this study showed that Philippine nurses used all three modes—preservation, accommodation, and repatterning—to attain cultural care congruence with Anglo-American nurses. This theme revealed the acculturation of Philippine nurses to minimize their cultural and care differences with Anglo-American nurses. In practice, this diversity theme was found to work this way: First, Philippine nurses preserved their care value and caregiving practices related to providing physical comfort, maintaining relationships, understanding others, respect, and patience. Second, care accommodation was repeatedly evident as Philippine nurses learned technological care and other American practices and standards. Third, Philippine nurses repatterned some aspects of their traditional cultural values such as respect and deference to authority.

The above three patterns were discovered by the researcher being directly involved with nurses and by observing their intercultural encounters each day. These patterns also were elucidated by examining the expressed and manifest care acts and experiences of Philippine nurses who had been in the United States at three different periods of time, that is: (1) less than five years, (2) between five and ten years, and (3) over ten years. The study of Philippine nurses over these time periods was instructive and provided much insight about their acculturation struggles and their actions and decisions to fit their care values and caregiving practices with the care values and caregiving practices of Anglo-American nurses.

There were 14 Philippine nurses who had been in the United States less than five years, with five belonging to the key informants' group and nine belonging to the general informants' group. These Philippine nurses represented the core of the theme "obligation to care." They took their work very seriously and were eager to learn and eager to please. However, they also experienced the most conflict with the host culture's values. Many were acutely aware of their foreign status. One Philippine nurse stated, "When you are a foreigner, it is hard to be a leader. I feel that the Americans are saying, why should I listen to this upstart?" Perhaps because of the language barrier, because they were unsure of themselves, and because they considered themselves still learning, they released their energy by emphasizing physical care and other activities deemed less desirable by Anglo-American nurses. Their attention to these activities and their self-effacing manner contributed to the previously described theme of "obligation to care."

There were seven nurses in the five to ten years category, five of whom were key informants and two of whom were general informants. These nurses were more exuberant and vocal compared with the first group. When the Anglo-American nurses mentioned exceptions to their characterization of Philippine nurses as "non assertive," five nurses in this group were described as "assertive nurses." These Philippine nurses were fluent in English, expressed their disagreements directly, and were less subservient to physicians than the first group. They had mastered the technical requirements of their job but continued to stress the importance of providing physical comfort, maintaining relationships, and showing respect and patience.

Five Philippine nurses, who had been in the United States for over ten years, were general informants and no formal and intensive observation-participation data were available. Nevertheless, all five nurses volunteered in-depth interviews lasting over an hour, and two of them were observed informally by the researcher. These nurses seemed to have a much broader perspective of their lives and their work. Many had concerns about their children and the values they were learning in school and society at large. They stated that they wanted their children to appreciate and preserve Philippine culture, but they also wanted them to be part of mainstream American culture. At work, these nurses appeared comfortable and at ease. They had attained the respect of other nurses on the unit by demonstrating competency and by virtue of having been around for some time. They knew many of the hospital employees and they carried out their work efficiently. These nurses differed somewhat from the five to ten years group in that they were more acculturated, had a friendlier relationship with administrators, and they related well with Anglo-American nurses. Nevertheless, they continued to profess "love for bedside nursing" and "hands-on patient care."

Universal Theme Findings

Two universal care themes were discovered that showed the significant influence of environment, social structure, and cultural values of the hospital on the nurses' care practices. These findings confirmed predictions in Leininger's theory that social structure, cultural values, language, and environmental contexts influence care and other human expressions. Most importantly, these care influencers had an impact on the health or well being of nurses involved in caregiving activities.

Universal theme one: A nursing shortage led to heavy workload, nurses' frustration and inability to provide professional nursing care ideal. In this qualitative ethnonursing research study, the phenomenon of nursing shortage was discovered to be acute and had a significant impact on the domains of interest. Although the nursing shortage was one reason why nurses from different cultures were recruited to work in the United States, it remained a serious frustration for the nurses. In fact, it was the reason nurses gave for not providing "total patient care," the expressed professional nursing value ideal of both Anglo-American and Philippine nurses. The nurses affirmed the importance of caring for the total person by meeting the "physical," "emotional," "social," and "spiritual" (only one Anglo-American mentioned "cultural") needs of patients. They asserted that concern for the total person provided the perspective from which they administered nursing care and expressed their care for patients. Nurses' concern for the total person, however, was little observed in daily nursing activities. Both nursing groups attributed their inability to provide their stated nursing care ideal to the nursing shortage. Nurses expressed frustration because they did not have enough time "to spend time talking with patients," "to get to know patients more," "to be connected," "to show concern," or "to do little extra things for the patients."

Universal theme two: Institutional norms, standards, and regulations strongly influence nursing practice. This finding demonstrated the prevailing norm related to the dominance of medicine, curing ethos, and institutional rational-legal requirements on nursing practices. Carrying out of cure orders of physicians remained a high priority in the practice of nursing. Regulatory agencies such as The Joint Commission for Accreditation of Hospital Organizations (JCAHO) stipulated certain standards that the hospital observed in order to maintain accreditation and to be eligible for third-party reimbursements. Bureaucratic traditions also prevailed, but were softened by the strong caring and family atmosphere promoted by the administrators. The hierarchical organization and the demand to protect life in situations which were unpredictable and prone to emergencies contributed to numerous bureaucratic requirements. The nurses performed the tasks assigned to them, they reported to their immediate superiors, and they adhered to set policies and procedures. This finding reaffirmed the powerful influence of institutional cultural norms and standards on nurses' caregiving practices.

CONCLUSIONS AND IMPLICATIONS

Major findings included the four diversity themes and two universal themes presented above. Space does not permit a full discussion of these findings from the rich tapestry of daily work life and language which substantiate the theory of Culture Care. The diversity themes clearly illustrated the influence of worldview, social structure, and cultural values on the care values and caregiving practices of nurses. Some care values and caregiving practices of nurses were cognitively learned in their education and training, but some were more directly traceable to their worldview, social structure, and traditional cultural beliefs and values. The delineation of professional and generic care, however, was sometimes difficult because nursing education or the professional preparation of nurses occurred within specific cultural environments. The culture in which nursing education occurred influenced the values, directions, practices, and priorities of care. Consistent with, and supportive of, Leininger's theoretical framework, this study also showed that situations, events, and environmental contexts have a strong and potent influence on nurses' caregiving practices. The critical nursing shortage frustrated both groups of nurses, impeded the practice of total patient care, and contributed to some observed uncaring events. The hospital's bureaucratic requirements tended to standardize practice so that idiographic cultural tendencies were obscured.

This study demonstrated the importance, relevance, and meaningfulness of Leininger's theory of Culture Care to discover and explicating the meanings and interpretation of care values and caregiving practices from the perspective of nurses from different cultures. The theory was substantiated by use of qualitative criteria of credibility, confirmability, meaning-in-context, recurrent patterning, saturation, and transferability. The study showed that culture, social structure features, language, and environmental context influence generic and professional care values and practices. As predicted by the theory, cultural differences generated conflicts that influenced nurses' practice and, possibly, patient care outcomes. The examination of cultural care congruence from the perspective of nurse-to-nurse care congruence showed the adaptability of the theoretical concept to study the fit or congruence between culturally different nurses in caregiving roles. This study supported and substantiated the importance of using the theory to study caregiver and care-recipient congruence with nurses of diverse or similar cultures.

Study findings demonstrated the need to include and emphasize transcultural nursing with care focus in nursing curricula and nursing service areas. Nurses participating in this study showed a lack of knowledge and understanding of transcultural nursing and the meaning and expressions of culture. With worldwide communication and increased migration and travel, it is increasingly important for nurses to not only know and understand culture, but also transcultural nursing knowledge in order to provide culture-specific care practices. For nursing educators in other countries, there is a need to discover and value indigenous care beliefs and practices and examine them in relation to professional caregiving values and practices. Migration and "brain drain" may be decreased if indigenous cultures begin to examine the strengths of their own care values and caregiving practices and take pride in them. Indigenous care values and practices may be overlooked or undervalued unless nurses are prepared in transcultural nursing.

In the practice setting, the findings of this study offer practical suggestions for easing cultural differences and cultural conflicts. Hospitals which employ nurses from different cultures need a plan for addressing and meeting the language and cultural adjustment requirements of the nurses they recruit to the United States. They should be cognizant of the language difficulties and, most importantly, the differences in cultural beliefs, values, and lifeways. Nursing service personnel need to provide programs to facilitate language and intercultural nursing care process. These intercultural programs need to be directed to both foreign and American-born nurses. Such programs should address cultural care diversities, ways of developing cultural awareness, sensitivity and knowledge, and creative ways to promote cultural care preservation or maintenance, cultural care accommodation or negotiation, and cultural care repatterning or restructuring between nurses of different cultures. Most importantly, the theory of Culture Care is essential to guide nursing care education and practice to advance the scientific and humanistic dimensions of nursing.

This study is the first ethnonursing qualitative investigation to identify Anglo-American and Philippine nursing care patterns and themes. It provides a preliminary epistemic base for future studies about care values and caregiving practices of nurses from diverse cultures. However, it must be recognized that in the complex and dynamic nature of culture care, the interrelated influences of worldview, culture, and social structure features on care must be carefully assessed over time and within particular culture and environmental contexts. Additionally, culture care inquiry requires a research methodology that is cognizant and sensitive of cultures' pluralistic, comprehensive, integral, reflexive, and hermeneutic qualities.

REFERENCES

Aamodt, A. (1972). The child view of health and healing. In M. Batey (Ed.), *Communicating nursing research: The many sources of nursing knowledge* (Vol. 4, pp. 38–54). Boulder, CO: Western Interstate Commission for Higher Education.

Aguino, N. S., Trent, P. J., & Deutsch, J. (1982). Factors related to foreign nurse graduates' test-taking performance. *Nursing Research, 28*(2), 111–114.

Arbeiter, J. S. (1988). The facts about foreign nurses. *R.N., 51*(9), 56–63.

Arensberg, C. M., & Neihoff, A. H. (1975). American cultural values. In J. P. Spradley & M. A. Rynkievich (Eds.), *The nacirema*. Boston: Little, Brown & Company.

Asperilla, P. F. (1986). Cultural characteristics of the Filipino: origins and influences. *Journal of New York State Nurses Association, 17*(1), 16–20.

Baugh, A. C. (1957). *A history of the English Language* (2nd ed.). New York: Appleton-Century-Crofts.

Barnett, M. L. (1966). Hiya, shame, and guilt: Preliminary consideration of the concepts as analytical tools for Philippine social science. *Philippine Sociological Review, 15*(4), 276–281.

Benner, P., & Wrubel, J. (1989). *The primacy of caring: Stress and coping in health and illness*. Menlo Park, CA: Addison-Wesley.

Beyers, M. (1979). *Exploration of factors affecting the achievement of licensure for foreign-educated nurses*. Unpublished doctoral dissertation, Northwestern University of Chicago.

Byerly, E. L., Molgaard, C. A., & Snow, C. T. (1979). Dissonance in the dessert: What to do with the golden seal? In M.M. Leininger (Ed.), *Transcultural nursing care: Culture change, ethics, and nursing care implications. Proceedings from the fourth national transcultural nursing conference* (pp. 114-133). Salt Lake City: University of Utah.

Carroll, J. J. (1972). The traditional Philippine social structure. *Silliman Journal, 19*(1), 81-88.

Casino, E. S. (1982). *The Filipino nation: The Philippines, land, peoples, a cultural geography.* Denbury, CT: Grolier International.

Curran, C. (1989). *Overview of the nursing shortage.* Paper presented at Robert Packer Hospital School of nursing, Sayre, PA.

de la Costa, H. (1965). *Readings in Philippine history.* Manila: Bookmark.

Drew, N. (1986). Exclusion and confirmation: A phenomenology of patients' experiences with caregivers. *Image: Journal of Nursing Scholarship, 18*(2), 39-43.

Du Bois, C. (1955). The dominant value profile of American culture. *American Anthropologist, 57,* 1232-1239.

Eggan, F. (1971). Philippine social structure. In G. M. Guthrie (Ed.), *Six perspectives on the Philippines.* Manila: Bookmark, 1-47.

Enriquez, V. G. (1986). Kapwa: A core concept in Filipino social psychology. In V. G. Enriquez (Ed.), *Philippine world view.* Singapore: Institute of Southeast Asian Study, 6-19.

Guthrie, G. M. (1971). The Philippine temperament. In G. M. Guthrie (Ed.), *Six perspectives on the Philippines.* Manila: Bookmark, 49-83.

Horn, B. (1978). Transcultural nursing and childbearing of the Muckleshoot people. In M.M. Leininger (Ed.), *Transcultural nursing: Concepts, theories, and practice,* 223-238.

Hsu, F. L. K. (1955). *Americans and Chinese.* London: Cresset Press.

Hunt, C., Pal, A., Collier, R., Espiritu, S., de Young, J. E., & Corpuz, S. F. (1963). *Sociology in Philippine setting.* Quezon City: Phoenix Publishing House.

Karnow, S. (1989). *In our image—America's empire in the Philippines.* New York: Random House.

Kendall, K. (1979). Maternal and child nursing in an Iranian village. In M. M. Leininger (Ed.), *Transcultural nursing* (pp. 42-46). New York: Masson International Nursing Publications.

Kluckhohn, C. (1949). *Mirror for man.* New York: McGraw-Hill.

Landa-Jocano, F. L. (1966). Rethinking "smooth interpersonal relations." *Philippine Sociological Review, 14*(4), 282-291.

Landa-Jocano, F. L. (1972). Filipino social structure and value system. *Silliman Journal, 19*(1), 59-79.

Leininger, M. M. (1970). *Nursing and anthropology: Two worlds to blend.* New York: John Wiley & Sons.

Leininger, M. M. (1976). *Health care dimensions: Transcultural health care issues and conditions.* Philadelphia: F. A. Davis.

Leininger, M. M. (1977). Culture and transcultural nursing: meaning and significance for nurses. In *Cultural dimension in baccalaureate nursing curriculum.* New York: National League for Nursing, 85–105.

Leininger, M. M. (1978). *Transcultural nursing: Concepts, theories, and practices.* New York: John Wiley & Sons.

Leininger, M. M. (1979). *Transcultural nursing 79.* New York: Masson International Publications.

Leininger, M. M. (1980, October). Caring: A central focus of nursing and health services. *Nursing and Health Care,* 135–143.

Leininger, M. M. (1981). The phenomenon of caring: Importance, research questions, and theoretical considerations. In M.M. Leininger (Ed.), *Caring: An essential human need.* Thorofare, NJ: Slack, 3–16.

Leininger, M. M. (1984). Care: the essence of nursing and health. In M.M. Leininger (Ed.), *Care: The essence of nursing and health.* Thorofare, NJ: Slack, 3–16.

Leininger, M. M. (1985). *Qualitative research methods in nursing.* New York: Grune and Stratton Inc.

Leininger, M. M. (1988). Leininger's theory of nursing: Cultural care diversity and universality. *Nursing Science Quarterly, 1*(4), 152–160.

Leininger, M. M. (1990). Ethnomethods: The philosophic and epistemic bases to explicate transcultural nursing knowledge. *Journal of Transcultural Nursing, 1*(2), 40–51.

Luna, L. (1989). *Care and cultural context of Lebanese Muslims in an urban U.S. community: An ethnographic and ethnonursing study conceptualized within Leininger's theory.* Unpublished doctoral dissertation. Detroit: Wayne State University.

Lynch, F. (1970). Social acceptance reconsidered. In F. Lynch & A. de Guzman (Eds.). *Four readings on Philippine values* (IPC Papers No. 2). Quezon City, Philippines: Ateneo de Manila Press.

Maroun, V., & Serota, C. (1988). Demanding quality when foreign nurses are in demand. *Nursing and Health Care, 9*(7), 361–363.

Mason, L. (1955). The characterization of American culture in studies of acculturation. *American Anthropologist, 57,* 1264–1279.

Miraflor, C. G. (1976). *The Philippine nurse: Implications for orientation and in-service education for foreign nurses in the United States.* Unpublished doctoral dissertation, Loyola University, Chicago, Illinois.

Neivaard, A. C. (1987). Communicating climate and patient care: causes and effects of nurses' attitudes to patients. *Social Science and Medicine, 24*(9), 777–784.

Pascacio, E. M. (1971). Communication breakdowns. *Silliman Journal, 18*(3), 312–319.

Pilette, K. L. (1989). Recruitment and retention of international nurses aided by recognition of phases of adjustment process. *The Journal of Continuing Education, 20*(6), 277–281.

Ray, M. (1984). The development of classification system of instituting caring. In M. M. Leininger (Ed.), *Care, the essence of nursing and health*. Thorofare, NJ: Slack.

Rokeach, M., & Ball-Rokeach, S. J. (1989). Stability and change in American value priorities. *American Psychologist, 44*(5), 775–784.

Rosenbaum, J. (1990). *Cultural care, cultural health, and grief phenomena related to older Greek Canadian widows within Leininger's theory of culture care*. Unpublished doctoral dissertation. Detroit: Wayne State University.

Slater, P. E. (1976). *The pursuit of loneliness: American culture at the breaking point* (rev. ed.). Boston: Beacon Press.

Spradley, J. P. (1979). *The ethnographic interview*. New York: Holt, Rinehart and Winston.

Thompson, T. (1990). *A qualitative investigation of rehabilitation nursing care in an inpatient rehabilitation unit using Leininger's theory*. Unpublished doctoral dissertation. Detroit: Wayne State University.

Tripp-Reimer, T. (1982). Barriers to health care: variations in interpretation of Appalachian client behavior by Appalachian and non-Appalachian health professionals. *Western Journal of Nursing Research, 4*(2), 179–191.

Veroff, J., Douvan, E., & Kulka, R. A. (1981). *The inner American. A self-portrait from 1957 to 1976*. New York: Basic Books.

Visintainer, M. (1986). The nature of knowledge and theory in nursing. *Image: The Journal of Nursing Scholarship, 18*(2), 32–38.

Wenger, A. F. (1988). *The phenomenon of care in a high context culture: the old order Amish*. Unpublished doctoral dissertation. Detroit: Wayne State University.

Yraola-Westfall, E. (1986). Tagalization of Spanish and English. A case study of code switching and mixing. *Dissertation Abstract, 47*(4), 1309-A.

4

The Culture Care Theory and the Old Order Amish

Anna Frances Wenger

This chapter will discuss Leininger's theory of Culture Care Diversity and Universality and Hall's concept of culture context to discover and explicate the nature, meanings, and expressions of care with the Old Order Amish. Culture-specific care for the Old Order Amish also will be discussed relative to Leininger's modes of nursing actions and decisions.

Leininger defines theory as a systematic and creative way to discover something or to account for a phenomenon for which little is known (Leininger, 1988; Alexander et al., 1989). Care is an elusive and complex phenomenon which is embedded in the fabric of a culture. Leininger's Culture Care theory provides a framework for the study of care in many varied cultures, but is applied here to a specific culture.

Leininger (1978, 1981, 1985, 1988) has held care as the essence of nursing. The challenge for this investigator and other contributors to

This research was partially funded by a Sigma Theta Tau Lambda Chapter grant, a Miller-Erb Fund grant and Goshen College faculty research grants.

the development of transcultural nursing knowledge is to discover care beliefs and values and practices in specific cultures, and then to show the relationship of care to the health and well being of families, communities, institutions, and nations. Historically, care has had a linguistic and practice emphasis within the field of nursing. Ironically, systematic research into the meanings, functions, and expressions of care and caring has been done only in the past two decades by a small cadre of care scientists.

Leininger (1978) has theorized that care is essential for any culture to survive. She states that "human caring is a universal phenomenon, but expressions, processes, and patterns vary among cultures" (1981, p. 11). Care expressions are developed and communicated within each culture in ways that promote the survival of that group. One can further theorize that when humans care for themselves and others so as to maintain their health and well being, their cultural values and beliefs about health and illness influence the caring modalities that they prefer. Moreover, such patterns of human care must be understood not only from the people who express them, but from their social structure, worldview, and cultural context in order to provide what Leininger has called culture congruent care.

RESEARCH QUESTIONS AS DOMAINS OF INQUIRY

The research questions which guided this study follow:

1. What are the meanings and expressions of care to the Old Order Amish as high-context culture?

2. What are the functions of care within this high-context culture?

3. What social structure factors, environmental context, and cultural lifeways influence the culture of the Old Order Amish and their use of folk and professional care services?

4. What generational or family differences exist in the expressions and meanings of culture care in the Old Order Amish culture?

These questions provided focused areas of inquiry for this qualitative study. They were of interest to the researcher and congruent with Leininger's theory to discover care expressions and functions. Leininger (1988) holds that this "theory can guide researchers to discover naturalistic inquiry patterns and expressions of cultural care within diverse environmental contexts and social structures" (p. 154).

IMPORTANCE OF THE STUDY

The present study gains importance as it increases the body of knowledge regarding the phenomenon of care. Since Leininger (1966) did the first transcultural care study with the Gadsup people in New Guinea, there has been a slow but steady increase in the number of studies on care in different cultures (Aamodt, 1978; Boyle, 1984; Glittenberg, 1978; Horn, 1978; Leininger, 1969, 1984b, 1985b; Luna, 1986; Panfilli, 1985; Wenger, 1985). The study reported here was the first to focus specifically on the relationship between culture care and high-culture context of a particular culture. The insularity of high-context cultures and boundary maintenance practices which separate insiders from outsiders have made it difficult to understand the indigenous care beliefs of concern. Thus, care knowledge related to high-culture context will contribute to the growing body of transcultural and general nursing knowledge. Since the goal of the Culture Care theory is to provide culturally congruent care, this study was designed to discover ways that this might be achieved by the three modes of decision making posited in the theory.

CULTURAL CARE THEORY AND HIGH CULTURAL CONTEXT: THE CONCEPTUAL FRAMEWORK

The conceptual framework for this investigation was based on Leininger's theory of Culture Care Diversity and Universality (1985c, 1988) and Hall's conceptualization of high-context culture (1976, 1983). Culture Care theory provided the researcher a broad general framework in which to discover care meanings, expressions, and functions by focusing on social structure, environment, and language contexts, and professional and folk health care systems. Leininger's (1988) Sunrise Model provided a holistic conceptualization to show the interrelated cultural care dimensions of worldview, social structure factors, cultural values, and folk and professional health systems within language use and environmental context. Social structure factors predicted to influence care and well being included economics, education, politics, kinship, religion or philosophy, technology, and cultural values. Although these factors are interrelated within a given culture, Leininger predicted that variability and diversity exist in the way that specific social structure factors influence care and health.

Environmental context and language were held by Leininger to be important for understanding social structure factors. Environment referred to the social, physical, and geographical setting in which care was expressed. It included family, friendship, neighbor, church district, and Amish and non-Amish relationships. Language also was held to be important to understand care expressions. In this study, it was found that the Amish informants were better able to discuss the meaning of care in *Deitsch*, the German dialect which they use in everyday communication in their culture, than in English, which was their second language and the contact language for outsiders. The interviews were conducted in English, with *Deitsch* being used to elaborate on the linguistic meanings of care.

Leininger posited that general and specialized care are provided by folk health practitioners and that folk (generic or indigenous) and professional care systems may exist side by side, sometimes in conflict with each other. One of the research questions focused specifically on the folk and professional health care systems. The three modes in the Culture Care theory predicted to guide nursing decisions and actions—culture care preservation, culture care accommodation, and culture care repatterning or restructuring—were examined in this study. These modes were predicted from the total knowledge generated from the study about the Amish culture.

Edward T. Hall's conceptualization of high-context culture also was used within Leininger's Culture Care theory. Hall (1976) developed the concept of high and low context, holding that in real life, context and meaning can be seen only as different aspects of a single event

(p. 90). Hall identified general characteristics of high- and low-context cultures which refer to the nature of the context dependency in human–environment interchange. Table 1 presents a comparative list of these characteristics.

For example, persons in high-context cultures are deeply involved with each other and share much cultural knowledge and experience. By contrast, persons in low-context cultures tend to share fewer life activities, have more variability in cultural lifeways, and accept change more readily.

This study focused only on the high-context features of the Old Order Amish. The notion of high-context culture as conceptualized by Hall (1976, 1983a,b) was congruent with Leininger's (1985c, 1988) Cultural Care theory in that both theorists hold that cultural contexts vary and affect all aspects of persons' lives. Hall stated that there is variability in culture context within the conceptualization of high- and low-context cultures, and Leininger held that cultural care differences

Table 1
Hall's Characteristics of High- and Low-Context Cultures*

Characteristics	High Context	Low Context
Relationships	long-term	minimal acquaintance
Shared life activities	many	few
Meaning of message	implicit in context	explicit in transmission
Linguistic code	restricted	elaborated
Variability in cultural lifeways	more	less
Intergenerational kinship knowledge	more	less
Social control and support	high	low
Sociocultural boundaries	insider/outsider distinction marked	blurred
Integration of new situations	take more time	more quickly completed
Rate of change	slow	rapid

* Table developed by author (Wenger, 1991) with information from Hall (1976, 1983).

and similarities are related to cultural context. Therefore, it was posited by the researcher (Wenger, 1988) that the phenomenon of care would be explicitly known in high-context cultures.

LITERATURE REVIEW

Ethnographic and ethnonursing studies lend support to Leininger's contention that patterns of care, as viewed by the insider, can be learned and do vary among cultural groups. Leininger's ethnoscience research on the caring and curing behaviors of the Gadsup people of New Guinea in the early 1960s led the way for other nurse researchers to explore and analyze culture care. Culture care constructs have been identified in cultures such as Muckleshoot Indian (Horn, 1978), Arab-American (Luna, 1986), Mexican-American (Leininger, 1984; Panfilli, 1985), African-American (Leininger, 1984; Smith, 1985), and Soviet-Jewish immigrant (Wenger, 1985). It has been found that worldview, language, environment, and sociocultural factors, as well as historical events, influence culture care patterns and experiences.

There has been little deliberate focus on culture context in the research process, although many researchers refer to the importance of context. Leininger (1970) first wrote about the culture context approach in relation to Spanish-Americans and nursing care. Ragucci (1979), a nurse anthropologist, contends that many studies on cultural transformation owing to urbanization have focused on social structure and value changes, whereas her study dealt with the persistence of traditional beliefs and practices of rural people as they adapt to the urban context. McKenna (1979) suggests that cultural context may be a major influencing factor in the retention of some familiar health care practices from the rural cultural context for North American Indians who relocate in urban settings.

No studies were found in the literature that related Hall's high-context conceptualization to culture care. In fact, most of Hall's (1976, 1983a,b) research has had to do with communication theory. In the present study, the conceptualization of culture context and culture care was much broader than communication. A major assumption of this study was that high-context cultures reflect that people interact in interdependent lifeways using social roles and language styles that make care expressions meaningful and functional. The prediction held was that care beliefs and practices in high-context cultures, although difficult for outsiders to identify and understand, would be highly integrated and supported by the high-context features of the Old Order Amish (Wenger, 1990).

ORIENTATIONAL DEFINITIONS

Orientational definitions were adapted from Leininger's Cultural Care theory and Hall's conceptualization of high-context culture. They are stated as follows:

Culture Care—*the meanings and expressions known by Old Order Amish that support and enhance a sense of personal, family, and community well being, assisting them in improving human conditions, or in facing disabilities or death.*

High-Context Culture—*context-dependent actions and words within the human–environment interchange characterized by kinship and language expressions that tend to bind people together with signs of cohesiveness and increase their awareness of themselves as insiders.*

ETHNOHISTORY

In keeping with qualitative ethnonursing research, a brief ethnohistory is provided for a general orientation to the study. It is based on already available historical studies and general observations on the Old Order Amish. The Old Order Amish, technically known as the Amish Mennonites (Old Order), constitute an ethnoreligious group who live in settlements in 20 states of the United States and in Ontario, Canada (Hostetler, 1980). There are approximately 100,000 Amish in the United States of America, of which 75 percent live in Ohio, Pennsylvania, and Indiana (Krabill, 1989). They are usually recognized by non-Amish for their distinctive dress, selective use of modern technology, resistance to change, cohesive family and social structure, use of a German dialect among themselves in everyday speech, rejection of formal education beyond the elementary level, nonparticipation in government or political activities, propensity for farming as a preferred occupation, nonparticipation in war efforts and isolationist rules and regulations which separate them from the surrounding dominant culture (Hostetler, 1980; Huntington, 1981; Krabill, 1989).

The Old Order Amish are a variant within the Anabaptist movement which originated in Switzerland in 1525. They were part of a religious movement that viewed baptism of adult believers as a symbol of commitment to live peaceably, loving their neighbors in accord with the guidelines of the Early Church, as described in the New Testament (Hostetler, 1980). As a result of severe persecution and martyrdom, the Amish and other related groups migrated to the United States in the eighteenth and nineteenth centuries. They came in search of religious freedom and a place where they could practice their beliefs in a setting providing access to land on which to grow their crops and live their lives peaceably.

In the New World, they settled in new agricultural lands in Pennsylvania, Ohio, Indiana, and Canada. Many later migrated westward to Illinois, Iowa, Kansas, and Missouri. They settled in areas where they could form constellations of church districts that were in close geographical proximity to Mennonites and other groups who shared their beliefs of living a simple life in accordance with their understanding of the Bible. No Amish remain in Europe today.

The Old Order Amish live in settlements that are divided into church districts similar to rural parishes. The church districts are usually composed of 30 to 40 families in each district. This size allows for personal interaction and for reasonable distances that can be traveled by horse and buggy, their accepted mode of transportation (Huntington, 1957; Hostetler, 1976). The charter of the Amish community "encompasses basic beliefs and a body of tradition and wisdom that guide the members in their daily lives" (Hostetler, 1980, p. 75). Some of the basic cultural values include honesty, order, personal responsibility, obedience to parents, church and God, nonresistance, and perception of the human body as the temple of God. These values are significant in all spheres of life, including beliefs and practices related to health and illness. Obedience and conformity to the community's rules of discipline are indicators of loyalty to God (Huntington, 1981). These rules also stipulate the ways in which members are permitted to inter-act with non-Amish people.

The Amish worldview incorporates an understanding of boundary maintenance between Amish and non-Amish and a general avoidance which exhibits varying degrees of permeability (Huntington, 1987). "They view themselves as a Christian community suspended in a ten-sion-field between obedience to God and those who have rejected God in their disobedience" (Hostetler, 1980, pp. 75-76). Marriage, family, children, and a disciplined life are highly valued (Hostetler & Hunting-ton, 1971).

RESEARCH METHOD

For the present study, ethnography, ethnonursing, and life history methods were chosen because of the need to establish an epistemologi-cal base of nursing knowledge about culture care from the emic per-spective (i.e., from the people's point of view) (Leininger, 1985b). Ethnography was chosen to provide a documented account of current lifeways of the Old Order Amish. Ethnonursing was used to explicate and document specific nursing care data from both emic and etic perspectives, within Leininger's Culture Care theory. The life history method (Langness, 1965; Leininger, 1985a) provided specific longitudi-nal meaning-in-context data about care beliefs and practices and gener-ational differences in care practices. Life histories also were used to help confirm information about care from key and general informants. The use of these three methods within the qualitative paradigm pro-vided ways to identify and study recurring patterns and themes and in relation to qualitative criteria, such as saturation and credibility of data.

INFORMANTS

The study focused on the lifeways of Old Order Amish families whose children attended one of the 21 Old Order Amish schools in a settle-ment located in the third largest such settlement of the Old Order Amish in the world (Hostetler, 1980). Using all the families represented in the school was congruent with their cultural values of blurring individual distinctions in favor of focusing attention on the group, in this case, families served by the school. Individual informants could refuse to participate, but they were more likely to participate if their participation was the result of a group decision. The following criteria were used in selecting the school: (1) 12 to 15 families are represented in the school; (2) the teacher was respected in the Amish community; (3) the teacher had taught there at least three years; (4) the school board did not oppose the study; and (5) the bishop did not oppose the study.

The informants included 13 key informants and 34 general Old Order Amish informants. Key informants were members of the culture who possessed the most knowledge and experience about the domain of inquiry. Mothers of the 13 informant families were chosen as key informants because, in most cultures, health care information is passed from one generation to the next by women. The general informants included 10 fathers, 34 children, 5 grandmothers, 2 grandfathers and 2 Amish healers. A total of 69 Amish children were present at some time during the interviews and contributed in varying ways to the discussion. General informants participated in some, but not all discussions. General informants were used to help confirm data from key informant interviewing and participant observation as generally representative of Amish cultural lifeways. In addition, contact was made with three of the 15 Amish healers mentioned by the informants. Two healers were observed while giving treatments, and discussions took place on three separate occasions.

ENTRY INTO THE FIELD

Entry into the field took three months, with much of the time spent in waiting and determining the appropriate strategies to enter successfully into the community and become accepted. Initial contact was made with the author of the local Amish directory for the settlement, which was followed by contact with the chairman of the statewide Amish school committee. This was followed by contact with the chairman of the local school board, with teachers of the selected school, and with the bishop in whose church district the selected school was located. An invitation was received to meet with the parents who were to become the informants at a parent-teacher meeting in the schoolhouse. This approach permitted the study to move ahead with all persons involved being fully informed, and with the researcher learning to adapt to their cultural lifeways in the process.

DATA COLLECTION

Data were collected over a three-year period of time, beginning in June 1985. Intensive full-time interviewing and participant observation in selected community activities took place from January to April 1986. During the initial period and the latter phases of the study, involvement with the community was on a part-time basis.

Participant observation, a major part of the study, involved purposeful observation of the people, activities and environment for the purpose of studying specific social and cultural phenomena (McCall & Simmons, 1969; Spradley, 1980). Leininger's ethnonursing method called for observation, participation, and reflection phases that provided specific ways to obtain detailed data. These phases are different from the traditional anthropological approach (Leininger, 1985b). Table 2 shows the model with the allocated time phases used in this study. It includes observation (25 percent), observation-participation (50 percent), participation (20 percent), and observation-reflection (5 percent).

These phases in the continuum of observation-participation are directional, not discrete, with much overlapping of activities. In this study, some observation and participation activities included attending church services, auction sales, quilting bees, funerals, singing practice, hospital visits, school functions, baptism service, and visits to traditional healers.

Four ethnographic and ethnonursing interviews focusing on topic and subtopic domains were held with the 11 key informants and two each with two of the key informants. The focus of the interview was with the mother. In all but one family, the father also was involved at least part of the time. Fathers participated in 39 percent of the interviews. Children also were present in 80 percent of the interviews.

Life histories done with five grandmothers in the family population focused on life health-illness histories, using Leininger's life health history guide. These grandmothers were selected because they were members of eight of the informant families, and could provide the context for comparisons of generational differences and confirmation

Table 2
Observation-Participation and Reflection Phases*

Phases	I	II	III	IV
NAME	OBSERVATION	OBSERVATION PARTICIPATION	PARTICIPATION	OBSERVATION & REFLECTION
Relative Time Period	June–October 1985	October–December 1986	January–April 1986 Full Time	September 1986- June 1988
Types of Activities	Observing informants and contextual situations			
			Attendance at church services, funerals, school activities	
	Talking with other researchers, persons related			
	Reading documents on Amish in historical libraries (in USA & Canada)	Participation in monthly quiltings		Interviews with a few key informants
		Interviews with key informant families		Occasional meetings with some informants in hospital, school activities, singing session
	Finding study location and informants		Interviews, observations with Amish healers	
	Developing recording system and computer data program		Involvement with one family's health care activities with medical center, hospital, Amish healers, and folk remedies	Confirming observations with experts in Amish research and ethnography
				Writing report

* Based on Leininger's Sequenced Phases of Observation-Participation-Reflection Field Method (Leininger, 1985b, p. 52).

of data from other informants. They also were selected to gain in-depth insights about culture care from an intergenerational perspective.

DATA RECORDING SYSTEM

A recording system was used that included a field work journal and a condensed and expanded account (Leininger, 1985; Spradley, 1980). The field work journal contained a record of personal perceptions that were taken into account in the continuing process of analysis. A record of observations and interviews written down during or immediately following a research contact situation was kept in the condensed account. The expanded account is a fuller notation that was recorded usually within 24 hours of the research contact time. In all written records, a coding system was used to identify the informants and the relationship within the extended family.

A computer program using Data Base IIIPlus was developed for the microcomputer in order to process data. This menu driven program was developed from the Leininger-Templin Data Management System, a software system to transcribe, code, and classify ethnographic and ethnonursing field data (Templin, 1985). This was an earlier version of the currently available Leininger-Templin-Thompson Qualitative Ethnoscript Software system (Leininger, 1990a). Leininger's field research codes for Ethnoscript were used, with four codes added that were specific to this research.

DATA ANALYSIS

Since this study extended over a three-year period, many findings were discovered, but owing to space limitations, only major findings are reported here. Leininger's Four Phases of Ethnonursing Data Analysis were used for the continuous comparative analysis throughout the study. In addition, Leininger's Evaluation of Qualitative Criteria for data analysis were used. Criteria used were credibility, confirmability, meaning-in-context, recurrent patterning, saturation, and transferability (Leininger, 1990b). A description of these criteria is provided on pages 112–114. These criteria are extremely important to support or refute findings.

The first phase involved collecting and documenting raw data. This field note was recorded after a first interview with two key informants during a discussion on the meaning of care:

> "Children learn by seeing. They must see parents and older people showing care. They must see it. They will learn to respect it if they see it in others." While we talked, five children ages 4 to 19 were in the room. They listened and talked, but never interrupted. The parents spoke kindly to and about the children.

This section was categorized as "teaching children" during the first phase of analysis. Later it was coded "ethnocare," "child-adolescent practices," and "kinship social structure." These codes are examples of categories in the Leininger Ethnoscript codes.

During the second phase, code descriptions and categories were identified from the raw data. Intensive interviewing and participant observation were taking place at this time. Data were studied for similarities and dissimilarities. Confirming information and establishing the credibility and accuracy of data were major tasks here. An example of a check for credibility in the field notes following an interview with a key informant family follows:

> They get some colds. Do not take vitamins regularly. The mother said, "I guess we should." They use 500-C chewable vitamin in tabs. The children each ate one.

In an interview, another family mentioned that they were buying herb pills and vitamins from the family mentioned above, stating that that family sells these products. During a later interview with the former family, the mother's injury from a recent fall was discussed. The following was then recorded in the field notes:

> I asked her if she went to the chiropractor when she fell. She looked at me, paused and then said, "Yes, I did. I don't know what you think of chiropractors." I told her I think they can help with some things. . . . Then she said, "I also use herbs. I don't know what you think about that." We talked then about what she uses.

As trust developed, the researcher found that more accurate information was gradually disclosed.

The third phase focused on pattern analysis. From the second phase data base, recurrent patterns emerged and were identified. One recurring pattern that was noted was the attention given to arranging occasions and activities where people regularly came together in various age groups and relational constellations. In addition, people often discussed activities in which they responded to needs within the family, the church district, the settlement, and in the broader Amish community in the United States and Canada. These data were then organized into a chart of community care activities and further analyzed.

The fourth phase focused on abstraction of the major themes, and other general research findings. The formulation of themes and theoretical statements was a major creative task of the researcher. For example, a recurrent theme identified related to community care actions, and was named "anticipatory care." Anticipatory care referred to care whereby persons develop cultural assistive or supportive patterns that allow them to maintain high-context relationships and knowledge about each other's "caring" needs. For the Amish, anticipatory care was grounded in their strong beliefs about serving others and putting other persons and their needs above one's own personal needs.

PATTERNS AND THEMES

The data analysis resulted in the formulation of patterns and themes about culture care which were derived from raw empirical data (Phase I) to descriptors (Phase II), to patterns (Phase III), and finally to the abstracted major themes. These themes reflect findings to address the research questions that were focused on the meaning, expressions, and functions of care, and factors that influenced the use of folk and professional care services along with generational or family differences in ethnocare. The four cultural care themes were: (1) centrality of care in Amish worldview and social structure, (2) anticipatory care in high-context daily life, (3) active participation in care situations, and (4) principled pragmatism in Amish culture care.

Centrality of Care in Amish Worldview and Social Structure

This emic theme of care as "being Amish" was central to the development of the Amish personal and group identity. The Amish identity which self-consciously separates them from the dominant culture was reinforced through the Amish social structure. The size of the church district was deliberately limited to a number that allowed individuals to know each other personally. One informant summarized this theme as follows: "We care for each other because we are concerned. Our people belong together. It is what keeps the community together." The pattern of giving and receiving care in an environmental context that is socially structured in congregational units (church districts), and that encourages close interpersonal relationships, was congruent with and confirmed both Leininger's Culture Care theory and Hall's high-context concept. Leininger (1988) predicted that culture care has meaningful functions and structural patterns that were derived from worldview, social structure, and environmental contexts of a culture. According to Hall (1976), a high-context culture was one that encourages close interpersonal relationships.

Credibility for the analysis that care is a central theme of being Amish was established through confirmation of the descriptors with both key and general informants. Although only a few informants used the word "obligation" when discussing care, they talked about needing to care and wanting to express their care in helpful ways. Of the 13 key informant mothers, three expressed uncertainty about knowing whether their care actions would be adequate or appropriate in some instances. Saturation of the data was evident when all the informant families fully and repeatedly identified care in the family, church district, neighborhood, and the larger Amish community as essential to the life of the Old Order Amish people. Using the Pennsylvania German dialect in discovering and then back-translating into English proved an essential way to increase the accuracy of the data and increase the informants' comfort in the interview as they discussed the emic meaning of care, and to establish credibility of the researcher's data, especially of emic meanings. Table 3 presents a semantic analysis of care in *Deitsch* and English.

Table 3
Semantic Analysis of Care in *Deitsch* and English

Types of Care		
achtgewwe *bekimmere* *hiede* *abwaarde*	>	is a type of care
Ways to Care		
to help, to serve	>	is a way to care (*achtgewwe*)
to think about, to be concerned for, to have respect for	>	is a way to care (*bekimmere*)
to watch over, to protect, to tend	>	is a way to care (*hiede*)
to wait upon, to serve	>	is a way to care (*abwaarde*)
Ways to be Amish		
to care for our parents to offer help generously to accept help with humility to consider others' needs above our own	>	is a way to be Amish

To be Amish means to express care by giving help generously and accepting help with humility. Four specific types of care emerged: *achtgewwe*, *abwaarde*, *hiede*, and *bekimmere*, which are strict inclusion semantic relationships (Spradley, 1980). For example, to help and to serve in the sense of being aware of someone's needs and then acting on that person's behalf are inclusive meanings of *achtgewwe*. The four types of care are categorized according to type and meaning. This categorization of the meaning of the four types was expressed by 12 key informants with agreement by all general informants who were present in the discussions.

Achtgewwe, *abwaarde*, and *hiede* were associated with attitude that leads to action. Care as *bekimmere* also was expressed by thinking about a person and was therefore different from the other three terms, in that it did not require action. To think about a person was a way of being present and, therefore, a way to express care. *Achtgewwe* (to help) and *bekimmere* (to have concern for) were most frequently mentioned first as linguistic terms, with 100 percent of the informants using these terms. *Achtgewwe* will be discussed briefly in terms of semantic meaning and centrality of care theme. The same analysis has been done with *bekimmere* and *hiede*. Both *achtgewwe* and *abwaarde* mean "to serve," but there a distinction arose between in the meaning of "to serve." "To serve" in the sense of *achtgewwe* meant to be aware of someone's needs and then to act, whereas the term *abwaarde* meant to minister to someone by being in their presence and serving them, such as when someone is sick in bed. *Achtgewwe* meant helping in whatever way is appropriate because persons are responsible to and for each other. This responsibility was most evident and persistent within the family, such as with children and grandparents. The responsibility to help others extended outward from the immediate family to the church district, the neighborhood (Amish and non-Amish included), and the Amish as a total group extending from Pennsylvania to Montana.

Since the meanings of care were discovered to be related to the emic meaning of being Amish, the focus shifted to enculturation of care in the cultural lifeways in order to describe worldview and social structure factors related to care. It was predicted that if care was a way to be Amish, then learning Amish lifeways involved an enculturation process of learning to care. Informants were asked to "Tell about how people learn to care" or "How children are taught about care." Documented from their responses was the process by which care knowledge became an integral part of the culture.

From repeated participant observation and interviews, the researcher discovered that Amish children learn by modeling after parents and other adults. Parents, in particular, intend that their actions will be scrutinized by the children. Children are expected to obey their parents, and that includes following modeling behavior of parents, grandparents, and others in the Amish community. Emic comments made during interviews with eight key informant families emphasized seeing, hearing, doing, and talking activities, which influenced the child's development in the process of becoming fully enculturated. The following descriptors are given as examples: (1) "Children learn by doing." (2) "They must see it (care) in others." (3) "Children learn by watching adults." (4) "They will learn respect if they see it in others." The following care set was identified as a pattern representative of this theme: (1) giving care involves both obligation and privilege; (2) receiving care involves both expectation and humility (Wenger, 1991).

Role expectations include care obligations to family, church district, neighborhood, and the wider Amish community. Parents were obligated to teach their children to work and consequently how to care. Obligation to care was not perceived as a burden, but as a privilege. Informants discussed the personal benefits of caring, including that of feeling good. A characteristic response was, "I just feel good when I am helping others." Indeed, the ability to help others is considered a privilege. Persons who are healthy, who have material resources, and are able financially to help view these as gifts from God. The counterpart to the obligation and privilege of giving care is the expectation that care is available whenever it is needed throughout one's life. This expectation to receive care was coupled with humility, a deeply held positive value. Humility referred to a personal submission to God's will and thought for others before oneself. Amish persons were aware constantly of others who may need care more than they themselves do.

Leininger (1978, 1988) states that social structure features are discovered within environmental and language contexts, and that language and environment interface in the study of the phenomenon of care. In the present study, the Amish view of care was found to be so much interrelated with everyday life, language expressions, religious values, and kinship structure that the strength of the Amish culture was clearly dependent on a holistic integrative view of culture care. The characteristics of high context identified by Hall (1976, 1983) contributed to this theme of the centrality of care in Amish culture by providing the consistent and continuous personal and intergenerational contacts that encourage shared culture care values, beliefs, and practices to promote well being of the people.

Anticipatory Care

Anticipatory care was discovered to mean care whereby persons develop cultural patterns that allow them to maintain high-context relationships and knowledge about other persons' needs, thus developing the ability to sense people's care needs (Wenger, 1991). The importance of "knowing about each other," of "keeping the community together," and of fulfilling the biblical mandate to "bear one another's burdens and so fulfill the law of Christ" (Bible, Galatians 6:2) requires an anticipatory stance regarding community care. Old Order Amish actively created and maintained the context for community care. A complex network of social event patterns provide situations where people can visit, help, and learn about care needs and nurture attitudes about culture care. This involves proactive care with members of the culture anticipating care needs within the extended family and community.

Freindschaft, the three-generational extended family network, was a care pattern expressed in the daily awareness of Amish families through visiting, helping, and generally knowing about each other. Personal contact or correspondence with members who live in other districts or even in other states is expected. The extended family functions as the social structure through which family members express care most frequently and intimately, thereby strengthening the family and maintaining high-context relationships.

Community care was a pattern that supported the theme of anticipatory care. Community care was expressed through culturally sanctioned care activities, as listed in Table 4.

Patterns for helping and visiting are known and practiced throughout the Amish community. Greeting cards and small gift showers reminded persons of the care network to which they belonged. Since most Amish do not participate in insurance plans, money showers are sometimes needed to cover catastrophe costs for illness or natural disasters. The general concept of community care actions were represented in these two emic examples: (1) "Our people belong together. Caring for each other is what keeps the community together." (2) "Helping others is a time for bringing relatives together. It is a time for visiting. It is good for people to get together. It is how we care for each other and know about each other."

Active Participation

Amish are actively involved in care situations pertaining to them as individuals, family, and community. *Active participation* was defined from the data as involvement in care activities that promote individual,

Table 4
Community Care Activities Discussed by Informants

Activities	Expressions	Indicators for Care
Showers	Greeting cards	For elderly, ill persons in church district in response to requests in Amish newsletter
	Money gifts	After extended illness
	Neighbor	After illness, death, accident
Surprises	Towel (with gifts sewn on it)	After accidents, major or extended illnesses
	Boxes (with small gifts enclosed)	Same as above
	Sunshine books	After accidents, illness and for elderly
	Visits	Birthdays
Helping	Bring food, do farm work, care for children, clean house, help with visitors, repairs on property, care for animals, make telephone calls	During illness, death, and dying After accidents Following natural disasters
Visiting	Elderly and widows in church district neighbors and the extended family	On special holidays, regular weekly or biweekly schedule, on personal days, such as birthdays and anniversaries

family, and community well being on a daily basis. This theme was abstracted from the following seven major patterns: (1) persons are expected to help themselves, which involved care through self and others within the social structure of the culture; (2) health care choices included a broad array of professions, folk, and alternative care options; (3) getting and giving health care advice was highly valued; (4) Amish wanted to participate in health care decisions which affect them; (5) folk, professional, and alternative care services were often used simultaneously; (6) there were family differences in the participation of various kinds of professional, folk, and alternative care options, and (7) the use of care services was generally dependent on social structure factors such as cost, transportation, caring attitudes of the care provider, and family preferences.

Folk, or generic care, referred to care provided in the family or by Amish healers. All Amish informants in this study used herbs, home remedies, foot treatments as well as *brauche*, a folk healing art called "powwowing" in English, which was commonly practiced years ago among Pennsylvania Germans (Hostetler, 1980; Yoder, 1972; Studer, 1980). Informants referred to it as "warm hands." Families differed in the extent to which they used folk care such as *brauche*, but all families used it at some time and especially for children. Many alternative care services were mentioned, including chiropractic, reflexology, and iridology. All informant families had family physicians and dentists.

Folk, professional, and alternative care services were used simultaneously. Cost, access, transportation, and advice from family and friends were the major factors influencing health care choices. Folk care, especially *brauche* and foot treatments, provide occasions for social interactions, and generally increased those interactions. High context was found to be promoted through the process of seeking counsel and advice about health care options and giving and receiving folk care services.

Principled Pragmatism

This theme was discovered to mean a course of action based on cultural values or principles with day-to-day consequences. For example, a mother may be planning to take her child to the family physician, but she may instead take the child to a *braucher*, because transportation was available that day to go to the *braucher*. Going to the *braucher* was more accessible, less expensive, and *brauche* was an acceptable treatment mode. These cultural values guided her action in a pragmatic way in that particular situation. This theme was abstracted from the following three major patterns: (1) Amish do what needs to be done to promote family and community well being; (2) health care actions are frequently based on the results obtained by family and friends or trusted authorities, such as those advertising in the Amish newsletters; and (3) when cultural infractions occur, care is expressed in ways that help to retain persons within Amish culture.

Hall (1976) postulated that high-context cultures exhibit internal flexibility which allows for considerable bending of the system because the bonds between people are so strong. This high-context feature accounted for the expressions of Old Order Amish care identified when cultural infractions occur. It was predicted that the complexity of the Old Order Amish care system would tend to strengthen and stabilize the culture and promote healthy lifeways. The Amish view of culture care included: (1) a wide range of health care options; (2) a high value in seeking counsel from each other; (3) a focus on day-to-day consequences; and (4) shared knowledge of accepted rules of behavior (*ordnung*) based on their understanding of Biblical truth. These cultural care values supported the theme of principled pragmatism. The patterns related to this theme supported Leininger's theory which states that worldview, social structure, cultural values, language, and environmental context influence culture care patterns, expressions, and functions.

GENERATIONAL AND FAMILY DIFFERENCES

Family cohesiveness and intergenerational relationships were found to be highly valued and nurtured in the Old Order Amish culture. However, despite the pervasiveness of shared or more universal knowledge among Amish families and between generations, differences existed. One pattern noted to support Leininger's theory of care diversities was diversity in family health care expressions. Informant families reminded the investigator on several occasions that families do things differently. One informant stated after learning about another family's response to immunizations, "So you are finding out we are not all alike." The major family differences in culture care focused on the use of folk care practices and choice of care providers. Although *brauche* was used by all informant families, some families used *brauche* to a greater extent than others. Some families were more interested in using herbs and foot treatments than others. These preferences were often shared in the extended family network and were passed from one generation to the next. This finding supported Egeland's (1967) analysis in a study of health behavior among Old Order Amish in Pennsylvania.

Family preferences for selection of care providers was influenced by the previous generation. Other things being equal, the maternal kinship influence was greater than the paternal influence. But the paternal influence became more evident if the geographical distance was greater between the family and the maternal grandparents than the paternal grandparents. Several informants reported going to the same family physician and dentist which their parents used.

Generational differences were more frequently noted by the grandparent informants than by the parent informants. Grandmothers reflected on changes in culture care in three generations: their parents, themselves, and their children. Changes were reported in the use of home remedies and herbs. In the grandparent generation, herbs were grown and dried for medicinal teas and poultices, whereas the key informant generation purchased bottled herbs in tablet form. The increased use of commercial herb tablets was believed to be partially due to the increased use of herbs in the dominant Anglo-American culture. The cost of health care and increased interest in prevention of illness and health promotion in the dominant culture were held to have influenced the Amish culture and to have increased the frequent use of herbs and of professional health services. Home remedies such as poultices and ointments were used infrequently by this parent generation.

Three grandmother informants discussed their recipes for various folk remedies. One grandmother kept her remedies at the same place her grandmother kept them when she lived in the *daadi haus* more than 70 years ago. This informant prepared grease and herb-soaked cloths (*rote laufa lumba*) to be used as poultices for each of her daughters when they married. However, the daughters did not use them and the grandmother related how this practice will not be continued to her grandchildren's generation.

Generational differences were reported in perinatal care. Whereas in the grandparent generation most babies were born at home, in the parent generation most babies were born in the hospital. However, the number of home births was now shown to be increasing again. This was attributed to the increased cost of hospital care and influences from the dominant culture regarding home births and use of midwives. The general interest in health and self-care in the dominant culture has affected the Amish culture. The Amish place a high value on health and thus may be more aware of health care trends in the dominant culture than in areas other than health care. Nevertheless, as change occurs slowly in a high-context culture, the generational and family differences in culture care are minimal.

MAJOR FINDINGS AND THEORETICAL STATEMENTS

The major findings from this investigation focused on four themes: (1) culture care at the core of the Amish worldview and social structure; (2) anticipatory care which creates a high-context care environment; (3) active participation in culture care which daily promotes individual, family and community well being; and (4) principled pragmatism which guides culture care choices. *Deitsch* and equivalent English terms for care were emically discovered, including the semantic range of help, serve, wait upon, protect, tend, think about, concern for, respect, and presence. Furthermore, it was found that Amish use professional, alternative and folk care services simultaneously. There were family differences in their preferences for and consistency in their use of specific types of health care services. Finally, four high-context features were identified that tend to have major influence on culture care: (1) long-term interpersonal relationships, (2) shared cultural knowledge, (3) frequent intergenerational contacts, and (4) boundary maintenance. Although family and generational differences in culture care were discovered, they were minimal.

From these findings seven theoretical statements were formulated. The following are offered here for consideration of future studies related to culture care, high-context culture, and the Old Order Amish.

1. Culture care will be closely related to worldview, sociocultural factors, environment, and language contexts in a high-context culture.

2. Culture care will be found to be central to the worldview and social structure of the Old Order Amish as a high-context culture.

3. Members of a high-context culture will be actively involved on a regular basis in different forms and expressions of culture care.

4. Old Order Amish will develop cultural patterns that encourage frequent and sustained relationships and shared knowledge about culture care which promote individual, family, and community health and well being.

5. In a high-context culture such as the Old Order Amish, there will be signs of flexibility, so that deeply held care values and beliefs can be upheld at times of cultural crisis in order to promote family and community well being.

6. Understanding the influence of high-culture context on Old Order Amish culture will increase the effectiveness of transcultural nurses to care for this cultural group.

7. Old Order Amish will participate actively in using folk, professional, and alternative care options that fit their religious and cultural values and beliefs.

These statements should serve as the basis for future studies discovering similarities of culture care of Amish in other locations: Amish with non-Amish high-context cultures, Amish with the dominant Anglo-American culture, and high-context with low-context cultures.

MODES OF DECISION MAKING AND AMISH CULTURE CARE

Findings from the worldview, social structure, cultural values, and environmental context had direct implications to guide nursing care for the Old Order Amish. The three modes in the Culture Care theory which were predicted to guide nursing actions and decisions were readily identified. These will be discussed using a few examples from the data in this study.

Culture Care Preservation/Maintenance

Culture care preservation should be a major consideration for nurses in providing congruent care to Old Order Amish. The extended family, neighborhood, and church district care actions must be understood and encouraged by nurses caring for Amish clients. There are many social events that create a context for people to learn about care needs, in addition to the publication of care needs in the Amish newsletters. The enculturation of care patterns in the Amish culture was exemplary. Modeling care behavior, with its concomitant various expectations related to age, gender, and role, is likely the most important aspect of culture care preservation. The enculturation of care and caring actions is essential for survival of the Old Order Amish in their high-context culture. As new generations learn the care expectations which are culture-specific for the Old Order Amish, they reinforce their identity as members of the culture.

Culture Care Accommodation and/or Negotiation

Professional nursing actions can be established if nurses learn how to provide culture care accommodation or negotiation practices with the Old Order Amish. Hospital regulations for visiting privileges must be relaxed in order to accommodate Amish families' transportation to and from the hospital. This is important as Amish are dependent on hired drivers and often travel in groups to reduce costs. In addition, Amish express care by being present with each other, and many family members will expect to visit the hospitalized person. Nurses should consider ways to accommodate their teaching methods to take into account and to respect Amish religious values and cultural learning styles. For instance, some Amish may want to be excused when a prenatal film is shown, since they object to watching television and films. Nurses may want to incorporate role modeling concepts into health promotion teaching to accommodate different cultural learning styles. The demonstration and return demonstration of instructions are important for this culture, which is oriented to learning by observation and role modeling. A major area of accommodation lies in the need for nurses to learn about Amish use of folk and alternative care. Negotiation may be needed to accommodate those Amish who use folk and professional care simultaneously. In some situations, it may be appropriate for the Amish healer to come to the hospital in order to treat the client. Since Amish do not carry medical insurance and do not own motorized vehicles, nurses should consider cost and travel requirements for health care interventions and scheduling appointments. Interventions requiring the use of high technology may be objectionable to Amish due to high cost or because of their nonacceptance of the particular technology. In general, Amish accept modern technology within the hospital setting if the client benefits from the treatment. However, any treatment which must be done in their homes cannot require electricity or will need to be converted to gas power. Amish want to be involved in their health care and thus will welcome the opportunity to negotiate for their personal and community well being.

Culture Care Repatterning/Restructuring

Changing lifeways and adopting new or different care patterns is difficult in any culture. For the Amish, change must take place slowly and through the appropriate cultural structures in order for it to be culture congruent. Health promotion actions with the Amish would need to include nutritional consideration because their diet tends to be high in carbohydrates and sugars. Another area of concern is the simultaneous use of folk, alternative, and professional care. Although some accommodation is needed to allow Amish to choose among options they consider beneficial, there are some care modalities which may have deleterious effects. When an open and trusting relationship is developed between the nurse and Amish clients, the latter will more readily discuss their full range of health care preferences. Amish culture care would be enhanced with an enlarged knowledge base of human physiology and health care. Amish do not attend school beyond ninth grade or age 16. It was reported by two informants that in many of their schools, health is not adequately taught. These proposals for repatterning would need to involve the Amish and change should progress at a slow rate, which is congruent for their culture.

SUMMARY

This chapter discussed knowledge about culture care and culture context in relation to Old Order Amish culture. Leininger's theory of Cultural Care Diversity and Universality and Hall's concept of high-context culture were used to study culture care of the Old Order Amish. This study provided new findings about the culture, especially as related to culture care and high context. These findings also are important to guide nurses and other health care professionals in providing culture-specific care to the Old Order Amish. Leininger's Cultural Care theory has provided a comprehensive theoretical framework to explicate embedded care constructs and patterns of daily living within this culture. Hall's concepts helped to value and discover the importance of high context within the Old Order Amish culture and its relation to the phenomenon of care.

REFERENCES

Aamodt, A. M. (1978). Socio-cultural dimensions of caring in the world of the Papago child and adolescent. In M. M. Leininger, *Transcultural nursing: Concepts, theories, and practices*. New York: John Wiley & Sons.

Alexander, J. A., Beagle, C. J., Butler, P., Dougherty, D. A., Andrews Robards, K. D., & Velotta, C. (1989). Madeleine Leininger: Cultural care theory. In A. Marriner-Tomey (Ed.), *Nursing theorists and their work* (2nd ed.). St. Louis: C.V. Mosby, 146–163.

Boyle, J. (1984). Indigenous caring practices in a Guatemalan Colonia. In M. M. Leininger, *Care: The essence of nursing and health*. Thorofare, NJ: Slack, 123–132.

Egeland, J. A. (1967). *Belief and behavior as related to illness: A community case study of the Old Order Amish* (Doctoral dissertation, Yale University). Dissertation Abstracts International, X, 1967.

Gardner, K. G., & Wheeler, E. (1981). The meaning of caring in the context of nursing. In M. M. Leininger, *Caring: An essential human need*. Thorofare, NJ: Slack.

Glittenberg, J. (1978). Fertility patterns and child rearing of the Ladinos and Indians of Guatemala. In M. M. Leininger, *Transcultural nursing: Concepts, theories and practices*. New York: John Wiley & Sons, 417–432.

Hall, E. T. (1976). *Beyond culture*. Garden City, NY: Anchor Press.

Hall, E. T. (1983a). Personal communication.

Hall, E. T. (1983b). *The dance of life: The other dimension of time*. Garden City, NY: Anchor Press.

Horn, B. M. (1978). Transcultural nursing and child-rearing of the Muckleshoot people. In M. M. Leininger, *Transcultural nursing: Concepts, theories and practices*. New York: John Wiley & Sons, 223–237.

Hostetler, J. A. (1980). *Amish society* (3rd ed.). Baltimore: The Johns Hopkins University Press.

Hostetler, J. A., Huntington, G. E. (1971). *Children in Amish society.* New York: Holt, Rinehart and Winston.

Huntington, G. E. (1957). *Dove at the window: A study of an Old Order Amish community in Ohio* (Doctoral dissertation, Yale University). Dissertation Abstracts International, 26, 04.

Huntington, G. E. (1981). The Amish family. In C. H. Mindel & R. W. Habenstein (Eds.), *Ethnic families in America* (2nd ed.). New York: Elsevier.

Huntington, G. (1987, November). *Cultural interaction during times of crises: Permeable boundaries and Amish cultural success.* Paper presented at the annual meeting of the American Anthropological Association, Chicago.

Krabill, D. B. (1989). *The riddle of Amish culture.* Baltimore: Johns Hopkins University Press.

Langness, L. L. (1965). *The life history in anthropological science.* New York: Holt & Rinehart.

Leininger, M. M. (1966). *Convergence and divergence of human behavior: An ethnopsychological comparative study of two Gadsup villages in the eastern highlands of New Guinea* (Doctoral dissertation, University of Washington). Dissertation Abstracts International, 27, 06-B.

Leininger, M. M. (1969). *Study of the health-illness system of Spanish-Americans in an urban community.* Unpublished manuscript.

Leininger, M. M. (1970). The culture context of behavior: Spanish-Americans and nursing care. In M. M. Leininger, *Nursing and anthropology: Two worlds to blend.* New York: John Wiley & Sons, 11–127.

Leininger, M. M. (1978). *Transcultural nursing: Concepts, theory and practices.* New York: John Wiley & Sons.

Leininger, M. M. (Ed.) (1981). *Caring: An essential human need.* Thorofare, NJ: Slack.

Leininger, M. M. (1984). Southern rural black and white American lifeways with focus on care and health phenomena. In M. M. Leininger, *Care: The essence of nursing and health.* Thorofare, NJ: Slack, 133–159.

Leininger, M. M. (1985a). Life health-care history: Purposes, methods, and techniques. In M. M. Leininger, *Qualitative research methods in nursing.* New York: Grune & Stratton.

Leininger, M. M. (1985b). *Qualitative research methods in nursing.* New York: Grune and Stratton.

Leininger, M. M. (1985c). Transcultural care diversity and universality: A theory of nursing. *Nursing and Health Care, 6*(4), 209–212.

Leininger, M. M. (1988). Leininger's theory of nursing: Cultural care diversity and universality. In R. R. Parse (Ed.), *Nursing science quarterly*. Pennsylvania: Williams & Wilkins.

Leininger, M. M. (1990a). Leininger-Templin-Thompson ethnoscript qualitative software program: *User handbook*. Detroit: Wayne State University Press.

Leininger, M. M. (1990b). Ethnomethods: The philosophic and epistemic bases to explicate transcultural nursing knowledge. *Journal of Transcultural Nursing, 1*(2), 40–51.

Luna, L. (1986). *Health and care phenomena among Lebanese Arab American Muslims*. Unpublished field study. Wayne State University College of Nursing, Detroit.

McCall, G. J., & Simmons, J. L. (1969). *Issues in participant observation*. Reading, MA: Addison Wesley.

McKenna, M. (1979). An ethnoscientific approach to selected aspects of illness behavior among an urban American Indian population. In M. M. Leininger (Ed.), *Transcultural nursing care: Cultural change, ethics and nursing care implications*, Proceedings of the Fourth National Transcultural Nursing Conference (pp. 140–165). Salt Lake City: University of Utah College of Nursing.

Panfilli, R. (1985). An ethnocaring and transcultural nursing study of urban Mexican-American families. In M. Carter (Ed.), *Proceedings of the tenth annual transcultural nursing conference*. Salt Lake City, Utah: University of Utah Press, 8–28.

Ragucci, A. T. (1979). The urban context of health and illness beliefs and practices of elderly women in an Italian-American enclave. In M. M. Leininger (Ed.), *Transcultural nursing care of the elderly: Proceedings from the second national transcultural nursing conference*. Salt Lake City: University of Utah College of Nursing.

Smith, P. (1985). Black adolescent motherhood: Studies in ethnonursing. In M. Carter (Ed.), *Proceedings of the tenth annual transcultural nursing conference*. Salt Lake City: University of Utah Press, 38–53.

Spradley, J. P. (1980). *Participant observation*. New York: Holt, Rinehart and Winston.

Studer, G. (1980). *Powwowing: Folk medicine or white magic?* Pennsylvania Mennonite Heritage, 3(3), 17–23.

Templin, T. (1985). *Users Manual for the Leininger/Templin Ethnographic Data management System*. Unpublished manuscript. Wayne State University, College of Nursing Center for Health Research.

Wenger, A. F. (1985). Learning to do a mini ethnonursing research study: A doctoral student's experience. In M. M. Leininger, *Qualitative research methods in nursing*. New York: Grune & Stratton, 283–316.

Wenger, A. F. (1988). *The phenomenon of care in a high context culture: The Old Order Amish* (Doctoral dissertation, Wayne State University). Dissertation Abstracts International, 50/02-B.

Wenger, A. F. (1991). The role of context in culture-specific care. In P. Chinn (Ed.), *An anthology of caring*. New York: National League for Nursing, 95–110.

Yoder, D. (1972). Folk medicine. In R.M. Dorson, *Folklore and Life*. Chicago: The University of Chicago Press, 191–215.

5

Culture Care Theory with Mexican-Americans in an Urban Context

David B. Stasiak

The discovery and analysis of the beliefs, meanings, and expressions of care and health of urban Mexican-Americans in a large midwestern community comprise the focus of this ethnonursing study. Major significance was given to the study of Mexican-American folk health care practices to obtain data for developing appropriate nursing practices related to cultural care preservation, accommodation, and restructuring. Hopefully, this study will help to increase the body of nursing knowledge now available and guide nurses to provide culturally congruent nursing care to Mexican-Americans.

SIGNIFICANCE OF THE STUDY

This study gains significance for several reasons. First, discovering the dimension of care within Mexican-American culture, with its specific meanings and expressions, will enable nurses to understand how care influences the health or well being of the people of concern. Appropriate to this study is Leininger's theory of Culture Care (1979, 1985, 1988), the only theory of nursing of its kind. As such, this study will examine Leininger's culture care predictions and ways to make culture care specific in providing beneficial, satisfactory, or therapeutic well being for Mexican-Americans. To date, culturally congruent nursing care for Mexican-Americans has prompted only limited exploration, especially in regard to folk care meanings and expressions. As Mexican-American culture becomes a dominant culture in the twenty-first century, nurses will be called on to care for more clients from this cultural heritage. Providing such care will require an adequate knowledge base.

DOMAINS OF INQUIRY

The central domain of inquiry for this study was on the meanings and practices of folk (generic) care and professional health care as viewed by Mexican-Americans. The study itself grew from my interest in different cultures while doing graduate transcultural nursing coursework. While conducting an earlier community nursing assessment in the same community in which I later did the study, I discovered that Mexican-American residents resisted the use of a local hospital for this reason: The professional health care providers at the hospital had limited sensitivity to and knowledge of the cultural needs of Mexican-Americans. With transcultural nursing preparation, I began to realize the importance of transcultural nursing and the need to study such concerns. Consequently, I raised the following questions: Where and how did Mexican-Americans obtain care? What would happen if folk caring practices were used by nurses and other health care professionals to give quality nursing care? What differences could be identified between generic and professional care values and practices? In what ways would generic and professional care promote the health or well being of Mexican-Americans? Would Leininger's theory of Culture Care help explain why Mexican-Americans would not use the hospital? These questions seemed important to help nurses discover and understand the cultural beliefs and philosophical bases of care for Mexican-Americans. Indeed, such an understanding would be essential for nurses to provide culturally congruent and beneficial care as promoted by Leininger's (1978, 1985) work in transcultural nursing.

ETHNONURSING RESEARCH QUESTIONS

Although the above questions initially stimulated my interest in the present study, three further ethnonursing research questions were developed to guide the research.

1. Using Leininger's theory of Culture Care Diversity and Universality, what cultural care (emic) values and constructs were used by Mexican-Americans in a designated urban community?

2. What generic folk practices influence the care or caring, and health practices of Mexican-Americans?

3. Are the three predicted modes in Leininger's theory—cultural care preservation, accommodations, and restructuring—useful to provide culturally congruent nursing care to Mexican-Americans of a designated community?

THEORETICAL FRAMEWORK

Leininger's theory of Culture Care Diversity and Universality (1979, 1985, 1988) posits this central position: culturally congruent care is essential for clients for their well being or to gain and remain healthy. The theory rests on several theoretical premises which are used to describe, explain, predict, and interpret nursing phenomena. The following premises were used to guide this study (Leininger, 1988):

1. Care is the essence of nursing and the distinct, dominant and unifying feature of nursing.

2. Mexican-American culture has generic folk care values, beliefs, and practices that can influence professional cultural care practices.

3. Worldview, social structure, cultural values, language, environment, and folk and professional health systems influence expressions and practices.

4. Culture care meanings and patterns influence Mexican-Americans' well being and health status and can guide nurses to provide culturally congruent professional care practices.

Orientational Definitions

In keeping with the ethnonursing and qualitative method, orientational rather than operational definitions were used.

Mexican-American refers to those individuals of Mexican descent who identify themselves as Mexican-American citizens.

Care (noun) "refers to phenomena related to assisting, supportive, or enabling behavior toward or for another individual (or group) with evident or anticipated needs to ameliorate or improve a human condition or lifeway" (Leininger, 1988, p. 156).

Folk (generic) care (well-being) system refers to traditional or local indigenous health care beliefs and practices performed by local practitioners that are well known to the culture and which have special meanings and uses to heal or assist people to regain well being or health, or to face unfavorable circumstances (Leininger, 1988).

Professional care refers to those cognitively learned and practiced modes of assisting others that are obtained through formal professional schools of learning (Leininger, 1981).

REVIEW OF THE LITERATURE

Beliefs and Practices Influencing Health

Leininger (1970, 1978) and Kleinman (1980) relate that each culture makes decisions regarding their health or well being: decisions about which foods to eat and how to prepare those foods; how to handle stresses, aches, and pains; whom to consult when one does not feel well; how to care for others and self; and which medicines or herbal preparations to use. Leininger identified that such decisions are strongly influenced by the social structure, worldview, cultural values, ideals, beliefs, and practices passed down by families, traditions, and cultural groups. Moreover, persons with acute or chronic illness may regard themselves, and are regarded by others, as innocent victims of malevolent forces (Martinez & Martin, 1966). In such cases, family and friends may indulge patients, allowing them to be passive and to expect support through the human process (Kleinman, 1980).

Mexican-Americans often extend the thought *ayudate que Dios te ayudara* (help yourself and God will help you), by placing the responsibility for care and caring with the entire family and God (COSSMHO, 1988). As such, the family is essential to promote the caring that leads to health. Notions of balance and harmony, while not held by all Mexican-Americans, may be relevant to understanding a Mexican-American's interaction with the professional health system (Maduro, 1983).

Another belief specific to Mexican-American culture and supportive of their theory of disease and treatment (Clark, 1970; Leininger, 1970, 1978) concerns the importance of balance and harmony between hot and cold foods, substances, and liquids. According to hot and cold theory, diseases are caused by humeral imbalance (Clark, 1970). Foods and medications are thought to cure diseases by restoring the balance between certain hot or cold substances. For example, a hot illness is curing by balancing it with cold medications and foods; cold illnesses are treated with hot substances (Murillo-Rhode, 1979).

Perrone, Stockel, and Krueger (1989) identify various types of plant sources used as teas and liniments, and other methods to promote caring, curing, and well being of Mexican-Americans. Ortiz de Montenello (1975, 1990) empirically tested and proved the chemical and pharmacologic effects of several plant sources used with Mexican-American folk healing practices. This anthropologist established that the medicinal effects of selected plant sources used by Mexican-American's in folk practices have some therapeutic benefits to heal or to regain health and well being.

Spiritual and Folk Healers

Some Mexican-Americans seek the services of spiritual and folk (generic) healers who offer contact with God and the supernaturals without the intervention of the traditional Catholic church (Devine 1982). Nonetheless, the traditional church and folk healing coexist. Folk healers in the Mexican-American culture do play a major role in healing, caring for, and curing others. They include generic healers (*curanderos*, *curanderas*), herbalists (*yerberas*), midwives (*parteras*), massage therapists (*sobadoras*), and witches (*brujas*) (Perrone, Stockel, & Krueger, 1989).

Curanderas have the highest status of folk healers among Mexican-Americans. *Curanderas* know about different types of home remedies and herbs and have skills in treating certain physical conditions that require special mental powers (Perrone, Stockel, & Krueger, 1989). Gomez and Gomez (1985) identify that *curanderas* are customarily consulted for the treatment of five traditional folk illnesses, including: (1) the evil eye (*mal ojo* or *el ojo*), (2) surfeit (*empacho*), (3) fallen fontanelle (*caida de mollera*), (4) magic fright (*susto*), and (5) hexes (*mal puesto* or *mono clavado*). *Curanderas* commonly employ massages, compresses, and packs that contain flowers and herbs. In addition, while a *curandera* works there is chanting and collective prayers.

A *yerbero* or *yerbera* is an herbalist who works with herbs alone, and does not place his or her hands on people. A *patera* is a midwife, but may also use herbs during the course of prenatal care. She may be a *yerbera* and a *curandera* as well. A *sobodora* is a specialist in massage therapy, especially as it applies to ailments of the stomach or digestive tract (Perrone, Stockel, & Krueger, 1989).

Finally, Mexican *brujeria*, as practiced and recognized by many Mexican-Americans, is a mixture of Aztec Myths, Catholic ideologies, and European witchcraft (Devine, 1982, p. 100). Contrary to Catholic views, however, *brujeria* centers around a female instead of a male diety. Perrone (1989) identifies that most *brujas* voluntarily take up the practice of *brujeria* after entering a "Faustian pact with the devil" (p. 181). She further describes that *brujas* analyze dreams, have premonitions, read cards, and indulge in other areas of black arts. *Arbularias* are considered benevolent healers of the effects of witchcraft. The healer helps the client with his or her own prayers, support, and religious sacrifices.

Human Care and Mexican-Americans

It was in the late 1960s that Leininger began the first nursing study involving the human care of Mexican-Americans in an urban city. This transcultural nursing research, published in 1970, drew attention to differences and similarities in care values, beliefs, and practices between Mexican-American and Spanish-Americans, but especially between the beliefs and practices of nursing professionals who were not Mexican-American and generic folk carers and curers. In 1983, in Detroit, Leininger continued her ethnonursing study of Mexican-Americans guided by her theory of Cultural Care and discovered that dominant care constructs of key and general informants were (1) filial love, (2) family support, (3) succorance, (4) respect, and (5) attention to (Leininger, 1990). In addition, there were many social-cultural values, structure, and environmental factors influencing their wellness and illness states as reported in this unpublished field study.

Panfilli (1983), also a transcultural nurse, did an ethnonursing study and discovered specific care constructs of Mexican-Americans in an urban community quite similar to Leininger's findings. Being with one's family, succorance, and filial love were dominant themes.

In 1988, Dugan also confirmed the care construct of *compradrazago*, a caring phenomenon defined by Mexican-American informants as a means to promote unity among family members and fictive kin. The construct of family care again substantiates by credibility and confirmability criteria the findings of Leininger, and Panfilli, who identified family care involvement as a dominant Mexican-American care value.

RESEARCH METHOD

As stated, this study employed qualitative ethnonursing research methods to discover, describe, and explain the beliefs, meanings, and expressions of care of Mexican-Americans living in an urban midwest community in the United States. The study also was designed to examine Leininger's theory of Culture Care with Mexican-Americans. The researcher collected all data, with Leininger's mentorship, during eight months in the field.

Collection of the Data

Data were collected using the Observation-Participation-Reflection (OPR) guide with interviews in a Mexican-American community in Metropolitan Detroit. Data collection was performed in a structured format using four phases identified by Leininger (1985), including (1) observation, (2) observation with some participation, (3) participation, and (4) reflection. Several of Leininger's ethnonursing enabling tools and guides were used as well, including: Observation-Participation-Reflection guide, Acculturation Profile guide, Interview Inquiry Form, Field Journal guide, and Stranger-Friend guide (see Chapter 2). The Leininger-Templin-Thompson Ethnoscript Qualitative Software Program (LTT) (1988, 1990) was used for processing, categorizing, and retrieval of data.

Brief Ethnohistory of the Mexican-Americans

In keeping with ethnonursing research methods, I studied available anthropological, nursing, and other literature on Mexican-Americans. A brief overview follows to help the reader's understanding of Mexican-Americans. However, because the ethnohistory of the Mexican-American is extensive, readers will need to refer to transcultural nursing and other cultural anthropology readings.

In or around 1494, Spanish colonizers arrived in Mexico, bringing with them Spanish culture, language, and Catholicism (Bierhorst, 1984). Davies (1982) explains that in 1598, nine years before Jamestown and 22 years before Pilgrims landed on Plymouth Rock, Duan Juan de Onate began colonizing New Mexico. During the 1600–1800s, Spain extended its dominance to what is known today as Mexico, California, Texas, Florida, New Mexico, and Arizona. In 1821, the United States of Mexico gained independence from Spain. During the 1820s, Mexico agreed to let North Americans settle in what is now Texas, on the condition that those settlers remain loyal to Mexico and adopt Catholicism as their religion of choice (Samora 1961). Between 1836-1948, North American settlers established the Republic of Texas (1836), and then defended it in the "Mexican War" (1846-1848). As a result of the Treaty of Guadalupe Hedalgo, Mexico ceded a huge territory to the United States: what is known today as Arizona, California, Texas, New Mexico, Utah, and parts of Colorado, Nevada, and Wyoming (Moore & Pachon, 1985). Although the treaty provided protection for the new Americans of Mexican descent of their civil, linguistic, religious, and cultural rights, as well as of their land and property, few, if any, of these provisions were honored (Falicov 1982).

The community chosen for the present study began to develop post-World War I as many Mexicans migrated from Mexico and the southwest United States to the midwest. These individuals found employment in Michigan sugar beet fields, with the railroads, and in automobile factories. Valdes (1982) describes how Henry Ford of Detroit, Michigan, recruited Mexican workers to his automobile plants to develop a production staff and an overseas operation. A variety of federal government programs also encouraged importation of Mexican workers to assist industries with continuing a supply of seasoned helpers (Moore & Pachon, 1985). Such employment opportunities were significant in determining where Mexicans settled in this community.

Preparing and Entering the Community

Following the ethnonursing research method, I began the study with what is called a "windshield assessment," an exploratory drive through the community to see the different areas and agencies. On several occasions, I also walked through the Mexican-American community to meet the people I would be studying in person, and I drove and walked through the community to get an appreciation of their worldview. Fluent in Spanish, I was able to conduct the study using both Spanish and English. Although a number of businesses were located in this "Mexican Village," as it was known, other businesses were cut off from the central area of the town by a freeway. This intrusion by freeway into the hegemonic life of the community was a source of concern in maintaining cultural unity. Within the Mexican-American community, there also were industrial sites including printing, chemical, and trucking, a rubber company, as well as maintenance and messenger service enterprises, and taverns. Set directly in the middle of the Mexican-American community were large trucking stations, customs and immigration operations for nearby Canada, duty free shops, a bait shop, and barber and hair salons. Neighborhood homes were built before 1925 and were in fair condition. Two large Gothic-style Roman Catholic churches also were located in the Mexican-American community. Each parish had its own elementary school which many children from the community attended. The community had a block of popular Mexican restaurants which were frequently attended by many Anglo-European area residents. In addition, many grocery stores in the community had various herbs, candles, and materials used for folk practices, as well as foods commonly included in the Mexican-American diet.

Key and General Informants

As this was a mini-ethnonursing study focused on a specific area of inquiry (Leininger, 1985, p. 35), five key and ten general informants were purposefully selected. As researcher, I had done 15 one- to two-hour interviews with key informants and 11 interviews less than one hour with general informants. I met my informants in their homes so as to more fully appreciate and learn from them as well as to participate in their activities as the study progressed. All informants consented to participate and seemed genuinely interested.

The five key informants included three females and two males, with a mean age of 45.4 years, and a mean educational level 13.8 years. The ten general informants included five females and five males, with a mean age of 52.1 years, and a mean educational level of 11.6 years. Fourteen of the 15 informants were second generation Mexican-Americans, with one informant being of the first generation. The marital status of the 15 informants included six single informants, six married informants, and three who had been widowed. All 15 informants were Roman Catholic and of middle and lower economic income.

ANALYSIS OF THE DATA AND FINDINGS

The Leininger Phases of Ethnonursing Analysis for Qualitative Data was used to analyze the data. This guide has been presented earlier and will not be discussed fully here (see Chapter 2). With this data analysis method, the first phase consisted of studying the raw emic data by reading and rereading the descriptive observations and participatory data. In the second phase, I identified descriptors and components, studied data to find similar or dissimilar statements that could be coded or classified to further understand the domain of inquiry. In the third phase, I scrutinized and identified data to discover patterns of behavior while looking for evidence of saturation, consistencies, and credibility of data. The fourth phase required synthesis and abstraction of ideas from the previous phases to formulate themes and major research findings (Leininger, 1990). The analysis began on the first day of data collection and continued to the end of the study. From the analysis, four universal themes identifying commonalities and one diverse theme among informants in the study were discovered. Finally, nursing implications were developed through the use of confirmed themes of fourth phase and grounded in the three other phases (Leininger, 1990, p. 50). It is important to note that Leininger's five qualitative criteria of credibility, confirmability, meanings-in-context, recurrency, and saturation were used to support the findings.

Universal Theme One

Caring was expressed as love of family and neighbor (filial love). Spiritual ties included compadrazgo *(fictive kin) and invocations to the power of God and Blessed Mother to heal by the use of prayer.* This theme was developed from the first phase of analysis from verbatim descriptors. For example, "Usually the mother will care for the ill family member." A key informant said, "Care involves the entire family, including the *padrinos* and *madrinos*. There is always a crowd of people when someone is ill. We use a lot of [family] hugging and kissing. Care is an extended family process." Two general informants stated, "I usually pray to Our Lady of Guadalupe. She is the sign of unity. She will help us." "On the whole, Latino's are not trusting people to strangers. They don't easily trust medical care professionals." Respect was shown with this recurrent statement: "You must speak our language, address us formally, and maintain eye contact while you talk to us."

Table 1 identifies Mexican-American care values that were identified by key and general informants.

In the Mexican-American key and general informants, it was clear that caring involves all family members. Extended family members express care as a close social group, and they especially rely on a caring ethos in times of need. An extended family may include fictive kin (*compadres*) who act like parents or a caring guardian to specific families. God parents or *padrinos* or *compadres* have a special link with the parents which was built on spiritual ties known as *compadrazgo*. God parents not only have an obligation toward their God child, but also show caring expressions of filial love, support, and guidance for the parents. The relationship of filial love is built on and through marriage, religion, extended family friendship, and need. Thus the religious and spiritual systems are closely linked together and are a powerful influence on care and caring modalities. These findings support the other research findings: Clark (1970), Leininger (1978), Panfilli (1983), and Dugan (1988).

All key and general informants considered it was desired and a great value to be with others, particularly those who are lonely or in need. One informant related this commonly held expression, saying "*te acompano en tus sentimientos*" (I am with you as you are feeling now). Sometimes when Mexican-Americans find it is necessary to take care of or help a sick person, this act of care for others and being with

Table 1
Mexican-American Care Values of Key and General Informants

Care Value Meanings	Informants	Percent
Obtaining and giving *respeto* (respect)	14	90
Involvement of the family	13	86
God is omnipotent	13	86
Filial love	12	80
Succorance—attention to direct assistance	12	80

becomes a charitable act and has precedence over participation in, for instance, a Sunday liturgy. *Caring for others* was clearly evident in study findings as being attentive to others, assistive, and supportive. Informants provided only very limited emphasis on self-care.

All informants saw God as omnipotent or *todopoderoso*. This power of God reflected their appreciation and value of the greatness and majesty of a supreme being. Several informants held that God does not maltreat without cause; unfaithfulness to God may lead to illness or other bad circumstances.

The majority of Mexican-American informants had a great love of Mary as mother of Jesus, and as their spiritual mother. She was talked about and referred to with different titles and names, such as Our Lady of Guadalupe, Madonna of the Street, Our Lady of Mount Carmel. Mary was viewed as caring and as an extension of filial love, showing especially maternal care for Mexican-Americans and in their diverse life situations or circumstances. This the first theme of care of filial love was an integral part of kinship and religious or spiritual beliefs, values, and practices.

Universal Theme Two

Care means "everything or almost everything" (*todo o casi todo*) was the second common or universal theme discovered. Here, care also meant being with family, eating certain foods, and well being (*bienestar*). This theme was derived from verbatim descriptors and patterns, and could be found in raw data expressions. For example, several key informants said, "Health is everything or almost everything [*todo o casi todo*]." Another informant said, "Health is having well being [*bienestar*]. You have to have a balance. Health means eating the right foods."

Table 2 presents Mexican-American key and general informant health beliefs and values.

The findings from all informants revealed that being healthy was dependent on care expressions and meanings. Being healthy means support from the entire family and extended family, including fictive kin. Health was usually defined in Spanish as *bienestar*, which was translated by informants as a state of well being. Eating proper foods and maintaining balance in the foods they ate also was identified as

Table 2
Key and General Informants' Health Beliefs and Values

Health beliefs, values and meanings	Respondents	Percent
Being with one's family (as caring)	14	90
Involving one's family to promote health and well being by being caring	14	90
Living a harmonious or balanced life through caring relationships	13	86
God's blessing	13	86
Everything or almost everything (*Todo o casi todo*)	12	80

being healthy. The latter included a proper balance of hot and cold foods and liquids. Thus the second theme showed that health meant well being (*bienestar*) and was influenced by and buttressed within the concept of care.

Universal Theme Three

That *folk practices and rituals were essential to promote caring and healing among Mexican-Americans* was the third common or universal care theme expressed by informants and from the researcher's observations and participant experiences. There were several verbatim statements from key informants to confirm this theme. For example, a typical or recurrent statement from key informants was:

> I watched my aunt do incantations in front of my son when he had evil eye [el ojo]. She rubbed my son down from the top of his head and all around his body with an egg she took out of the refrigerator. She lit candles before a statue of St. Therese. She took a glass of water and broke the egg into the water. The egg became solidified. His fever broke. Amazingly, he fell sound asleep and was normal.

Another key informant stated,

> One [illness I saw] was the evil eye or mal ojo. If a person looked at the baby in a wrong fashion, the baby would get extremely ill and would get a fever. Bad ear aches were also treated by my mother

Table 3
Key and General Informants' Illnesses
and Generic Folk Care Beliefs and Treatments

Illness	Folk Treatment
Ear ache	Cornucopia (*alcatraz*) of newspaper in ear lit on fire producing a suction
Evil eye (*mal ojo*)	Incantations, massage, lit candles, raw egg in water glass
Vomiting	Beaten eggs, nutmeg, canned milk
Colic	Catnip tea (*estafiente*); bay leaf, wintergreen and sugar tea (*yerba bueno*); massage infant with oil and place flannel on abdomen
Hiccups	Red flannel on forehead
Diarrhea	Drink rice water
Indigestion (*empacho*)	Massage to body with oil ("snap noise"); castor oil and orange juice

with a newspaper rolled into a cone or cornucopia. The newspaper would be lit on fire and air would come into the bad ear. You would feel a suction. Then mom would put cotton in your ear. It worked. Also, the cone used for ear aches is called an alcatraz.

A general informant stated, "*susto* [illness] happens if you get frightened. *Brujas* [witches] can cause *sustado* or *susto*. They also cause *mal ojo* [evil eye]."

Table 3 summarizes common folk beliefs and illnesses described by the informants with their generic folk treatments.

Universal Theme Four

Findings from this theme revealed that generic folk care was readily identified by all informants and came from the use of proper rituals and folk treatments. This finding supported Leininger's (1990) theory that folk care expression exists in this culture and reflected a caring ethos. The theme *professional care providers are seen as care providers and as an extension of God* was abstracted from informant statements but also from patterns of observed behaviors among Mexican-Americans. For example, several informants said:

> *I say prayers to the Blessed Mother to be with me during my surgery and to allow me to trust those giving me my care.*
>
> *I believe the nurse taking care of me is truly an extension of God, truly one of his instruments. We are people composed of a physical body, a psychological component, and a spiritual being with a connectedness to the earth, and to other spirits/souls. Power to heal comes from God and the Saints.*

Key and general informants believed that God gives healing power to health care providers. They had experiences with professional care providers. The informants said that during hospitalization or while they were making decisions regarding health outcomes, they prayed to a favorite saint, such as Our Lady of Guadalupe, or to God in his many manifestations. During these health experiences, all informants said they received comfort. In addition, anxiety was decreased by speaking Spanish to family members or to health care providers knowledgeable in the Spanish language. Thus this theme of care confirms from many informants that professional care providers, as informants see them, are extensions of God and that beneficial care comes from petitions or prayers to God.

During data analysis, confirming evidence arose that care was strongly influenced by kinship, religion, cultural values, worldview, and language uses with Mexican-Americans. Informants placed less emphasis on political, legal, or educational variables as influencing care. This was of particular interest theoretically as Leininger speaks to variables of the social structure factors on care. However, the dominant factors of kinship, religion, and cultural values prevailed. It also is important to note that generic folk care beliefs and practices were strong influences on care and influenced the well being (*bienestar*) or health of the people. Finally, the care themes abstracted from the raw data included recurrent patterns that, again, served to substantiate Leininger's theory of care expressions and meanings regarding the social structure of the generic folk care system.

Care Diversity

Leininger (1985) posits that "there are diverse expressions, meanings, and action patterns" of human care. Therefore, in Leininger's theory predictions of diversities within universal themes of a culture in h man care expressions, patterns, and practices exist. In the prese study as well, a diverse theme and diverse patterns were identifie for the role sanctioned for *brujas* (witches) in the community. Foi example, some informants spoke openly about *brujas*, while others demonstrated fear over talking about the actions of brujas. One key informant stated, "Don't underestimate the power of a *bruja.*" While some *brujas* were described to have magical powers by using certain prayer rituals, altars, and incantations, some *brujas* were described as using a variety of folk methods, including massage, folk herbs, liniments, rituals, and incantations.

TRANSCULTURAL CARE AND THE MODES OF ACTION AND DECISION

Leininger (1978, 1985) predicted caring—via cultural care preservation or maintenance, cultural care accommodation or negotiation, and cultural care repatterning or restructuring—would guide or enable professional nurses to promote culturally congruent nursing care. In Table 4, the researcher identifies care modes with Leininger's predictions based on care findings generated from the social structure, cultural values, language, and worldview. Leininger predicted that the use of care expressions and practices of a culture could lead to provision of culturally congruent care through consideration of the three modes of action and decision. They are presented in Table 4 with thought to appropriate actions for each mode of care which can be studied further to provide cultural care practices that are satisfying and beneficial for transcultural nursing work with Mexican-Americans.

In order to provide culturally congruent care as the goal of Leininger's Culture Care theory, a brief discussion of culture-specific care is offered.

Table 4
Summary of Transcultural Nursing Implications
for Mexican-American Cultural Congruent Care

Care Preservation or Maintenance
  Preserve generic folk practices to provide effective care
  Maintain kinship involvement and relationships as caring modes
  Maintain use of religious signs, symbols, and rituals
  Support religious beliefs in God as extension to help care providers
  Preserve folk beliefs and practices as caring ways
  Use Spanish language to provide comfort care
  Maintain filial love practices and expressions to promote care

Care Accommodation or Negotiation
  Support confidence (*confianza*) and respect (*respecto*) in providing care
  Accommodate involvement of family to give succorance or direct care
  Negotiate community values or protective care with professional staff who
    have different values
  Accommodate and use generic folk rituals with indigenous spiritual healers
  Accommodate and facilitate the use of prayer with professional nursing care
    practices for healing

Care Restructuring or Repatterning
  Restructure areas where professional nurse and generic folk practices are not
    in harmony or incongruent
  Establish new patterns unknown to professional nurses about Mexican-
    American health care needs and context

Care Preservation or Maintenance

A variety of generic folk practices including the use of herbs, teas, liniments, and oils are often used by the Mexican-American client, their family members, or generic folk healers. They need to be preserved by nurses to facilitate healing through caring modalities with folk practices. The nurse should be careful not to demean or criticize the Mexican-American client or family for the use of folk practices—they are generally beneficial. If curtailed, this could lead to the use of folk practices in a more covert manner. The nurse should be aware that folk treatments in the form of herbal teas and roots have proven pharmacologic and psychocultural benefits. The professional nurse also should be aware that there may be some generic or indigenous folk medicines that may be in conflict with professional medicines and treatments, and so the nurse must be attentive to these differences and protect the client. The nurse protects the client by informing him or her of the potential or actual danger of taking medications that work against each other and cause harm. Or the nurse may protect the client by changing a professional treatment or medicine of limited help to the client after discussing the matter with the physician and client.

Cultural care preservation or maintenance can be provided by nurses preserving generic folk practices by maintaining the use of religious signs, symbols, and various religious rituals and practices, including the uses of religious statues, saying the rosary, using prayer cards, and holy medals.

Eighty-six percent of the informants studied emphasized that nurses must use the Spanish language in order to understand the Mexican-American and the meanings behind foreign terms. All informants were pleased that the researcher could speak Spanish and understood the meanings shared with him. If the individual cannot understand or speak English, then an interpreter should be sought to facilitate communication. Routine written educational materials also should be printed in English and Spanish. With Mexican-Americans becoming a major cultural group in North America in the next century, nurses need to prepare themselves in Spanish.

Care Accommodation or Negotiation

Cultural care accommodation or negotiation would be promoted by nurses developing confidence (*confianza*) with and respect (*respecto*) for Mexican-Americans. That *confianza* develops over time is a particular challenge for nurses today because of mandated shortened hospital experiences by third-party payers and other health insurance program mandates. *Respecto* may be obtained by talking directly to the Mexican-American client, maintaining casual but not intense direct eye contact with him or her and family while talking to them or giving care. Mexican-Americans prefer to be addressed in a formal fashion, including the use of Mr., Mrs., or Miss, or *Señor, Señora,* or *Señorita.* It could be considered disrespectful to address a client by his or her first name without obtaining permission to do so. Accommodating family members and involving them with care of the Mexican-American client is an absolute essential. During periods of critical illness, a nurse should be prepared to accommodate immediate family, relatives, fictive kin, neighbors, and generic folk healers in the health care setting, including flexibility in visiting hours. The nurse should be prepared to accommodate the overt community expression of emotions. Most important, the nurse will need to accommodate the use of spiritual healers by calling a religious priest or making an attempt to provide time and necessary items used by indigenous spiritual or folk healers. The nurse also needs to be alert to possible harmful effects from folk practices. Should the nurse identify possible harmful effects, then he or she would attempt to negotiate with the individuals involved to promote a practice that is not harmful from the vantage of our present professional knowledge. Finally, the use of morning and evening prayer, and prayer before meals, should be accommodated from individual clients and families.

Care Restructuring and Repatterning

According to Leininger (1988), cultural care repatterning or restructuring "refers to those assistive, supportive, or enabling professional actions or decisions that help clients change their lifeways for new or different patterns that are culturally meaningful and satisfying or that support beneficial and healthy life patterns" (p. 156). From my perspective and in light of above findings, there would seem to be less need to restructure or repattern care. Most care and health beliefs seem to be beneficial for Mexican-American's culturally congruent care. Minimal cultural care repatterning or restructuring was viewed as necessary when the other two action modes were followed.

CONCLUSION

This study focused on the domain of meanings and practices of folk (generic) care and professional health care as viewed by Mexican-Americans. Leininger's (1990) theory of Culture Care was used to guide the investigation and, finally, nursing practices for culturally congruent care. Four major universal themes were confirmed from the data of this ethnonursing research: (1) caring is expressed through love of family and neighbor (filial love) and spiritual ties including *compadrazgo* (fictive kin), and through invoking the power of God to heal by the use of prayer; (2) care means *todo o casi todo* or everything or almost everything, being with family, eating certain foods, and *bienestar* or well being; (3) folk practices and rituals promote caring and healing among Mexican-Americans; and (4) professional health care providers are seen as an extension of God.

The culture-specific and dominant care constructs were *filial love, well being, respect, confidence,* and *succorance.* These care constructs with cultural themes were held to be essential to provide culturally congruent nursing care using the three action modes identified in Leininger's theory. Transcultural nursing implications include preservation of folk practices, use of Spanish, and use of religious signs, symbols, and material cultural goods with nursing care. Accommodation techniques include earning *confianza* (confidence) and *respecto* (respect), which require deference to family and community values, and accommodating caring actions of folk and spiritual healers. Minimal restructuring of care practices was found to be necessary if the first two modes of action were used. Use of these modalities by nurses will facilitate the administration of culturally congruent care to Mexican-Americans, and could lead to client care satisfaction and beneficial health care, which is the goal of Culture Care theory and that of transcultural nursing. Illnesses occur when care is not practiced.

In general, Leininger's theory of Culture Care and the ethnonursing qualitative research method were essential in explicating the covert and subtle aspects of cultural care of Mexican-Americans. The theory with the premises and Sunrise Model guided the researcher in discovering generic care phenomena, in developing and guiding the discovery of knowledge, and in creative thinking within the three modes of providing culturally congruent care. Culture care universalities (or commonalities) and diversities among informants were discovered with the use of the theory and confirmed the theoretical premises with the use of qualitative criteria to analyze the data.

REFERENCES

Bierhorst, J. (Ed. and Trans.) (1984). *The hungry woman.* New York: William Morrow.

Clark, M. (1970). *Health in the Mexican-American culture: A community study.* 2nd ed. Berkeley: University of California Press.

COSSMHO (The National Coalition of Hispanic Health and Human Services Organization). (1988). *Delivering preventive health care to Hispanics: a manual for providers.* Washington, DC: COSSMHO.

Davies, N. (1982). *The ancient kingdoms of Mexico: A magnificent re-creation of their art and life.* New York: Viking Penguin, Inc.

Devine, M. V. (1982). *Brujeria: A study of Mexican-American folk magic.* St. Paul, MN: Llewellyn Publications.

Dugan, A. B. (1988). Compadrazgo: A caring phenomenon among urban latinos and its relationship to health. In M. M. Leininger, (Ed.), *Care: The essence of nursing and health,* Detroit: Wayne State University Press.

Falicov, C. J. (1982). Mexican families. In M. McGoldrick, J. K. Pearce, & J. Giordano (Eds.), *Ethnicity and family therapy.* New York: Guilford Press, 134–163.

Gomez, G. E. and Gomez, E. A. (1985). Folk hearing among Hispanic Americans. *Public Health Nursing, 2*(4), 245–249.

Kleinman, A. (1980). *Patients and healers in the context of culture: An exploration of the borderland between anthropology, medicine and psychiatry.* Berkeley: The University of California Press.

Leininger, M. M. (1970). *Nursing and anthropology: Two worlds to blend.* New York: John Wiley & Sons.

Leininger, M. M. (1978). *Transcultural nursing concepts, theories, and practices.* New York: John Wiley & Sons.

Leininger, M. M. (1981, September). Transcultural nursing: Its progress and its future. *Nursing and Health Care,* 365–366.

Leininger, M. M. (1985). *Qualitative nursing: methods in nursing.* Orlando, FL: Grune & Stratton.

Leininger, M. M. (1983). Unpublished field study.

Leininger, M. M. (1988, November). Leininger's theory of nursing: Cultural care diversity and universality. *Nursing Science Quarterly, 1*(4), 152–160.

Leininger, M. M. (1990, Winter). Ethnomethods: the philosophic and epistemic bases to explicate transcultural nursing knowledge. *Journal of Transcultural Nursing, 1*(2), 40–51.

Leininger, M. M. (1990, April). *Proceedings of the Third Annual South Florida Nursing Conference,* Miami, Florida.

Leininger, M. M., Templin, T., & Thompson, T. (1988). *TLT. Software and coding data system for the Leininger, Templin, and Thompson field research ethnoscript.* Detroit: Wayne State University.

Leininger, M. M., Templin, M. T., & Thompson, T. (1990). *Leininger-Templin, Thompson ethnoscript qualitative software program user's handbook:* Detroit: Wayne State University.

Maduro, R. (1983, December). Curanderismo and Latino views of disease and curing. *The Western Journal of Medicine, 139*(6), 868–874.

Martinez, C. & Martin, H. W. (1966). Folk disease among urban Mexican-Americans: Etiology, symptoms, and treatment. *Journal of the American Medical Association, 196*(2), 147–164.

Moore, J., & Pachon, H. (1985). *Hispanics in the United States.* Englewood Cliffs, NJ: Prentice-Hall.

Murillo-Rohde, I. (1979). Cultural sensitivity in the care of the Hispanic patient. *Washington State Journal of Nursing — Special Supplement, 25*–32.

Octavio, I. R. V. (1965). Charismatic medicine, folk-healing and folk-sainthood. *American Anthropologist, 67*, 1151–1173.

Ortiz de Montellano, B. R. (1975). Empirical aztec medicine. *Science, 188*, 215–220.

Panfilli, R. R. (1983). *An ethnocaring and transcultural nursing study of urban Mexican-American families.* Unpublished master's thesis. Detroit: Wayne State University.

Perrone, B., Stockel, H. H., & Krueger, V. (1989). *Medicine women, curanderas, and women doctors.* Norman, OK: University of Oklahoma Press.

Samora, J. (1961). Conceptions of health and disease among Spanish-Americans. *The American Catholic Sociological Review, 22*(1), 314–323.

Valdes, D. N. (1982). *El pueblo Mexicano en Detroit y Michigan: A social history.* Detroit: Wayne State University.

6

Culture Care Meanings and Experiences of Pregnancy and Childbirth of Ukrainians

Irene Zwarycz Bohay

Although pregnancy and childbirth research on several United States' minority cultures appears in the literature, information on pregnancy and childbirth phenomena of the Ukrainian culture is scarce. Therefore, this research study focused on discovering pregnancy and childbirth care of Ukrainians in the metropolitan Detroit area with respect to intergenerational care values, beliefs, and practices within Leininger's (1988) theory of Culture Care Diversity and Universality. Discussed as well are ways that culture-specific care practices could be used by nurses to maintain health with Ukrainian individuals and family members and to improve nursing care.

The domain of inquiry was the cultural care meanings and experiences of Ukrainian mothers in pregnancy and childbirth. The following questions guided this domain of inquiry: What are the meanings and experiences of care of Ukrainian mothers in pregnancy and childbirth? What are some of the Ukrainians' intergenerational ethnocare differences or similarities in pregnancy and childbirth care? What gender differences or similarities prevail in cultural care values and practices of Ukrainian women and men related to pregnancy and childbirth? Using Leininger's three modes of culture care action and decisions, what are the ethnonursing implications to guide nurses to provide congruent care of Ukrainian parents during pregnancy and childbirth?

The rationale and significance of this study was to identify recurrent and patterned care lifeways of the Ukrainian people in order to guide nurses in providing culturally congruent nursing care. Knowledge from this study could provide a way of predicting and guiding ethnonursing care for Ukrainian people. As Leininger (1985a) has stated, "patterns of care are generally more satisfying to clients when they are expected and predicted to fit their lifeways" (p. 40).

In this chapter, then, I will present some major intergenerational pregnancy and childbirth care findings within Ukrainian culture. In addition, I will identify ways that culture care can be used to maintain culturally congruent care within the tenets of Leininger's theory of Culture Care. Use of the theory and nursing care implications of Ukrainian couples during pregnancy and childbirth also will be presented.

LEININGER'S THEORY OF CULTURE CARE

Leininger's (1988) theory of Culture Care explains and predicts human care patterns of cultures and nursing care practices. The purpose of the theory is "to describe, account for, interpret, and predict cultural congruent care" (p. 155). The goal of this theory is to provide culturally congruent care. Through the use of Leininger's theory and the Sunrise conceptual model, then, nurses can discover (1) meanings of care specific to a single culture and (2) specific care meanings of a culture so as to provide meaningful care that fits the client's cultural needs. As Leininger (1988) has stated, if you study the meanings, forms, and expressions of cultural care you can better understand care and predict the health or well being of individuals, families, and cultures. Leininger further contends that from the worldview, social structure components, and environmental factors, three modes of culture care decisions and actions can be predicted to guide nursing care: (1) cultural care preservation or maintenance, (2) cultural care accommodation or negotiation, and (3) cultural care repatterning or restructuring.

With the use of Leininger's Sunrise Model (see Chapter 1), the top part of the model focuses on the worldview, social structure, and cultural factors with attention to the language expressions and environmental context. These dimensions are held to be powerful and important influencers on care and health. With the Sunrise Model, the theory also focuses on discovering the influences of folk and professional health and nursing systems on human care and health. Through an inductive study of all these factors, the theorist predicts that as human care patterns become evident they will serve to guide nurses in providing culturally congruent nursing care practices.

Assumptions

The theory of Culture Care Diversity and Universality (Leininger, 1984, 1985b, 1988) rests on several assumptions which guided the present study within the qualitative paradigm:

1. Human care is universal; yet there are diverse expressions, meanings, patterns (or lifestyles), and action modalities.

2. Human care patterns, conditions, and actions are based largely on cultural care values, beliefs, and practices of particular cultures, and on the universal nature of humans as caring beings.

3. Care expressions, patterns, and lifestyles are influenced by different cultural contexts.

4. Care phenomenon can be discovered by examining social structure, language, environmental context, and the worldview of cultural groups.

5. Care behaviors, goals, and functions vary with social structure and specific values of people from different cultures.

6. Care is largely culturally derived and requires culturally-based knowledge and skills for beneficial, meaningful, and efficacious nursing care.

Orientational Definitions

Orientational rather than operational definitions were used in this qualitative ethnonursing research study (Leininger, 1985a; Lincoln & Guba, 1985). These major definitions and the above theoretical assumptions guided research in the specific domain of this study as well as in any new or unknown phenomena discovered during the research process. The following terms as defined by Leininger (1988) and myself provided a general orientation to study the theory within the Ukrainian culture and regarding pregnancy and childbearing care experiences:

1. *Culture* refers to the learned, shared, and transmitted values, beliefs, norms, and life practices of a particular group that guides thinking, decisions, and actions in patterned ways (p. 156).

2. *Ukrainian culture* refers to those people who value and trace their origin to the homeland of Ukraine.

3. *Care* (noun) refers to phenomena related to assisting, supportive, or enabling behavior toward or for another individual (or group) with evident or anticipated needs to ameliorate or improve a human condition or lifeway (p. 156).

4. *Cultural care* refers to the cognitively known values, beliefs, and patterned expressions that assist, support, or enable another individual or group to maintain well being, improve a human condition or lifeway, or face death and disabilities (p. 156).

5. *Worldview* refers to the way people tend to look at the world or universe when forming a picture or value stance about their life and the surrounding world (p. 156).

6. *Social structure* refers to the dynamic nature of interrelated structural or organizational factors of a particular culture (or society) and how these factors function to give meaning and structural order, including religious, kinship, political, economic, educational, technological, and cultural factors (p. 156).

7. *Health* refers to a state of well being that is culturally defined, valued, and practiced and which reflects the ability of individuals (or groups) to perform their daily role activities in a culturally satisfactory way (p. 156).

8. *Pregnancy (antepartum)* refers to a female condition or state of being with child (having a developing human embryo or fetus in the body) and the time period preceding childbirth.

9. *Childbirth (parturition)* refers to the experiences involved with the phenomenon of giving birth to a neonate.

10. *Professional health system* refers to professional care or cure services offered by diverse health personnel who have been prepared through formal professional programs of study in special educational institutions (p. 156).

11. *Cultural care preservation or maintenance* refers to those assistive, supportive, or enabling professional actions and decisions that help clients of a particular culture to preserve or maintain a state of health or to recover from illness and to face death (p. 156).

12. *Cultural care accommodation or negotiation* refers to those assistive, supportive, or enabling professional actions and decisions that help clients of a particular culture to adapt to or negotiate for a beneficial or satisfying health status or to face death (p. 156).

13. *Cultural care repatterning or restructuring* refers to those assistive, supportive, or enabling professional actions or decisions that help clients change their lifeways for new or different patterns that are culturally meaningful and satisfying or that support beneficial and health life patterns (p. 156).

14. *Culturally congruent care* refers to the creatively designed nursing decisions and actions that fit the lifeways of individuals, families, or groups so as to provide meaningful, satisfying, and beneficial care to clients (p. 156).

LITERATURE REVIEW

In a review of the literature regarding Ukrainian pregnancy and childbirth phenomena, only limited information was found. Until the late 1970s, much of the literature focused on early child care behaviors, feeding, early infant and child-rearing practices, and mother and infant interactions. For example, Klaus and Kennell's (1976) well-known research on maternal-infant bonding had a noticeable influence on many professional nurses in the nursing care of mothers and infants during the immediate postpartum period. There also were several articles on transcultural infant and child rearing practices (Leininger, 1970, 1978a, 1979; Horn, 1979; Kendall, 1979) as discussed in the next section. In the 1980s, social support systems, cultural factors, and psychological influences on pregnancy were areas of focus or problematic concerns for health professionals in infant and early child care. In the early 1980s, however, research on parenting began to increase (McBride, 1983, p. 65), and transcultural nursing courses on the lifecycle (birth to old age, including parenting roles) launched in the mid-1960s by Leininger grew in interest. As a result, nursing schools began to focus on family-centered nursing and parenting.

Interestingly, the father's participation in pregnancy, childbirth, or parenting in the United States did not become prominent in the literature until the latter part of the 1970s. In America and Canada, fathers have been traditionally viewed as biological contributors to the creation of a human being (Hamner & Turner, 1985, p. 8), but since the late 1970s fathers are playing a more active role in pregnancy and childrearing. Currently, fathers and their role in pregnancy, childbirth, postpartum, bonding, and parenting issues are being studied, but mainly in the United States and Canada. The comparative role of fathers and mothers in Western and non-Western cultures in nursing was limited except for the work of transcultural nurse researchers. The Ukrainian role of parents in pregnancy and childbirth with a focus on care was not found in the research literature.

TRANSCULTURAL NURSING

During the 1960s, Leininger initiated transcultural nursing studies with her research on the cultural patterns and values of the Gadsup people of the Eastern Highlands of New Guinea as well as on early-infant and later-child care phenomena. Thus began the transcultural nursing contribution to the literature on pregnancy and childbirth. This was followed by Kendall's (1968) exploratory and ethnographic study on infancy, early childhood, and school-age childrearing practices in an Iranian village. Several years later, Horn (1975) studied the transcultural phenomenon of childrearing practices of the Muckleshoot people, Northwest American Indians living in the Seattle area. In 1976, Leininger edited the first transcultural nursing publication on maternal-child nursing, *Proceedings from the First National Conference on Transcultural Care of Infants and Children*. In 1979, in a later edition of those proceedings, Sevcovic presented a study of the traditions of pregnancy that influence maternity care of the Navajo in relation to the antepartum, the parturition, and the postpartum. Thus transcultural nurse researchers were the first to study cultural differences among divergent groups with regard to pregnancy and childbirth with the goal of increasing cultural awareness of health professionals and understanding of cultures and the phenomenon of care. This transcultural research was ultimately directed to establish a body of knowledge to help nurses provide culturally meaningful and congruent care to clients who enter the health care system or receive home care. The present study is another means to add to the body of transcultural nursing knowledge that uses Leininger's theory to study culture care.

RESEARCH METHODS

Ethnonursing and life history comprise the research methods used to discover the care meanings and experiences related to pregnancy and childbirth of Ukrainian parents . Such qualitative paradigm methods were chosen to assist in explicating meanings and expressions of naturalistic and *emic* data unobtainable by quantitative methods (Leininger, 1985a).

As Leininger (1985a) has stated, the goal of the ethnonursing method, which she developed initially to study her Culture Care theory, is to discover largely unknown phenomena and knowledge about a particular domain of study. Ethnonursing focuses on documenting, describing, and explaining nursing phenomena related to care, health, prevention, and recovery from illness, as well as other unknown nursing phenomena derived from the data. Since the present researcher sought data primarily from informants' viewpoints, this method was ideal and appropriate to explicate emic care data.

As part of the ethnonursing method, Leininger (1985a, p. 52) developed sequenced phases of observation-participation-reflection in order to provide the researcher with an accurate means and a realistic way to get culture care data. The observation-participation experience involved the description, explanation, and accurate documentation of what transpired. The sequenced phases of this enabling tool were important guides in researching parental care in a systematic and careful way.

In the course of the ethnonursing method, two major types of interviews were used: open-ended and semistructured. The open-ended interview encouraged the informant to share ideas, worldviews, and information about the domain or questions under study. The semistructured interview, actually a combination of open and closed interviews, were instrumental in obtaining both definitive and unexpected kinds of information from informants (Leininger 1985a, p. 55).

Leininger's Life Health History enabler was another qualitative research means chosen to study the stated domain. This enabler was used to assess the lifestyle, health, and care patterns of selected informants and their relationship to health and care practices and health maintenance within the culture being studied from a lifespan viewpoint. The life history was an important means to obtain qualitative data related to pregnancy and childrearing and to identify and document health and lifecycle care patterns of people who used professional health care systems (Leininger, 1985a, p. 120). A life health history, biographical in nature, was obtained during the data collection process. Two interviews of two-and-one-half hours each were held with the life health history informant, for a total of five hours. The researcher used an open-ended interview focused on the developmental periods of childhood, adolescence, and middlescence to discover culture care with intergenerational aspects.

INFORMANTS

In keeping with qualitative ethnonursing method, informants were purposefully selected from the metropolitan Detroit community based on specific criteria. Key informants were selected both for their first-hand knowledge of Ukrainian culture and their experience related to pregnancy and childbirth care. General informants were selected for their general reflective knowledge or experiences related to pregnancy and childbirth care, with recognition, however, that they could not provide as in-depth knowledge as expected of key informants.

Seven *key* informants (including one life health history informant) and six *general* informants were selected for study in their daily life environmental contexts. Ukrainian women were selected as key informants, because of their role as biological childbearers, and Ukrainian men were selected as general informants. Key informants ranged in years from 34 to 68; general informants ranged in years from 34 to 66. Six of the seven key informants had lived in the United States from 27 to 41 years with a mean number of 36.4 years. Only one of the seven key informants was born in the United States. General informants had lived in the United States from 34 to 41 years with a mean number of 38.4 years. Two of the six general informants were born in the United States. The arrival time for the informants to the United States coincided with the immigration of Ukrainians to the United States after World War II.

Table 1 depicts the age at which key informants gave birth to their first child, with an average age of 26 years.

The number of children delivered by all Ukrainian mothers in the study is shown in Table 2. The average number of children born to these mothers was three.

The number of children for Ukrainian male general informants was three and identified in Table 3.

All key and general informants had completed their high school education, several had pursued college courses, and one had completed a doctoral degree.

Table 1
Age at Which Key Informants Had First Child

Key Informants	Age of Having First Child
1	27
2	28
4	18
5	28
6	21
7	29
10	29

Table 2
Number of Children
Born to Female Key Informants

Key Informants	Number of Children
1	2
2	3
4	3
5	3
6	5
7	2
10	1

All interviews were conducted by the researcher who had been prepared in use of the theory and research methods under Leininger. The majority of interviews were conducted primarily in English. However, since the researcher could speak and read Ukrainian, some Ukrainian words were used during interviews by both researcher and informants for clarification. Two of the six key informants spoke Ukrainian throughout the interview, and one general informant spoke mainly Ukrainian with English to clarify responses.

Interviews took place in the informants' home setting or in a community environmental context that was familiar and naturalistic to them, and supportive of the ethnonursing research method. Five of the seven key informants were interviewed in their homes; the remaining two key

Table 3
Number of Children
for Male General Informants

General Informants	Number of Children
3	2
8	6
9	3
11	0
12	2
13	2

informants were interviewed in a local community service setting. Four of the six general informants were interviewed in their homes; the remaining two general informants were interviewed in a local community service environment. In-depth interviews and participant-observation with key informants averaged one hour and a half and two interviews. Interviews with general informants averaged one hour and a half and one interview.

Lincoln and Guba (1985) and Leininger (1985a) contend that the key to access of a culture is almost always in the hands of gatekeepers. It was a local Ukrainian gatekeeper who initially suggested three potential informants for the study, and two of the three informants met the criteria and were selected as key informants. This opened the door to select other key and general informants through spouse contact, key informant suggestions, volunteers who agreed to be interviewed when the study was mentioned by a key informant, and through direct approach of informants who met the criteria and volunteered to participate in the study. The researcher purposefully chose the key and general informants with thought to selection criteria.

DATA COLLECTION

Data collection followed the ethnonursing research method. Leininger's Observation-Participation-Reflection (O-P-R) enabler (see Chapter 2 for this enabler) was used prior to initiating interviews. The researcher followed the specified manner of using the enabler as described in this book. Leininger's O-P-R enabler was used to: (1) study people and their natural environments so as to discover and confirm beliefs and values with actions; and (2) assist the researcher in following a systematic, practical, realistic, and accurate way to make observations and participate with informants as part of the ethnographic research method (Leininger, 1985, p. 52). In general, with Phase I the researcher primarily focused on direct observation of the Ukrainian community environment. In Phase II, while the focus was still primarily observation of responses of those with whom the researcher had contact, it also included some participation by the researcher. In Phase III, mainly researcher participation with some observations took place. During Phase III, interview data were collected primarily in the informants' home environment, with the remainder taking place in the informants' community work setting.

In Phase IV, the researcher focused on reflection and confirmation of findings with key informants to establish credibility and recurrency of data. Informants helped to confirm the data meanings, patterns, and themes. From Phase I through Phase IV, the study took approximately six to eight months of intensive ethnonursing field research and data analysis with full documentation of data.

Informants were given copies (which included researcher's telephone number) of the verbal explanation and consent form for the study and time for clarification of any questions before signing the consent form. All informants agreed to participate. Informants were free to withdraw from the study at any time.

Two types of field notes were kept by the researcher. A *condensed* brief account was kept of all field notes that were taken in the field and during the actual interview or observations (Spradley, 1979, p. 75; Leininger, 1985a). An *expanded* field record, the full account of observations, participant experiences, and interviews, also was kept. The expanded field record included other primary source data on the domains of inquiry. Interview data were always recorded within 24–48 hours of the interview to assure accuracy of recall of the informant's viewpoint, beliefs, and practices as well as observations, questions, and reflections of the researcher. As an ongoing project, a fieldwork journal was kept by the researcher during all phases of the O-P-R process. It contained data such as nonverbal gestures and facial expressions, actions, symbols, rituals, descriptions of material cultural items, and the verbal interview data. The contextual data and the verbal interview data were kept separate in two columns to identify any patterns that emerged and to understand and distinguish more fully the people's emic lifeways from the researcher's *etic* views. The researcher's thoughts, biases, ideas, and reflections about the contextual and interview data were noted throughout the field experience. Field data were processed using the Leininger-Templin-Thompson Ethnoscript Software (see Chapter 2). This software enabled the researcher to process, code, and sort large amounts of qualitative data throughout the study by computer, whereas previously this systematic method was all done by hand.

DATA ANALYSIS AND FINDINGS

Findings from the data analysis with focus on the domains of inquiry in relation to the theory used are presented in this section. Leininger's Phases of Analysis for Ethnonursing for Qualitative Data was used because it helped to explicate theory dimensions and provided a rigorous and systemized method for data analysis. The method required a full analysis of the raw data moving to analysis of descriptors, patterns, and formulation of themes in the last part of the analysis. In conjunction with Leininger's method, a life history analysis, focused specifically on intergenerational emic patterns of living related to wellness, care, health maintenance, and critical life cycle events of the informant, was done. Upon completion of the study, a copy of the life history was given to the informant as well as a summary of the findings from the life history analysis.

ETHNOHISTORY OVERVIEW OF
THE UKRAINIAN CULTURE

In ethnonursing studies and the use of Leininger's theory, it is important to understand the historical factors at work in the cultures of concern. Thus, a brief ethnohistory of the Ukrainian culture follows. The term *Ukraine* is of Slavic origin and is connected with the word *Ukraina*, which literally means country. Until recently, Ukraine was a part of the Union of Soviet Socialist Republics (USSR). Currently, it is seeking to reorient its relationship as an independent entity in the new Union of Sovereign Soviet Republics. It remains the second largest republic in the new USSR with a population of 50 million people. Although Ukraine's territory accounts for a small percentage of the new USSR and its inhabitants for under one-fifth of the population, its soil yields approximately one-third of all Soviet agricultural production while its soil yields approximately one-fifth of the country's gross domestic product (Sikorski, 1990, p. 75). To the north and east are the Byelorussian and Russian Republics; to the west are Poland, Czechoslovakia, Hungary, Rumania, and the Moldavian Republic. The Black and Azov Seas are to the south of Ukraine.

The history of Ukraine began thousands of years ago, and for much of Ukraine's history, the countries of Russia, Poland, Lithuania, Turkey, Austria-Hungary, and Germany have tried to acquire Ukraine's territory with its human and unique physical resources. The emergence and continuity of an independent Ukrainian state for any great period of time has been hindered by centuries of wars, conquests, and colonization by successive invaders and oppressors (Stefaniuk & Dohrs, 1979, p. 3). With the advent of *perestroika* (restructuring) and *glasnost* (openness) in the latter part of the 1980s, dramatic changes regarding Ukraine's political status and religion have occurred at an accelerated pace. On July 19, 1990, the Government of Ukraine issued its Declaration of Sovereignty and *Rukh*, the democratic movement in Ukraine, has called for the complete independence of Ukraine. The recent demise of the rulership of the communist party has furthered this drive toward independence in a restructured Soviet Union. The legalization of the Catholic church in Ukraine is discussed in the next section.

Ukrainian mass immigration to the United States, mostly for political and economic reasons, came in several waves. The first occurred during Austro-Hungarian rule in the late nineteenth century. The majority of informants and all parents (except one) of junior informants (50 years old and younger) belonged to the final wave of mass Ukrainian immigration to the United States. Reasons for immigration included avoidance of religious, political, and economic oppression. This final wave of mass immigration occurred at the end of World War II when Ukraine fell into the hands of Soviet Russia. Specific social structure dimensions are highlighted next as part of Leininger's theory expectations to understand the people.

SOCIAL STRUCTURE INFLUENCERS AND FINDINGS

Worldview and Religion

Worldview and religion have long been closely linked together in the Ukrainian culture. Religion serves as a guide to daily living, interactions with people, and the center of social activities within the community. During the course of any year, the life of the Ukrainian people is in strict conformity to the holy seasons of the Catholic or Orthodox religion (Nahajewsky, 1975, p. 29).

In the Ukraine, religion, which reached its millennium in 1988, came from and was profoundly influenced by Byzantine or Greek Christianity (Orthodox). However, for long periods of time, it also received exposure from Catholic influences. As a result, when Ukraine entered the nineteenth and twentieth centuries, it was basically Orthodox in religion, but with a substantial number of Ukrainian Catholics in western Ukraine (Szporluk, 1979). In December 1989, Ukrainians throughout the world witnessed the revival of the Ukrainian Catholic church in Ukraine. Although this event has received much lip service throughout the media and the USSR, very little has actually occurred to normalize the status of the Catholic church in the Soviet Union (Gudziak, 1990, p. 417). Petitions to register Ukrainian Catholic churches have been ignored. Brutal religious repression continues by way of violence against and harassment of clergy and lay people.

In the United States, specifically in metropolitan Detroit, Ukrainians follow two types of religious orientations: Ukrainian Catholic and Ukrainian Orthodox beliefs and practices. Essential differences between the two orientations lie in dogma and canon law (Shevchenko Scientific Society, 1971, p. 214). The Ukrainian Catholic church has dogmas with papal authority and a single administrative center. The Ukrainian Orthodox church does not recognize the pope as its head, although many of its dogmas and practices are the same as the Catholic church. Another distinction of the Orthodox church is that its religious year follows the Julian calendar; the Catholic church follows the Gregorian calendar.

In metropolitan Detroit, there are three Ukrainian Catholic and two Ukrainian Orthodox churches. In this study, all informants were Ukrainian Catholic and attend Ukrainian Catholic church services. Essentially, religion still exerts tremendous influence on Ukrainian lives.

Family and Kinship

The family is highly valued in Ukrainian culture. Within the family context religion, lifeways, goodness, and respect for self and others are learned. In addition, the Ukrainian family is a significant contributor to emotional, sociocultural, and general holistic health.

It is the Ukrainian mother who maintains the organization of the household and is the axis around which members of the family revolve. Ukrainian mothers have traditionally remained at home during the childrearing years. From the key and general informant descriptors, two care patterns were identified in relation to the mother: (1) care is reflected in an all-encompassing *maternal obligation* toward family members, especially children; and (2) care is reflected in *maternal presence* during childrearing.

Informant descriptor data of the father's role in Ukrainian culture revealed interesting intergenerational differences in patterns of care meanings and expressions of the father over time. Traditionally, the Ukrainian father has been viewed as strict and as the disciplinarian in the family. Data from three senior female key informants and one young male general informant regarding care meanings and expressions showed "Care as a senior male role expectation of *strength, respect,* and *strictness* in childrearing"; and "Care as a male role expectation of *obligation for the provision of the necessities of life.*" On the other hand, all male general informants expressed "Care as reflected in male role expectation of *obligation for social, cultural, and religious consciousness in childrearing.*" These differences in gender and sex were clearly documented in observations and in verbal communication with key and general informants. Such diversities prevailed within the culture regarding care meanings and expressions.

The care pattern identified through informant descriptors of the children's role was "Care as reflected in children's role expectation of *obligation to ethnicity and nationality.*" Within the family structure, the children's role was observed to be this: to continue or prolong and conform to the cultural heritage and national life of Ukrainians. Children learn their cultural traditions, perpetuate them, and practice national lifeways over time.

Pregnancy Influenced by Education, Technology, Religion, and Kinship with Findings

The researcher observed and documented social structure factors that influenced care and health in daily life. Pregnancy and childbirth were an important part of the Ukrainian lifestyle, and particularly for fulfilling parental roles in having children. One senior female key informant stated: "Because we do value family life very much, there is a great deal of respect for the pregnant woman. There is family and community support."

During their pregnancies, all female informants sought professional prenatal care of physicians. It was interesting that the female key informants (age 50 years and older) had no preparation for pregnancy and childbirth; whereas the younger female key informants (under 50 years) had read about the Lamaze method, pregnancy, childbirth, and Cesarean section birth from professional and lay literature as well as talking to professional personnel—all in preparation for their pregnancy and childbirth experiences. All young pregnant female key informants had been through Lamaze classes. The researcher observed that the young female key informants were more aware of the physiology of their bodies, and they chose ways that they felt would give them a more positive outcome to the pregnancy. All three of the older female key informants spoke about the lack of information given to them by their physicians. One of the latter three key informants spoke about receiving a diuretic and a diet pill during a pregnancy. Another older key informant stated that she obtained a book on pregnancy and learned about this subject on her own.

Young female key informants discussed the prenatal tests they received during one or all of their pregnancies. The influence of technology with pregnancy was clearly stronger with younger female informants than the older female informants. The alpha-fetoprotein (AFP) test and ultrasound were commonly used and accepted tests by young informants. One young female informant had an amniocentesis following an abnormal AFP test.

Two of the three young key informants cited prayer as part of their pregnancy experience; whereas the majority of older key informants relied on prayer.

Care expressions by husbands of female key informants were reflected in psychophysical and learned cultural support and involvement to affirm: "Care as *presence of male spouses during pregnancy.*" This finding was very important to all female key informants. The researcher also observed that mothers of female key informants were involved during pregnancy by their active concern for the health of their pregnant offspring and unborn fetus.

Two intergenerational culture care differences were discovered during pregnancy. One was the intergenerational differences expressed with regard to what younger female key informants felt they were allowed to do during pregnancy as compared to their mothers or female ancestors. An example of this difference was found in the following statements by a young female key informant: "All these years you hear about women having kids in the steppe, but you get reprimanded for working too much. I feel I can do it all." The second intergenerational care difference was reflected in the lack of knowledge or preparation that older female key informants had or perceived they had for their pregnancy and childbirth experiences. Older female key informants felt they had virtually no preparation for their experiences. Physicians offered no information and questions were brushed aside with responses that made it clear that it should be the physician's concern and not the informant's. The younger female key informants actively sought to prepare themselves for their pregnancy and childbirth experiences.

Pregnancy and childbirth intergenerational care differences of the older and younger female and male informants revealed acculturation of younger informants into the American health system, use of technological advancements, as well as more health awareness than in the traditional culture. Male involvement in pregnancy and childbirth experiences reflected a very positive trend toward active care participation in the childbirth process and family caretaking of the child.

Childbirth Influencers with Technology, Kinship, Religion, Special Areas, and Findings

Study findings showed all female key informants delivered their children in a hospital setting. Only one child of an older female key informant was delivered in a hospital outside the United States. The latter female key informant's succeeding births occurred in United States hospitals.

At the time of delivery none of the husbands of the older female key informants were present at their children's births. An older male general informant voiced no disappointment over not attending his children's births. However, all younger general male and female key informants stated they had experienced the childbirth process with their spouses present at delivery. For the birth of one child where a Cesarean section was necessary, a young male general informant (the father) pressed to be present in the delivery room and was denied admittance. This male's overt emotional and verbal disappointment years later was still evident. For the male spouses, care patterns relied on the care constructs of *presence, support,* and *psychophysical involvement* during the childbirth experience. After delivery, the researcher observed that informants had care which was based on family support and assistance from several extended family members, husbands, or mothers of all female key informants.

With respect to the influence of technology, findings revealed that younger female key informants in labor favored its use. They would concentrate on breathing during labor, receive Pitocin to augment labor, receive some or no medication during labor, and have a fetal scalp electrode placed on the baby's scalp because of meconium-stained amniotic fluid. With the latter procedure, however, informants voiced anxiety. Young female key informants who delivered their babies by Cesarean section were given spinal anesthesia for deliveries. One older female key informant cited scopalamine for contractions, and spinal and general anesthesia were used during the vaginal births of these older female informants. Use of technological procedures were generally accepted without question by the women.

With respect to the influence of religion on childbirth, one young female key informant mentioned prayer during labor with her second baby following a previous miscarriage. However, older female key informants talked much about constantly praying before and after the birth of their children when a life-threatening situation arose in the neonatal period.

Baptism is a sacrament that the Ukrainian infant receives within the first few months of life. If the newborn is critically ill, the baptism will be performed as soon as possible after birth.

Breastfeeding practices were very common practice for Ukrainian mothers. The researcher observed in many homes and other daily living contexts with all male and female informants that breastfeeding is an expected and important part of childbirth well being. All older and younger female key informants breastfed their infants. These informants also stated that their spouses provided positive feedback favoring infant breastfeeding. The beliefs and reasons given by male informants about the advantages of breastfeeding included nutritional benefits, transference of antibodies to the infant, having healthier babies, the desire of closeness of the baby to mother, and the advantages of mother from a physiological basis to express her milk. The mothers viewed breastfeeding as caring by nurturing or promoting growth to the infant. Breastfeeding also reflected a cultural environment in which the infant grew up that included breastfeeding as a care lifeway, with male informants as integral parts of this highly-valued cultural socialization. Finally, findings revealed that breastfeeding expressed a strong health value for Ukrainian culture and for the newborn and infant for being "healthy is being breastfed." For the mother, breastfeeding contributed to her cultural and emotional well being.

It was interesting to discover that, although Ukrainian males traditionally have not been circumcised, female key and male general informants revealed three situations in which Ukrainian male offspring had been circumcised in recent years. These situations were: (1) if the male offspring was born in the United States and the physician said "it was necessary"; (2) if the male offspring was born to younger fathers who were circumcised in the United States; and (3) if the uncircumcised male offspring developed adhesions or infections of the foreskin.

With Ukrainian key and general informants, intergenerational differences were evident with respect to birth control. In the past as today, little or no communication between parents and their children regarding this topic took place. Older and younger informants were observed to differ in their birth control practices as well. The older generation (age 60 years and above) stated that their generation used rhythm, abstinence, withdrawal, condoms, or no type of birth control; whereas the younger generation of informants (below 60 years) stated that their generation used prophylactics, diaphragms, jellies, the pill, IUD, vasectomy, or tubal ligation for birth control. Interestingly, one older female key informant stated: "I don't think that a religious person would abort. If medically necessary, the adult has precedence over the fetus."

With respect to the ideal number of children for a Ukrainian couple, the researcher confirmed the general consensus for informants as between two and four in their family of procreation.

CARE THEMES DERIVED FROM MEANINGS AND EXPERIENCES IN USE OF THE THEORY

Table 4 illustrates the major themes of Ukrainian pregnancy and child-birth that were abstracted from the meanings and experiences of care of male and female informants using Leininger's Data Ethnonursing Qualitative Analysis Phases.

Culture care influencing health is a blueprint for human well being and determines what a culture will do to maintain its health status and care practices when illness appears (Leininger, 1979, p. 21). Dominant Ukrainian culture values included: (1) *health*; (2) *religious orientation to daily living*; (3) *involvement with family and community*; and (4) *humanism*. Dominant care constructs included: (1) *family presence*; (2) *closeness*; (3) *support*; and (4) *helping others*. Health values that support care were related to and derived from caring modes which included expressions of health through *mental, physical, and spiritual care practices*; health as *exercise*; *eating natural home-prepared meals*; and *breastfeeding*. Although these cultural care and health values and meanings were diverse, they were universally present in the researcher's observations of and related documented data on Ukrainian informants. As a result, confirmation of Leininger's theory of predicting diverse care meanings, expressions, forms, and practices arose and was documented as credible with all key and general informants. Moreover, the cultural care values were closely linked together as health promoting and leading to well being.

Table 4
Major Themes of Care of Female and Male Informants

1. Care is maternal acquisition of knowledge regarding pregnancy and childbirth.
2. Care is male presence, involvement, and support during pregnancy and childbirth.
3. Care is female family members' presence, support, and assistance during pregnancy and childbirth.
4. Care is family concern for health of pregnant woman and unborn fetus.
5. Care is breastfeeding.

Major care themes and related findings from this study and grounded largely in *emic* raw data, descriptors, and patterns are summarized below:

1. Care meanings and experiences for Ukrainian mothers and fathers were embedded in a religious, worldview, and kinship orientation that strongly guided their daily interactions with family and community members.

2. Care meanings, expressions, and experiences for Ukrainians were closely related to family and community obligations.

3. Care was strongly reflected in female family members' actions and decisions that were linked to health behaviors that promoted family and individual well being.

4. Universal care meanings, expressions, and patterns of living, which are preserved and maintained in the Ukrainian culture today, reflect care as family presence, closeness, support, and helping others.

5. Care diversities in care expressions exist with younger adults acculturated in American culture and contrast with older Ukrainians.

CARING AND NON-CARING NURSES

In this study, the researcher also explored with informants their views and experiences of a caring or non-caring professional nurse. Data analysis, as briefly presented here, revealed that both for male and female informants a caring nurse was viewed as being friendly, physically helpful to others, personable, benevolent, and gave explanations. For female informants, however, nurses were caring if they were more personable, meaning sympathetic, sensitive, took charge, and were empathetic to what those female informants were experiencing. Male informants gave descriptions of professional nurses as providing physical help such as bringing food, bringing a heating pad, and giving a back rub.

Both male and female informants described non-caring nurses as "just doing their job" and showing no interest in the informants.

While some male informants stated that the nurses showed no interest in them and conveyed laziness and coldness by their lack of responsiveness, female informants described these nurses as having no warmth in their eyes, a general lack of emotional involvement, no compassion, and were superefficient.

NURSING CARE MODALITIES AS GUIDES TO PRACTICE

Leininger's theory of Culture Care and use of the ethnonursing method proved valuable in discovering human caring as largely embedded in the social structure, worldview, language, cultural beliefs, and related areas. The three ethnonursing modalities of the theory that transcultural and other nurses should consider are apparent from this study of Ukrainian mothers and fathers with respect to pregnancy and childbirth. These modalities serve to guide health professionals in using the theory of Culture Care to provide culturally congruent care for health maintenance and well being of Ukrainian clients. Leininger's three modes of nursing decisions and actions used the knowledge discovered in the upper part of the Sunrise Model as guidelines to study and ultimately provide culturally congruent care—in this study for Ukrainian parents during pregnancy and childbirth. Such care modes will be discussed briefly with respect to the three modes stated in the theory.

Cultural Care Preservation or Maintenance

Cultural care preservation or maintenance would need to be considered along with the following understandings from the study findings: (1) Ukrainians have a religious orientation to care and health. Thus the nurse, when making decisions regarding care, would need to try and preserve as well as maintain religious beliefs and prayers during pregnancy, labor, and delivery. (2) Because care means *family closeness* in the Ukrainian culture, the nurse would need to involve family members during the pregnancy and childbirth experience, at the same time preserving and maintaining family care values of presence, support, and helping others. (3) Being healthy involves psychocultural well being and comes from caring family ways. The nurse would maintain care as being cheerful and acknowledge keen interest in the Ukrainian family unit during the childbearing phase of pregnancy care, especially in regard to their diverse health concerns. Thus, the nurse provides culture care preservation and maintenance actions and decisions. (4) With critically ill newborns, nursing actions would include baptizing the newborn as soon as possible after delivery and especially if death is imminent so as to reflect cultural care preservation and maintenance practices. (5) With critically ill mothers, a priest should be notified immediately to maintain and preserve religious practices and the long-standing cultural value of the central role of the mother as a care maintainer and stabilizer.

Cultural Care Accommodation or Negotiation

Cultural care accommodation or negotiation with regard to pregnancy and childbirth would guide nursing actions and decisions in the following culture-specific ways: (1) Spend some time with Ukrainian family members who are hospitalized or when going through the labor and delivery experience in the health system. (2) Nursing care should be viewed and expressed as helping others, by supporting and giving presence to their needs—for example, allowing the husband to be present during labor and delivery to help and support his wife as generic care. (3) Providing professional information to Ukrainians regarding pregnancy and childbirth as requested by the pregnant woman or couple or family member(s) as well as encouraging Ukrainian couples to express their health concerns, needs, and problems is important. (4) Care accommodation for breastfeeding is essential as a means of helping and supporting mothers as they breastfeed and especially to fulfill cultural care role expectations. (5) Care accommodation by *maternal presence* is important by allowing the newborn to be with the mother as much as possible in the hospital or health setting. (6) Care accommodation as facilitating *family presence* during the postpartum period would need to be recognized and especially as to provide nursing actions and decisions that would allow time for the mothers to be with family members.

Cultural Care Repatterning or Restructuring

In considering cultural care repatterning or restructuring, the Ukrainian informants were aware of the health care practices of the American health system, but they had had limited contact in using that system. Nonetheless, all young informants were interested in prenatal care and wanted the delivery of their child to take place within the American health care system. Attempts for repatterning or restructuring would be initiated by nurses being present and personable, showing respect for Ukrainian generic care values, and helping Ukrainians to use the American health care system appropriately. Nurses should keep in mind that mothers are the *health stabilizers* in the family, and it is the Ukrainian mother who will reach out for health care if congruent and needed. Prenatal, postpartum, well baby, and health maintenance visits in a health care setting are ideal times for nurses to build trusting relationships with these clients, share their knowledge, and provide information for health behaviors observed and in need of repatterning. Most importantly, nursing actions and decisions would need to be both *individualized* but with thought to *family patterns*. Since Ukrainians do things as naturally as possible with regard to their minds and bodies, meaningful culturally congruent patterned care would need to fit their expectations. Allowing time to build a trusting relationship over time would be important. Ukrainian clients need to feel secure and respected by nurses and others, and especially before changing traditional cultural values with older generation family members.

CONCLUSION

In conclusion, this study showed the importance of using Leininger's Culture Care theory to discover Ukrainian traditional and changing values, beliefs, and practices related to pregnancy and childbirth. As a nursing student in a master's degree program, I learned how to use the theory and particularly to value the importance of the theory to include social structure, worldview, values, environment, and professional health systems to discover anew cultural care concepts and practices that were unknown or vaguely known. The theory greatly expanded my views from looking at narrow or medical treatment and symptom variables to that of focusing on cultures and their human care meanings and expressions as powerful ways to understand and help people. The ethnonursing method and Leininger's enabler guides for data collection and analysis along with other specific features of the method were extremely helpful in studying and using the theory. Although I am of the Ukrainian culture, I discovered a wealth of new knowledge from the people that I was not fully cognizant of in my native and professional work. I will use these findings to guide my nursing practices and those of other professional nurses to give culture specific care that is congruent and fits the lifeways of Ukrainian people.

REFERENCES

Gudziak, B. A. (1990, July 13). The churches that would not die. *Commonweal*, 416–419.

Hamner, T. J., & Turner, P. H. (1985). *Parenting in contemporary society*. Englewood Cliffs, NJ: Prentice-Hall.

Horn, B. M. (1975). *An ethnoscience study to determine social and cultural factors affecting native American Indian women during pregnancy*. Unpublished doctoral dissertation. Seattle: University of Washington.

Horn, B. M. (1979). Transcultural nursing and child-rearing of the Muckleshoot people. In M. M. Leininger (Ed.), *Transcultural nursing: Proceedings from four transcultural nursing conferences*. New York: Masson, 57–69.

Kendall, K. W. (1968). *Personality development in an Iranian village: An analysis of socialization practices and the development of the woman's role*. Unpublished doctoral dissertation. Seattle: University of Washington.

Kendall, K. W. (1979). Maternal and child nursing in an Iranian village. In M. M. Leininger (Ed.), *Transcultural proceedings from four transcultural nursing conferences*. New York: Masson, 27–41.

Klaus, M. H., & Kennell, J. H. (1976). *Maternal-infant bonding*. St. Louis: C. V. Mosby.

Leininger, M. M. (1970). *Nursing and anthropology: Two worlds to blend*. New York: John Wiley & Sons.

Leininger, M. M. (1976). *Proceedings from the first national conference on transcultural care of infants and children*. Salt Lake City: University of Utah, College of Nursing.

Leininger, M. M. (1978a). The Gadsup of New Guinea and early child caring behaviors with nursing implications. In *Transcultural nursing: Concepts, theories, and practices*. New York: John Wiley & Sons, 375–398.

Leininger, M. M. (1978b). Transcultural nursing: Concepts, theories, and practices. New York: John Wiley & Sons.

Leininger, M. M. (1979). Transcultural nursing care: Proceedings from four national transcultural nursing conferences. New York: Masson Publishing.

Leininger, M. M. (1984). Care: The essence of nursing and health. Thorofare, NJ: Slack.

Leininger, M. M. (1985a) Qualitative research methods in nursing. New York: Grune & Stratton.

Leininger, M. M. (1985b). Transcultural care diversity and universality: A theory of nursing. Nursing and Health Care, 6(4), 209–212.

Leininger, M. M. (1988). Leininger's theory of nursing: Cultural care diversity and universality. Nursing Science Quarterly, 1(4), 152–160.

Leininger, M. M., Templin, T., & Thompson, F. (1990). Leininger-Templin-Thompson ethnoscript qualitative software program: User's handbook. Detroit: Wayne State University Press.

Lincoln, Y. S., & Guba, E. G. (1985). Naturalistic inquiry. Beverly Hills: Sage.

McBride, A. B. (1983). The experience of being a parent. In H. H. Werley & J. J. Fitzpatrick (Eds.), Annual review of nursing research, (Vol. 2, 63–81). New York: Springer.

Nahajewsky, I. (1975). History of Ukraine. Philadelphia: "America" Publishing House of "Providence" Association of Ukrainian Catholics in America.

Sevcovic, L. (1979). Traditions of pregnancy which influence maternity care of the Navajo. In Leininger, M. M. (Ed.), Transcultural nursing: Proceedings from four transcultural nursing conferences. New York, NY: Masson Publishing, 86–102.

Shevchenko Scientific Society. (1971). Ukraine: A concise encyclopaedia. V. Kubijovyc (Ed.). Toronto: University of Toronto Press.

Sikorski, R. (1990, November 5). Why Ukraine must be independent. National Review, 74–77.

Spradley, J. P. (1979). The ethnographic interview. Chicago: Holt, Rinehart and Winston.

Stefaniuk, M., & Dohrs, F. E. (1979). Ukrainians in Detroit. Detroit: Wayne State University.

Szporluk, R. (1979). Ukraine: A brief history. Detroit: Ukrainian Festival Committee.

7

Culture Care of the Gadsup Akuna of the Eastern Highlands of New Guinea

Madeleine M. Leininger

"You are a different kind of a woman. Will you be our friend or our enemy?"

In the early 1960s, I left the United States of America and entered a strange new world in which there were very few familiarities or commonalities with the people, language, homes, food, land, and indigenous lifeways. There were no modern modes of transportation, telephones, appliances, electricity, indoor toilets, or running water. In general, there were no modern Western amenities or comforts which many Americans enjoy. Although it was an initial culture shock, it soon turned into a new world to discover, understand, and value.

When I entered the Gadsup village in the Eastern Highlands of New Guinea, I well remember how the people stared at me wondering perhaps where this white woman came from and why she might be interested in them. I, too, wondered about these villagers and why I

231

came to study people who had been known as "head hunters of the Highlands." Would I survive and how could I ever learn about their world? It was a uniquely different world in which the Gadsup people and their lifeways baffled me. Their concern was reflected in their conscious but unspoken reflection, "You are a different kind of a woman. Will you be our friend or our enemy?" For this Western researcher, it was this very different world that posed a tremendous challenge: how to study and understand these people who were so different from the world I left behind.

When I went to New Guinea in the early 1960s, I was a third-year doctoral student at the University of Washington and had chosen this largely unknown culture to do an ethnographic and ethnonursing study by living alone with the villagers for an extended time. As yet, there were no anthropological writings on this unknown Melanesian New Guinean culture. I was prepared with a suitable theoretical and research background from my graduate studies as well as in psychiatric mental health nursing and as an educator ready to study and learn about strange or unexpected behaviors. My decision to go to New Guinea and study this non-Western culture also was welcomed by the department of anthropology—it needed to be studied soon, before the Western world changed it.

Before I left the United States, I wondered what I could learn about transcultural nursing and human caring and health from a culture that had not been touched by Western ideologies and practices. I wondered how the people lived in their naturalistic environment and what their actual daily and nightly lifeways were. I wondered how these people could function without modern technologies. Then there were my theoretical and research nursing interests in which I was eager to study the meanings and expressions of human care and how care had influenced the people's health and well being. I wanted to study human caring and health within the total lifeways of non-Western people and in a culture where there had been little to no contact with Western people. I was curious how this non-Western culture lived and expressed their human care needs, remained well, became ill, or faced death. I had heard that the Gadsup had survived and maintained themselves quite well over an extended time. Principally, I wanted to learn about the caring ways of the people from their *emic* (or local insider's) view, and how they would contrast with our American and other Western lifeways. In addition, I was interested in the environment or ecology of the people and how these factors influenced Gadsup life-ways.

During my graduate studies, I had already conceptualized most of the major ideas, tenets and concepts of my theory of Culture Care Diversity and Universality, and so I wanted to examine systematically the theory with my ethnonursing qualitative research method in a relatively small community. Since the idea of developing a culturally-based theory and using a nursing research method was unknown in nursing in the mid-1950s and early 1960s, I thought the Gadsup culture would be an ideal initial study group. The idea of using such study findings as knowledge for the new field of transcultural nursing was exciting to me. In those days, too, although no theoretical research studies in nursing with a transcultural perspective were available, there were several non-nurse anthropologists, such as Esther Lucille Brown (1948) and Lyle Saunders (1954), who encouraged nurses to use social science ideas in nursing education. The specific linkage of cultural knowledge to nursing, however, had yet to be developed and used. With increased world travel and with nurses working in different cultures, I was convinced that they would soon need transcultural care and health knowledge to be effective in future multicultural nursing. Nursing also needed the ethnonursing research approach to learn *directly from the people* of the daily lifeways of culture and to discover the role of caring in relation to health and well being. For these major reasons and others, I chose New Guinea as the site for my field research.

In this chapter I will highlight my research work in New Guinea with my theory of Culture Care and with the use of the ethnonursing method which was specifically designed for the theory. Since the theory and the ethnonursing method have already been presented in Chapters 1 and 2, the focus will be mainly on the Gadsup Akunans and their culture care expressions in relation to the theory, research method, ethnohistory, and other dimensions of the Sunrise Model with research findings.

RESEARCH DOMAIN, PURPOSE, AND QUESTIONS

The domain of inquiry was the study of the meanings, expressions, and lived experiences of human care to the Gadsup Akunans. This domain was chosen to discover the epistemic and ontologic nature of human care and its relationship to health with Gadsup in their particular environmental context. The central purpose of this study was to generate new nursing knowledge by identifying, describing, explaining, and interpreting human care (and caring) from the Gadsup's *emic* viewpoints focusing on influencers of human care in relation to worldview, social structure, cultural values, ethnohistory, folk care, and environment of the people. The assumptive premises and hunches stated in the Culture Care theory were of central interest to me because of the need for new knowledge for the discipline of nursing and for the field of transcultural nursing. Ultimately, such knowledge and future findings from other cultures in the world could guide nurses to provide relevant knowledge as well as culture-specific nursing care practices related to ethnocare and ethnohealth. This study—the first nursing research endeavor toward the evolving study of the meaning and nature of human care from an emic viewpoint—also was conducted to fulfill doctoral requirements in anthropology focusing on the general lifeways of a culture and their social structure features.

The following questions, which guided this ethnocare and ethnohealth research, did not limit my discovery of other Gadsup findings related to my theory of Culture Care and the lifeways of the people.

1. What are the meanings, expressions, patterns, and lived experiences of human care to the Gadsup Akunans and the influences on their health and well being?

2. In what ways does the worldview, ethnohistory, social structure, culture values, language, and the local (folk) practices influence the health and illness patterns of the people?

3. What specific cultural care values, beliefs, and practices throughout the lifecycle tend to influence the health and illness lifeways of the people?

4. In what way does the physical environment (or ecology) influence human care, health, or illness patterns of the people?

5. Given the predicted three modes of decisions and actions in the Culture Care theory, what nursing care modalities will most likely provide culturally congruent care practices?

THEORETICAL FRAMEWORK, ASSUMPTIVE PREMISES, AND ORIENTATIONAL QUESTIONS

In conceptualizing the theory of Culture Care for this investigation, I used the major tenets, assumptive premises, and orientational definitions of the theory using the Gadsup Akunans as the study focus along with the Sunrise Model as a conceptual guide. Since the theory and the model have already been presented in Chapter 1, they will not be presented again except for specific perspectives related to the Gadsups.

Although I held that care was the essence of nursing, there were different values, meanings, patterned expressions, and structure forms of care that were important to discover so as to establish transcultural and other comparative care knowledge. I predicted that the values, meanings, patterned expressions, and experiences of human care and caring would be influenced by worldview, social structure, ethnohistory, environmental (including ecology), and folk care practices screened through the Gadsup language. I further predicted that care beliefs and practices would influence the health, well being, or illness expectations of the people. Since nurses function in different kinds of environments with people, I was interested in the environmental context and ecological factors and I predicted these aspects would influence care, health, and illness patterns. The concepts of environmental context and worldview were new in nursing at that time, yet I believed they were extremely important to nursing. Finally, the three predicted modes for action and decision were viewed with the idea that if a non-Gadsup nurse were to function in the village, culture-specific care would be essential to provide acceptable, effective, and satisfying care. The idea of culturally congruent care was predicted to be important for nursing care practices.

Essentially, I used the same assumptive premises as stated in my theory in Chapter 1 except for these additional statements:

1. In a non-Western culture where there has been limited external contact by Western peoples, human care knowledge would probably provide different epistemic and naturalistic care meanings and patterned expressions of a culture.

2. If non-technological care practices exist, they will provide new kinds of knowledge of insights about human caring.

3. The ecological context of a culture influences care meanings and health expressions.

Conceptualizing this study was difficult because there was no published literature or completed general *ethnographic* studies on the Gadsup of the Highlands of New Guinea. Therefore, I had to envision as best I could what possibly might be the lifeways of the people and prepare myself for the New Guinea culture area and its people.

REVIEW OF THE LITERATURE ON THE GADSUP AND CULTURE CARE

In the 1960s, no research studies had yet been completed on the Gadsup. The more general culture area in which the Gadsup live, the Eastern Highlands, had also had few contacts with Western ideas and people—the geography and many diverse cultures therein were largely awaiting investigation. In 1959, Dr. James Watson (1963), at the University of Washington in Seattle, saw this need and began a series of multidisciplinary studies in the Eastern Highlands of New Guinea where the Gadsup lived to obtain physical, geographic, linguistic, and cultural anthropological data. I was invited to participate in this microevolution multidisciplinary study of four cultures under Dr. Watson (1963), and chose to focus on the Gadsup. Other anthropologists also were phased in to study the other cultures in the Highlands over a ten-year period. Since the late 1960s and mid-1970s, a series of publications, the *Anthropological Studies in the Eastern Highlands of New Guinea*, have provided important information about some Eastern Highland cultures, including the Gadsup: McKaughan's (1973) linguistic studies on the Highland languages; Pataki's (1970) study on the ecology and geography of the Highlands; and Watson and Cole's (1977) study on the prehistory of the Highlands. In 1975, du Toit's study became available on the Gadsup but it did not focus on the proposed study dimensions and there was limited information on folk health practices. During and since this time, I have written about some different aspects of the Gadsup, but primarily from a nursing care, health, and lifecycle perspective (Leininger 1966a, 1970, 1978b, 1979, 1985).

Since this study was an entirely new focus in nursing and a different approach to establish a new knowledge for transcultural nursing, it had great potential for new knowledge in nursing and especially about non-Western cultures. Again, the nursing literature in this area was nonexistent when the study was initiated. McCabe (1960) had, however, begun to use a mental health training grant to incorporate selected social science concepts into an undergraduate program, but it was not a research study nor was it focused on human care. Later, Horn (1978) and Aamodt (1978) became interested in culture care and did research on the Muckleshoots and Papago. Since then, other care studies have been gradually done in nursing with Bohay (1988), Gates (1988), Rosenbaum (1990), Spangler (1991), Stasiak (1990), and Wenger's (1987) research focused on the theory of Culture Care and reported in this book.

ORIENTATIONAL DEFINITIONS

The orientational definitions for the theory are presented in Chapter 1 except for this definition of the Gadsup: *Gadsup* refers to a non-Western culture living in the Eastern Highlands of the Island of New Guinea in which their language, non-technological lifeways, material items, social structure, ecology, and lifeways set them apart from Western cultures in the world.

POTENTIAL SIGNIFICANCE OF THE STUDY

There were a number of potential significant features of this study for nursing and for other disciplines interested in human care and health. First, this was the first transcultural human care study done in a non-Western culture, in which the people had never seen or worked with a white single nurse researcher. This historical study opened the door for subsequent Western and non-Western transcultural nursing studies focused on comparative care, health, well being, and illness patterns. Second, the study provided the epistemic and ontologic base of *emic* nursing knowledge about the meanings, expressions, and experiences of human care, and their relationship to health, illness, and well being studied within the Culture Care theory. It was a first study in nursing to focus on the universals and differences within a specific culture and environment using Culture Care theory to explicate care and health knowledge in nursing. Third, the study provided the first longitudinal and comparative nursing study of cultural care, covering approximately one year in two villages, and by a nurse researcher prepared in anthropology and nursing to collect and analyze the data. This study also was the first diachronic research in nursing to determine how the culture(s) changed over time, an extremely important aspect in the understanding of culture changes and nursing. Fourth, this study involved the first use of the ethnonursing method with the theory of Culture Care. Even today, this approach remains a new idea and is just beginning to be studied for its importance in nursing. Again, the method was designed to study some of the most invisible and little known aspects of human care as the essence of nursing. Fifth, with the nurse researcher living one year in the same village, the ethnonursing method provided one of the longest and most continuous observational and participatory studies in nursing; a unique feature never before done by a nurse researcher. Sixth, the study, the first transcultural nursing study, was done by the first nurse anthropologist. It also provided multidisciplinary collaborative contributions to anthropology and other disciplines. Seventh, this study was an in-depth, inductive, ethnonursing comparative investigation within the qualitative paradigm. The researcher compared two village groups for differences and similarities in the same language, culture, and ecological setting and at the same synchronic time period. Due to space limitations, however, only one village (Akuna) is presented here. Nonetheless, this study remains today as the only intervillage comparative nursing study and offers a different approach to studying nursing phenomena.

RESEARCH METHODS, INFORMANTS, AND ENABLERS

The ethnonursing method was purposely developed and used to discover culture care meanings, expressions, patterns, and lived experiences of a non-Western culture with a focus on diverse influencers on health or well being. (See Chapter 2 for a detailed account of the method.) Although the ethnographic method (Leininger, 1985) also was used to obtain a detailed descriptive account of the total lifeways of the people, only the ethnonursing method will be discussed here. It also is important to state that while I studied two Gadsup villages in the early 1960s in the Eastern Highlands of New Guinea only the Gadsup Akunans data will be reported here.

After arriving in Akuna, I soon found myself surrounded by 260 Gadsup Akunan villagers who lived in an open grassland (kunai) ecological environment with a small forested area on the edge of their village. The Akunans spoke an Eastern Highland language with some dialect differences within and between Gadsup villages. I lived in a bamboo and grass hut which was given to me by the villagers. My 24-hour participation in the daily and nightly lifeways of the people provided a unique opportunity to study in considerable detail their lifeways and to obtain a comprehensive picture of practically every facet of their life. During my one-year stay, I had no major or extended leaves from the village except to go on occasion to a small trade town about 25 miles from the village.

After being in the village for about one month, I chose 35 key informants of both sexes for in-depth observations, participant experiences, and interviews. Since there were no calendars, clocks, or written records in the villages, the information sources were oral narrations, observations, and material culture items. I held at least four to five special interviews (often more) with all key informants. Among these key informants were ten children and adolescents of approximately 5 to 16 years of age. All remaining Gadsup Akunans, about 200 in number, served as *general* informants. I visited all villagers at least once, knew their names, kinship ties, and something about each one. The key informants met these criteria; (1) they expressed an interest in having four to five visits with me; (2) they had lived practically all of their life in the village and knew the day and night lifeways of the people; (3) they understood Melanesian Pidgin English or could communicate with a native translator; and (4) they were interested in talking about "their village ways" which included their worldview, social structure, and other components depicted in the Sunrise Model and bearing on Culture Care theory. I did not begin in-depth interviews with key informants until after the third month and only when the people were reasonably comfortable with me as a friend. This decision was extremely important in gaining the trust of a non-Western people whose culture was markedly different from my own.

I began the study by using the Observation-Participation-Reflection enabling guide (described in Chapter 2), a helpful adjunct in learning about the people's daily lifeways with a focus on care, health, and illness patterns. In my interaction with the villagers in their environment, I gradually learned their kinship ties, special roles, and responsibilities in the village. During this time, I took detailed field journal notes on the naturalistic and patterned lifeways of the children and adults as well as what constituted typical day and night activities. I became fully immersed in the people's lifeways, learning much about them through direct observation, gradual participation, and reflection to assess the meanings of what I saw, heard, and experienced. I observed their caring rituals, symbols, and some of their most covert, secretive practices about health care. As the villagers become more comfortable with me, they became my "teacher" and I encouraged them in this role so as to learn as much as I could about them. I showed interest in all villagers and their animals, trees, gardens, mountains, flowers, huts, rituals, and anything they identified as influencing their care, health, and well being. Gradually, they described their history, legends, myths, and material artifacts—bows, arrows, war shields, sorcerer's substances. Later they described their male and female ceremonial rituals and secrets that influenced their care and well being. I continued as a *learner* and *researcher*, letting the people teach me the what, why, and how of their culture, and according to their readiness to share ideas with me. The Gadsup taught me about their traditional non-caring enemies and caring friends, their past and current lifeways, and how these factors influenced caring, health, and illness patterns. My total immersion and involvement in their lifeways provided rich, dense, meaningful data from key and general informants. The inductive *emic* ethnonursing method was fully and continuously used with the Observation-Participation-Reflection Guide, which kept me focused and helped me to enter and remain in their world. It also was a valuable way to learn from and move with the people in their life rhythms rather than by more conventional Western modes.

The Leininger Stranger-Friend Guide (described in Chapter 2) was an extremely valuable enabling mode to assess my role as stranger and my movement into the village. I had developed the guide before going to New Guinea as a research aid conceptualized with the theory of Culture Care. It helped me to reflect on and gauge my behavior with the people as a stranger and as I became a friend. Unquestionably, the Akunans first saw me not only as a stranger, but as a potential sorceress, with all the distrust and distancing behaviors implied by that perception. Some villagers "tested me" in several ways to determine my reaction—for example, did I value their food, their children, and general lifeways? Was I a "good woman" like their women and how was I different? By the third month, I had become their friend and during my stay a "true friend." Indicators on the aforesaid enabler, such as sharing secrets and trusting, were important guides to measuring acceptance of my behavior to the villagers and their behavior to me. In addition, such indicators were important for my survival—these people had been known as "headhunters of the Highlands." In fact it was only a few years before I arrived that the Australian government had stopped open tribal fighting in the Gadsup villages. A stranger, however, was still considered as a potential sorcerer (male) or sorceress (female) and could cause illnesses, trouble in the village, and even deaths. As a single woman without a husband and children, it was natural that I would be considered as a potential sorceress. Although I disliked this role assigned to me, it was necessary to understand it both for my survival and for a successful field study. As a result the people felt they had to watch me closely when I first arrived, so that I would not cause them harm, or become an active, destructive sorceress. Likewise, I watched their behavior to protect myself and to communicate effectively and appropriately with them. Shifting from a potential sorceress to a true friend was a formidable challenge. I also was quite aware of the potential consequences should they have declared I was a malevolent sorceress or a "no good woman." Although this nursing and anthropological research involved such "high risk," I had confidence that I could gain their trust and friendship by being alert to my own actions so they were not misinterpreted as non-caring or harmful to the Akunans. My clinical skills in psychiatric mental health nursing kept me alert to unexpected nonverbal cue behavior even though some Gadsup nonverbal cues did not have the meanings similar to those found in America. It also was difficult to "read the people" due to language difficulties—only a few men could speak Pidgin English. It was only when they began to call me "their friend" and trusted me with secrets and confirmed what I had seen and heard, that I knew I had shifted from actual stranger and potential sorceress to true friend.

During my stay, I kept detailed, continuous, and extensive field journal notes. I sent copies of my journal to my home in the United States whenever I could find ways to mail them in order to preserve the data. I also used selected tape recordings for care narratives and used photographs of the people to document detailed and complex phenomena. The photographs were used as an enabling method to capture caring episodes and the diverse, daily environmental contexts that men, women, and children experienced. The photographs, while providing rich insight, also were intriguing. The people were initially frightened by the camera, but later treasured the photos for their dead ancestors. Other features of the ethnonursing method used are described in Chapter 2.

GADSUP LAND AND ETHNOHISTORY OVERVIEW: ENTERING AND LEARNING FROM THE PEOPLE

The Gadsup Akunans live on the Island of New Guinea, which is about 1,500 miles long, 500 miles wide, and only 6 degrees from the equator. New Guinea is shaped like a big bird with its tail straddling Australia and its head flying towards Asia (see Figure 1). It is one of the most densely populated islands in the world with nearly 600

Figure 1
The Island of New Guinea

Gadsup study area = ●

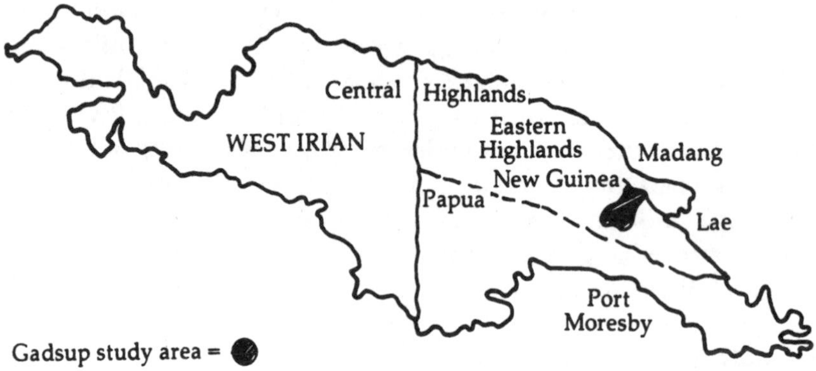

distinct cultures and many different languages (with dialect differences) and cultures. The Gadsup territory was an Australian Trust Territory and under Australian government until it became independent as Papua New Guinea in 1964 (Leininger, 1966a, 1966b).

The Akunans live in the Eastern part of the Eastern Highlands near the Markham Valley. The country is beautiful with green grasslands, large areas of new forest, and some distant high mountain ranges. The air was always fresh and clean with no industrial plants to pollute the environment. The mild temperature ranged between 58 degrees Fahrenheit at night and 85 degrees Fahrenheit in the daytime. Slight fluctuations occurred during the dry and rainy seasons. The average rainfall reported by patrol officers (while I was living there) was about 85 inches per year. The ecology revealed two major types of vegetation: grassland (kunai) which the Akuna village largely represented, and the more dense forest (bush) areas which the second village represented. The Akuna environment was covered largely with tall kangaroo grass (kunai) and had a few small streams about one mile from the village. There also were dense patches of pit-pit (a reed like grass), and a small forested area on the edge of the village.

The Akuna worked many vegetable gardens, their main source of food. From these gardens came sweet potatoes, taro, greens, corn, squash, beans, and other native vegetables. There were many varieties of sweet potatoes along with the very old taro plants. New gardens first were cleared by the men (slash-and-burn method) and turned over to the women who were the managers, producers, distributors, and controllers of the gardens. The women took much pride in working their gardens and involved young girls (from about seven years of age) to elderly women. When the elderly had "less muscle" to do garden work, they would stop such work and remain in the village plaza to care for children and provide surveillance of the plaza for all villagers.

The small forested area on the edge of the Akuna village was largely used and explored by men for hunting and to inspire young males to see the forest as "their male area of intrigue." In the forest area were betel nut, pandanus nut, fruit-bearing pandanus palms, breadfruit, banana palms (of great variety), and bamboo in addition to birds and animals. Fruit from several of these trees were used for food. Bamboo tree products were used for house building, cooking, and as containers for carrying water from the streams to the village each day. The Akuna children often found big edible mushrooms and seasonal nuts in the bush or forest area. The young boys and men would spend many hours in the forest hunting marsupials and birds, gathering nuts and mushrooms, and searching for other food sources. They also would collect tree materials to make their bows and arrows and music instruments. The forest area symbolized the man's world away from the women; the garden represented a woman's world and being away from men.

According to pre-historians, it is believed that the Gadsup area had been inhabited for thousands of years by their ancestors, also hunters and gatherers. There is continued speculation by anthropologists that the New Guinea people, especially the Gadsup, are a pre-neolithic culture. The many different languages and dialects spoken by the people across the Southern, Central, and Eastern Highlands of the Island of New Guinea are of interest as well as the variation in physical features and cultural lifeways of the Gadsup, and of the many other cultures who have lived in the Highlands for at least 800 years or more (Littlewood, 1972; Watson & Cole, 1977).

As the Cessna plane which first brought me to the Gadsup flew over the Eastern Highlands of New Guinea, I was struck by the dense forested area, the absence of highrise buildings, no paved roads or freeways, no billboards, and virtually no cars on the rough winding and narrow dirt roads. The ecology of the Highlands revealed much green vegetation, dense forest areas, and grasslands with high mountain ranges (some recorded at levels reaching nearly 12,000 feet) and the villages built on top of the mountain ridges. There were many active volcanoes that brought forth molten rich ash to nurture the green foliage, but there also were low intensity earthquakes (almost weekly) which the Gadsup feared.

When I first walked into the village of Akuna after a final 25-mile drive in an Australian landrover, I climbed over a wooden fence to the staring eyes of almost 15 dark bare-skinned people sitting around an earth oven in the village. Twenty or so bamboo and grass huts circled the village plaza. Most of the villagers were sitting around the earth oven talking and chewing on betel nut, and others (young children and adolescents) were walking about the village plaza. The wooden fence that surrounded the village divided a "lower" and "upper" village area which had sported several enclosed gardens nearby. At one end of the Akuna village was a church building, which I later found was built by

bottom) was used to cook food, as in aid in the care of children and pigs, and as a social center for talking, gossiping, and planning day or night activities. The women used small branches of trees and dry leaves for the open oven in which they cooked yams, taro, bananas, or sweet potatoes for their two meals—a light meal in the morning and a heavier meal at night. As most morning foods had been cooked the previous night, most villagers munched on the cold sweet potato, taro, sugar cane, or a slightly warmed over sweet potato.

After 10:00 A.M. every morning, the women went to their gardens carrying young infants in their string bags and on their heads along with a big handmade string bag filled with wooden garden tools, cold yams, sugar cane, and wood. A few girls (ages 9–12) remained in the plaza to care for their younger siblings or related kinschildren. They were assisted in their caregiving role by a few elderly adult men and women who watch over and protect the children and village. About 10:30 A.M., young boys and adult males strolled to the nearby forest area with their bows and arrows to hunt birds and small animals, collect mushrooms, and bamboo shoots, or to experience the mystical and powerful symbolism of the forest environment. Some men walked to nearby friendly villages to talk to their "fictive brothers or kinsmen" and then, after offering betel nut, foods or other village gifts, would return around 4:00 P.M. From about 10:00 A.M. until nearly 5:00 P.M., the village was empty except for very few people as the women were in their gardens, the men were "walking about" or making "big talk," and the small children were playing under the surveillance of older girls and the elderly. Teenage boys were free to go most anywhere and had virtually no role responsibilities. In contrast, teenage girls were either working with their mothers in the garden, collecting wood, or caring for their siblings.

Around 5:00 P.M., all the Akunans gathered around their earth ovens for the evening meal and to sing and talk about the day's happenings, a perfect time as well to care for children and to share general social experiences with other villagers. The women always prepared the evening meal in the big long oven and usually outside their hut and near those of their kinsmen or lineage. A typical evening meal consisted of baked yams, sweet potatoes, taro, breadfruit, native beans, greens, seasonal corn, squash, bananas, and sugar cane. If the men and young boys had been successful in the forest world, they may have brought back flying foxes, bird meat, and seasonal nuts. On very special occasions, wild and domestic pigs were cooked in the earth oven and especially for ceremonial lifecycle events, annual garden feasts, or for food sharing with friendly nearby villagers. The Akunans did not drink milk, soda pop, tea, or coffee, only water from the stream.

It is important to note that pigs were highly valued by all Gadsups. Pigs have long had symbolic meanings related to achieving social status, prestige, and economic gains. Pigs were owned, exchanged, and inherited individually and with lineages. It was interesting to observe the amount of care which small pigs received; the women often defined their role as caring for their children and their pigs. Small house pigs were raised in the huts by women who fed and stroked them until the pigs were able to forage for food outside the village. Attention was given to the foods pigs ate and ways to protect them. In general, pork was the only substantive protein eaten, if infrequently, and usually prepared only for special ceremonial occasions. Pigs, it must be noted, were generally few in number and highly valued for political and ceremonial exchanges, so their consumption required a special event. The more pigs a Gadsup had, the higher that Gadsup's social status, and pigs lost or stolen were often heated legal topics in village political sessions.

There was cassowary (W'uye) and emo (turkeylike) birds that also were trapped and used for ceremonial purposes. Emo eggs were large and green (about four times the size of a chicken egg). After gaining the villager's trust, these eggs were sometimes presented to me as a special gift, along with cassowary meat. It was of interest that I was given large delicious pineapples, huge white oranges, lemons, passion fruit, and many different kinds of bananas after they trusted me as a "true Gadsup friend." The Akuna men had obtained these fruits by walking great distances (about 25 miles to the Markham Valley). During my initial period in the village, however, when the Akunans watched and distrusted me, I received many dry old sweet potatoes, wilted greens, and virtually no fruit or desirable edible Akunan foods. Thus, one could assess my stranger-friend relationships by the quality and quantity of food given to me.

The eel, symbolic of male strength and viewed as a great delicacy, was another special village food eaten only by males. A male belief persisted that if females ate eel, they would become ill and especially if pregnant. Mushrooms and nuts were highly desired foods, but only available during certain seasons. These foods were often eaten as a mid-day snack with a cold yam or sweet potato. The big red seed of the pandanus tree was roasted in open fire and enjoyed while the villagers sat around the open earth pit visiting and gossiping about village affairs. All of these foods reflected the Gadsup's long history of food hunting, gathering, and having a small garden-forest subsistence economy. With no means to refrigerate or preserve such foods, they had to be collected daily and eaten. In light of foods eaten and village activities, I found no evidence of cancer, heart attacks, or strokes which I believe was related, in part, to their fresh foods, limited red meat, lots of vigorous garden work for women, and "walk abouts" for men.

At night, the Akunans would typically sit around the open fire hearth, casually talking or telling stories, laughing, singing, and gossiping about village affairs. Males often talked about their visits to nearby villages and the women talked about their gardens, children, small pigs, and other women matters. Male and female secrets, however, were never shared between sexes. They also talked about sorcery accusations, or threats of enemy villagers, and if someone was ill or dying. Ways to revenge sorcerers and prevent further illnesses and death were discussed in hushed, low-pitched voices. Sometimes men would get their bows and arrows and demonstrate how they fought in the "old days" and that they would be sorcerers. With the recent suppression of fighting, they were unable to engage in open warfare. As a result, sorcery, which seemed to replace the fighting, was more prevalent. Young male and female children and adolescents were always present at evening meals and for evening talks around the earth oven. Frequently, men and women would smoke or chew tobacco or betel nut. In the rainy season, the villagers stayed inside their family huts and talked about their dead kinsmen and caring ways about creation, myths, and about the general Gadsup lifeways that usually had caring and non-caring themes of protective care and well being.

Around 10:00 P.M., the small children villagers went inside their huts and slept on raised bamboo platforms. In keeping with past traditions and segregation of the sexes, the young boys and men went to their male huts. Earlier in the evening, however, the teenage girls and boys would walk about the village with young men trying to woo a girl for marriage. The girls and boys stayed together in groups as "companions" (about five or six), but these groups were not like gay or lesbian groups with sexual relationships.[1] The boys sang love songs to the girls in their family huts or as the girls sat in the village plaza. It was fascinating to hear teenage boys sing these love songs to the young girls without touching them. Sexual relations were reserved for marriage. The teenagers were always discrete, cautious, and used proper etiquette to be attracted to one another. Interestingly, the young girls remained in control of their decision of whom they would marry, and the boy was always thrilled and excited if "chosen" by the girl. While the parents made suggestions of whom they wanted their offspring to marry, they did not make the final decision. Rather, the girl makes the final decision after talking with her female kinswomen. In addition, if the bride price was arranged satisfactorily between the two families, the wedding ceremony would occur. All Gadsup marriages occurred around the ages of 16, 18, and even older with the mean age of 19 years. Because of a shortage of Akuna females, Akuna males had to seek marriage partners outside of Akuna. Accordingly, they would make "afternoon and night walks" to friendly villages to woo girls. Most Akuna marriages were exogamous (marrying women outside of their lineage or clan, but some married within the village if from another clan). Other details of the lifecycle are reported in other publications (Leininger, 1970, 1978b).

To complete the typical night, about midnight or later if there were no special ceremonies requiring dancing, drum beating, and feasting, the adult married men and women went to their huts to sleep. The village elderly usually went to bed earlier and after the young children went to sleep. Most nights in the Akuna village were active with villagers talking and singing in their huts, or with drum beating in the plaza. There were only three or four hours of silence from about 2:30 A.M. to 5:00 A.M.

CARE (CARING) WITH THE THEORY
SUNRISE MODEL DIMENSIONS

Worldview and Care

The Gadsup conceive themselves as having come from "one vine or root." They would often say, "We are *one* . . . We came from the *same* root and we are *all brothers* . . . We all speak the same language and believe the same things." These worldview statements guided how the Gadsup related and communicated to each other, involving a community caring ethos that supported the belief that they were of one origin. Gadsups spoke of a feeling of *interconnectedness* and *belonging* to each other as a tribe or clan over a long time span despite periodic intervillage feuds and fights. Most older Akunans were aware of their tribal identity (the largest sociocultural group), clan identity, subclan identity, lineages, and of course their extended families. These clan and subclan social ties were especially loose and fragile due to potential feuds and sorcery accusations. The lineage, which could be identified by most older men and women, included those closest in social ties and interdependency along with extended families that grew out of the lineage.

Another related worldview was that there were Gadsup villages that cared about each other and would provide protection in times of threat or losses. Enemy villages, which several called "non-caring" and which could bring harm to them by sorcery, also existed. There were periods of relation and tension with these changing views of the Gadsup world. Most importantly, they found it difficult to comprehend any world beyond that of nearby New Guineans and the fierce New Guinean fighters in the Highlands. None of the villagers had ever seen a map of the world, and none had attended a school or received a formal education. Only a few men had been to the New Guinea coast; hence, their worldview was quite small in scope. Most Akunans perceived Gadsup land as very big and their whole world. Such an ethnocentric worldview made it very difficult for Akunans to understand people who looked and acted so differently from them. As such, strangers were generally feared, and the question of where and how to place them, whether in their world or outside it, remained of concern to them.

Several key Akunan informants said, "We can have a peaceful and caring social world if we maintain good kinship ties, share foods, and perform our work . . . We must also follow the ways of our good ancestors." They also believed that they would have good health and stay well if they did not break any cultural taboos, values, and practices. When sharing their ideas about caring and health, it was clear that these went beyond individualism or self-care. Instead, they viewed caring as a way of doing good work and acts toward others and especially to other Gadsups in the Highlands. Most Akunans believed that a caring person should always watch out for others and try to protect them, especially those of close lineage and extended family members—mother's brother, father's sister, etc.—and other true Gadsup "brothers." They believed that caring relationships defined the particular value known as *community*. Feuds and sorcery accusations were non-caring and always threatening to the community. A non-caring Gadsup community did not act as "one vine and as true brothers." Instead, they acted in non-caring ways. Thus, caring and non-caring worldviews were closely linked together and were a source of concern that could greatly influence well being and health.

Care Embedded in Religious or Spiritual Dimensions

The Gadsup Akunans held that "true care" could be found in the way their ancestors lived in the past. They believed that when a person died their "*life essence lived on*" which became a moral, ethical, and spiritual guide to living villagers and especially to those closest to the deceased kin. Practically all key informants said, "My good ancestor continues to care for me and others here even though they are not here." When an Akunan was in trouble, they would petition to their ancestors to guide them to do good and help them get out of trouble. They were always cognizant that if one betrayed or acted counter to the cultural lifeways or norms of the ancestors that revenge and harm could come to them. They especially feared revenge or harm from a recent deceased ancestors whose spirit was very powerful, and so they were always deferent, cautious, and careful how they behaved immediately after a recent kin death, especially a "Big Man's" death in the village.

Although the Gadsup had no formal doctrine or organized religious beliefs, they did rely on their spiritual beliefs, which were rooted in their life essence and their worship of great ancestors in their daily lives, as guides. The spiritual caring components they spoke about were *surveillance* ("to watch over them"), *nurturance* (to help them grow as "good Gadsups"), and to provide *protective care*. These were embedded in their spiritual beliefs and served as a moral guide to prevent illnesses, harm from others, and sudden death.

Although the Lutherans and Seventh Day Adventists had tried to "teach the Akunans some Christian beliefs," they had a very difficult time. These church leaders tried to teach them about God, heaven, hell, and the devil, but these concepts were not in the Gadsup world-view nor in their spiritual ancestral views. The Gadsup found the ideas incongruous with their spiritual life and worldview perspectives. In fact, the Akunans felt at times they were coerced to attend services, learn Christian beliefs, and had a very difficult time accepting such imported ideas. They experienced cultural imposition conflicts that some felt were non-caring ways of the ministers. The Akunans ancestral spiritual guidance was far more important than trying to learn a foreign religion. Akunans said they always had to be attentive to the spiritual power of their deceased kin as this was a community responsibility so that people's health would not be adversely affected. Akunans would appease the ancestors by offering food, making petitions, and preparing special gifts to them in order to prevent revenge, illnesses, or unfavorable life conditions in the total Gadsup community. Grief expressions for a deceased "Big Man" of the village who had powerful life essences were observed. An elderly person who lived a full life was not grieved as much as a young child or "Big Man." The elderly and children had less powerful life spirits than an active middleaged man or woman. I often observed situations in which a quick burial of these powerful dead took place within a few hours to reduce unfavorable spiritual harm or threats to their well being and health status. Most importantly, Akunans firmly believed that one must always be attentive to and thus care for the dead as well as the living. To not do so exemplified a non-caring, bad person.

Kinship, Social Relatedness, and Caring Modalities

The kinship and social organizational structure of the Akunans proved to be very complex and difficult to study. From my interviews with the key informants and a number of other villagers along with many genealogies taken, I found most Akunans belonged to extended families, patrilineages, some loose subclans, and a few patriclans. Practically all informants saw their identify with the Gadsup tribe as the largest social organization. Most of the older Akunans felt strong ties to the tribe that made them "one people." The patriclan was recognized in the past as an important group that was involved in war activities, and most

could not trace their descent to specific kin. The few *subclans* identified were loose in their organizational features, but did constitute
groups good at feuds and some past warfare. Members of *patrilineages*
were able to trace their kinship ties with social alignments to specific
descent members some recalled, and who usually remained near the
extended family in an Akuna village. Members of *extended families*
were able to trace their social descent lines through the lineages and
lived usually in the same village. According to most key informants,
these "nesting" social structure groupings, especially the extended
families and lineages were quite important in the daily lives of the
Gadsup. However, all social structure groupings were said to be
stronger in the past before warfare was suppressed. Nonetheless, they
were identifiable by several older informants.

Discovering how important the extended families and lineages were
in marriages, feuding, political actions, lifecycle ceremonies (birth to
death), economic exchanges of food and pigs, and other material exchanges in the daily life of the people proved of great interest. I also
discovered strong ethnopsychological feelings and activities between
kinsmen that influenced caring and non-caring patterns related to
protection, keeping people well, and preventing sorcery. Kinship ties
influenced group cooperation, helping others with their work, caring
for others when in need, and food exchanges. These positive activities
helped to maintain village well being, solidarity, and protection.

While I found every Akunan had considerable freedom to make
choices and decisions, still these individuals were especially influenced
by the cultural values, beliefs, and practices of the extended family and
the lineages. The culture identity of the Gadsup Akunan as members
of the Gadsup tribe—viewed largely today as the large Gadsup community—was proudly talked about by adult male key informants and
some females. While individual decisions were made, they were influenced by kinship ties and the past Gadsup image with its deep historical roots. Although a full discussion of the kinship structure of the
Akunans is not possible here, the reader needs to realize that kinship
ties and the total social organization present were powerful means to
help Akunans feel not only united in some ways, but also "cared for"
and "cared about" in the village. It was fascinating to hear the villagers
talk about the ways kinship ties provided *protective care, surveillance
care,* and *nurturant activities* to support their growth, well being, and

community relatedness. The informants and my observations showed evident signs of Akunan *surveillance patterns* and of looking after one's "brothers" (including females) as supported by extended family members still today. Caring activities and attitudes were largely embedded in kinship ties and concomitant tacit behavioral expectations. Teasing out kinship and social structure features took considerable time along with confirmation of the credibility of such kinship ties. The Akunans were not ready to share spontaneously their social or kinship ties, and always wanted me to discover them first before adding any confirmation commitments. This was an interesting challenge, but through documentation of their genealogies and action patterns each day, it was possible not only to inductively confirm these patterns, but also to obtain a picture of how the villagers functioned in terms of social relatedness. Once I had identified the major features, several key informants said to me: "Now you know us and have it right. You speak true and know our ways. We have no more to tell you as you discovered our ways and we are happy." This search revealed how much they valued and kept kinship ties their secret *emic* information.

Non-caring behaviors were evident when kinship and social expectations were violated, cultural taboos overlooked, and role responsibilities neglected. Non-caring manifestations were usually altered by physical punishments to children, strong negative verbal responses to adults by the villagers, and open talks to those who violated cultural practices. When non-caring villagers caused trouble in the village, they were often denied a role in ceremonies, admonished by elders, and subject to being gossiped about by other Akunans.

Political Dimensions and Care

The Akunan "Big Men" (as they were called) were the active and respected political orators, decisions makers, and leaders for most internal and external village affairs. Political activities such as pig and food exchanges and dealing with sorcery accusations were in the hands of the "Big Men." These village concerns greatly influenced Akunan caring modes and their well being. Gadsup political activity largely focused on how one effectively and successfully dealt with crisis situations, maintained control, and handled local and intervillage affairs.

The "Big Men" had achieved their title and the prestige associated with it by being successful in "watching out" (surveillance) and "looking after" the political caring needs of the villagers. Exceptionally skilled in assessing group concerns, handling sorcery accusations, dealing with strangers, holding pig and food ceremonies, and in protecting the villagers, the "Big Men" had earned their title by repeatedly demonstrating good decision making, proper communication skills, as well as exhibiting bravery in fights and general leadership in the village. They were skilled in handling village problems by listening, seeking different viewpoints, and maintaining a caring attitude for all villagers with equal interest and good will. These political "Big Men," usually aged 45–65 years, had considerable village experience dealing with outside and inside village matters in diplomatic and successful ways. They were respected by most Akunans because they used and maintained the cultural values of egalitariansim, social control, protection, moral justice, and respect for all Gadsup people, land, and the past history. At no time did they manifest showy or ostentatious behavior. When conducting political sessions in the village plaza, they exhibited an equal interest in all attending but always kept the interests of the total Gadsup villagers in mind. They were exceptionally skilled in handling matters related to stealing pigs, women, food, property and discussing sorcery accusations. The political hearings which these political leaders conducted were always open to all Akunans and often times the entire village attended these sessions. The "Big Men" showed great acumen to handle tense matters in a protective caring way and with fairness and equal consideration to all.

Practically all key informants told me they valued the leadership of the "Big Men," but that they had often influenced their thinking prior to the village meetings while in the home hut. This also was an especially important women's secret—how to influence the male leaders without letting other males know. These women leaders gave accounts of how they discussed serious village matters and what they thought ought to be done while talking to their kinsmen or lineage leaders who were "Big Men." The women's viewpoints were taken into consideration in village political discussions and were used in some final decision's. Some of their ideas were confirmed with my observations. When the "Big Men" gave orations about village matters in the plaza, they expressed some women's ideas discussed prior to the meeting. At political meetings, the women usually sat in the outer circle with all the males sitting or standing in the inner circle and near the leader. The women seldom spoke out in public about the issue unless it was an older woman who knew the "Big Man" well. When asked about this behavior, the Akuna women said it was inappropriate to "talk out" at these meetings as it was the men who would be ultimately responsible for such big decisions and actions, and besides, they contended that they had already given their ideas to the political leader and "he usually used them."

Political actions and good decision making were extremely valued and important to the Akunans as it provided protection and security. Political activities with good leadership prevented serious intervillage feuding, fighting encounters, and curtailed ongoing discontent in the village. Key informants and all other villagers viewed this as "protective caring." Caring was embedded in the ways the people acted and made decisions in the village. Political caring was reinforced by the kinship system with social rules for protection and to prevent major inter-village problems from emerging. There were two men in the village, however, with different views on this matter. Both were silently jealous and wanted to be a "Big Man" leader. A threat to village solidarity and protection, these deviant men became known as "no goods." When the Akuna villagers became ill during the first Australian New Guinea election (Leininger, 1966b), these deviant men were viewed, in part, for the problems. In general, the "Big Men" were most effective in handling village and intervillage problems and to protect the people against threats of illnesses. Unquestionably, political caring increased group solidarity and helped the village to remain in control and maintain a positive image with other Akunans.

Economic Dimensions and Caring

Since the Akunans maintained their daily lives on a very lean subsistence economy, they were constantly attentive to the women who provided garden foods, their most reliable survival resource. Shortly before my arrival, the Akunans had begun to raise coffee trees on a few acres of land via a promotional campaign for cash income by the Australian government. Although the income from selling coffee beans was very small, it helped them to buy shorts, enamel pans, rice, canned fish, salt, tobacco, and several other items Akunans longed for at the nearest trade store. In addition, there was an exchange of money for pigs with nearby villagers usually for ceremonial food gathering or for marriage and birth ceremonies. Pigs also were used as bride wealth. The major economic sources for wealth or subsistence was the exchange of a small margin of extra garden foods, raising coffee beans, selling or exchanging pigs, and the men and women doing periodic roadwork for the Australian government. (With the latter activity, they were seldom paid. In my experience, women were never paid by the Austrialian government for their roadwork, even during the rainy season when roads were completely washed out and women did most of the work.)

Reflecting on the Akunan economy and caring, I discovered that health and well being were related to caring and non-caring patterns and that economics supported care behaviors primarily to maintain the villagers' health. There also were signs of caring patterns with women caring for small children and pigs. Intervillage exchanges of food symbolized Akunan ways of caring for their own people and other Gadsups. The women who controlled the gardens and distributed the foods demonstrated caring and non-caring expressions as well: caring with food reflected nurturance as care and providing for the health and well being of their extended families each day. Garden foods, the major substance source, was collected and shared with extended family members daily, but also with lineages on special village affairs. From such sharing came nurturant and protective caring. The women also showed non-caring behaviors when they would withhold food from their husbands, children, or other kinspersons for various reasons such as wife beating, breaking of cultural taboos, punishing children inappropriately, or neglecting their social roles involved with children and infants.

Technological Influences and Care

Since the Gadsup Akunans had no modern Western technologies, there was no use of such technologies for physical care. Instead, care was more sociocultural. The villagers had their own material or native garden and hunting technologies which included handmade tools such as wooden digging sticks, stone adzes and hoes, wooden bows, and stone arrows for hunting. In the past, there were war shields and special fighting equipment for intervillage warfare and head hunting for male honor and prestige. Women made their infant and garden string bags, their grass skirts, and pandanus mats for infants. Gadsup men made wooden vessels in which to place their cooked earth oven foods. They also made musical ceremonial instruments such as the small mouth harp, ceremonial drums, bamboo smoking pipes, big head pieces for *singsings* (dance festivals), and arm and leg amulets. Great care was demonstrated in making these cultural items in good artistic style and usually for practical and functional purposes. Cooperative caring and supportive village behaviors were important among the elders in making sex-linked artifacts as well. Such village artifacts were made as secret sex symbols. Through these activities, then, Gadsup villagers enjoyed their ceremonies, consumed healthy foods, and felt at home in their villages.

Educational, Language, and Caring Influences

The Akunans had only informal or local educational experiences. There was no formal educational system established for the children until the end of my field research. Informal education was largely an enculturation process of helping the child or adult to learn the Gadsup and particularly Akunan culture in order to live properly and survive. Many village kinspeople were involved in helping small children and young boys and girls become enculturated about Gadsup cultural values, taboos, and appropriate living and caring ways in order to avoid intra and intervillage conflicts or problems. Children and adolescents had positive role models to observe and work with throughout the lifecycle. *Experiential learning-in-context* was the major teaching and learning mode for all villagers at different periods in the lifecycle. Informal education was achieved by using real, concrete, and practical life situations, and by talking about Gadsup village events, incidents, and ceremonies. Children and adolescents were always free to be active participants in daily and most nightly community affairs. Very few facts of life were hidden from them. A rich oral history replete with legend and information necessary to be a true Akunan was available. In the early 1960s, however, their language had not been completely analyzed by linguistic experts—a major communication handicap for me. I spoke Melanesian Pidgin English and also learned some common language expressions. During the first few months, I focused on nonverbal communication and on intense observations and cue behavior to confirm with the people what I had seen and experienced. The Gadsups taught me that my nonverbal American gestures did not accurately communicate meanings to Gadsups. Learning Gadsup gestures with *meanings-in-context* was extremely important in my grasping and understanding Gadsup lifeways as well as for Gadsups in their understanding of me. It also was important to learn some Gadsup expressions of phrases for my survival, especially when I was feared as a potential sorceress who could cause village harm. Informal verbal and nonverbal learning between researcher and Gadsups occurred daily.

The Gadsups depended greatly on oral narratives to learn about their culture, their nearby world, and most everything of importance to them. As mentioned above, many oral Gadsup creation myths, historical legends, life histories, narrative events, and daily life experiences constituted some of the informal teaching and learning modes used. The Gadsup like these informal teaching and learning ways and often spoke of them as "our good ways." Caring expressions by being patient, helping others to learn, and being protective by being sure you understood the language was important. They also cared for others by sharing daily life experiences and special life events.

Caring expressions through informal educational experiences were manifested with caring behaviors related to knowing how to help others, anticipation of other's needs, learning to be a protective sharing Gadsup, groups, and by knowing how to help others to prevent unhealthy or illness conditions. Learning to avoid violating cultural taboos and discovering ways to be a "good ethical and moral Gadsup" were frequently emphasized by all key and general village informants.

Folk (Generic) Care and Health (Well Being) System

For years, the Akunans have relied upon their folk indigenous care system which they claim has helped them to keep well and healthy. The concept of care was used and known in their language and actions. While *care* and *caring* were used in different ways and with slightly different referent meanings, they generally referred "to *protective* and *nurturant ways* to enable Gadsups to grow, function, and survive" (Leininger, 1966a, 1970). Caring was primarily associated with the idea of a nurturant act of helping children and adults grow holistically; caring was not associated with an intellectual dichotomization of humans into mind and body or biopsychosocial beings. Instead, caring was documented by key and general informants as nurturant lifecycle activities related to growth and development experiences as part of living and being in the Gadsup Akunan world. In discussions with females, caring ideas came easier than in discussions with males, for caring was essential for infant survival and in raising healthy or well children. I observed caring acts of the mother and her female kinswomen in the village as they watched, protected, and held vulnerable newborns both by day and night. Women protected infants and children from external harm such as sorcery, cold air, and occasionally physical harm. Sorcery was always a threat to vulnerable newborn infants and children, especially by outside strangers who used substances such as feces, blood, or "not good foods." Maternal caring was expressed in infant breastfeeding, the mother intuitively and knowing the needs of her infant and small children. Stroking, rubbing, talking, and feeding infants were nurturant caring acts. The mother and her kinsmen watched and helped the children grow properly. Such nurturant acts continued throughout the early years of childhood, but changed in form and expression for males and females at about age ten. Nonetheless, caring activities from birth to old age were held as essential for the health or well being of the individual, family, and community despite slightly different processes and activities among the caregivers. Unquestionably, the women carried the heaviest responsibility for nurturant caring activities and attitudes.

While the Gadsup cared for individuals, they also always focused on the village group and what was happening to them. Caring activities for kinsmen and kinswomen were valued and expected in the village. If kin resided in another village, such as a daughter who was married and living in her husband's village (patrilocal), caring concerns prevailed for her. Caring was especially directed to families, lineages, groups, and to sociocultural institutions such as birth, marriage, and death ceremonies. The Gadsup emphases on "*other-care,*" as I referred to this in 1960, was a discovery important for its sharp contrast with present-day

American nursing "self-care" ideologies and practices (Orem, 1980). Several key informants stated, "We care for all Gadsups (referring to the "oneness and unity" concept as the broadest cultural identity of the Gadsup) just like we care for our children, small pigs, and others in our big families." Several key informants added, "It is important that we care for all kinsmen and all in our related groups (referring to the lineage) and to all in our big Gadsup community." Thus, caring was more group and other-care oriented than self-care oriented for individuals. When I asked, "How does caring help your people?", informants usually replied, "It keeps us together, well, and growing healthy . . . It helps to work in our gardens, hunt and do our village work." While the Gadsup did not neglect individuals and their care concerns or needs, the idea of a community and village care ethos prevailed.

In attempting to discover if there were any differences between care and health, the informants replied, "Health is being able to do our work each day . . . Health is being able to go to our gardens each day (females)." Others said, "When we can no longer do our daily work, we have to stay in this village like our elderly men and women, then we are not as healthy." They added, "We die when our muscles are no longer able to function or if a sorcerer or sorceress kills us." Many informants said, "If we care for our people with food, watching out for them (surveillance and protection), then we can protect them from sorcery and enemies . . . But we must also watch that they do not break village taboos, so they will remain well and be healthy." The concept of health, therefore, was differentiated from the concept of care as delineated above. Care and caring remained the powerful explanatory means to keep people well, healthy, and prevent illness in the village.

Folk care practices using local material substances that included ritual caring acts were more fully known to Akunan females than males. The women were able to identify the caring acts and ways they cared for villagers to prevent potential harm and the threat of illnesses or death. In contrast, males were far more oriented to curing acts and knew how to call on curers as specialists outside the village to deal with selected illnesses, major body injuries (fractures), or to cure powerful illnesses due to male sorcery. These findings were repeatedly confirmed and established as patterns of care and cure with ethnonursing and ethnoscience linguistic analysis of village data (Leininger, 1970). Findings from this fieldwork provided the first evidence that care and cure are gender linked and that there are different ways of caring and curing with females and males. Caring was viewed as largely a female role whereas curing was viewed as a male role in Gadsup land and throughout their long prehistory. (Parenthetically, this may be a precursor to early professional Western practices in nursing and medicines.)

While special medicines were used in Gadsup caring and curing practices, emphasis was given to caring ways as a means to prevent illness and maintain well being. This finding, confirmed repeatedly, helped me realize the great importance of care and caring, and the role of nurses as care providers and in illness prevention and health maintenance—an idea in direct contrast to the Western view of the nurse as a medicine dispenser, a handmaiden to physicians, or as some other "medical" technician. The Gadsup helped me to become keenly conscious of the significant role of women as caring experts.

Folk caring was symbolically expressed by selecting special foods for the pregnant spouse before, during, and occasionally after pregnancy. These food preferences surrounding pregnancy were known in the village, and it was the husband who often walked great distances to get such foods. In addition, mothers, brothers, mothers' sisters, and close kinsmen showed anticipatory and nurturant caring for pregnant women by buying or requesting special food from strangers or friends. Caring by mothers in breastfeeding their newborns and their young children (ages 2–5) were examples of caring as nurturance to help Akunans grow, be healthy, avoid illnesses, and become strong, healthy, and active men and women. These attributes also had economic benefits in the prevention of costly illnesses or death.

Folk caring modalities to prevent sickness and death and to protect the villagers from sorcery accusations and actions were documented and confirmed on repeated occasions. Many folk preventive carative measures were identified when villagers would alert other careless villagers about the disposal of their hair clippings, nails, and human excreta. They also watched for signs of the villagers violating cultural taboos or breaking village rules. Such actions were identified as noncaring behaviors and given negative sanctions by family or friends. Acts of surveillance, protection, and prevention measures were often documented within and outside the village to prevent illnesses (largely related to sorcery) or careless behaviors. Folk caring behaviors also were manifested at village ceremonies related to newborns, at marriage ceremonies, at village feasts, and at death ceremonies. For example, men's legs were pricked with leaves to reduce edema after hours of ceremonial dancing and during birth in the bush hut folk touching practices were used. Of course, many other folk practices were used as caring to promote healing and well being.

Unquestionably, the Gadsup were deeply interested in and con-cerned about *prevention* as an important caring modality. Modes of prevention were based on maintaining cultural norms and practices rather than focusing primarily on physical activities or psychological factors as emphasized in most Western health systems. Preventing chil-dren or adults from becoming physically ill or experiencing threats to health or to their lives could be prevented by maintaining cultural rules or norms. Adult key female informants often made these state-ments: "We must teach our children how to protect themselves so they won't get sick and die . . . We teach them our ways—the good ways to act . . ." "We love our children and we do not want them to die . . ." "We must *watch* (surveillance) that our infants and children do not have sorcerers making them ill and die . . ." "We also must help our adolescents not get into big intervillage trouble in our own village feuds as some adults get too angry and kill each other like they did in the past. . . ." "We teach them to obey our ways." These verba-tim statements and others supported evidence that watchfulness, pro-tection, and prevention were all important caring modes in Akunan life.

Primary caregivers were adult women and young girls (7–14 years). Acutely ill males with distended abdomens, sorcery pains, and back pain would occasionally go to experienced female caregivers even though they feared possible contamination with menstrual blood. The majority of males went to male curers in other friendly Gadsup villages for curing treatments related to breaking culture taboos, broken bones, arrow tip injuries, cuts, and other unknown conditions.

Every two to three months the Australian government provided the services of a public health nurse and a "doctor boi" (a native helper who spoke Pidgin English and English) at a health station nearly two miles away from the village. The Australian Patrol officers told the Akunan villagers "to bring their small children to these stations for medicines." Gadsup women were most reluctant to do this, however. They believed that the danger of their small child being exposed to sorcery and other cultural illnesses outweighed any possible benefit of a visit. Consequently, only five or six women would go, and then reluctantly, to the station. While with the nurse, the child was weighed and given immunizations. During these procedures, mothers and their infants and small children grew very frightened and they put a white powdered substance on the child's fontanel to protect the child from harm. The health nurse, usually not aware of the great fear of the mothers, was not too effective in her efforts. This nurse focused mainly on the physical condition of the child, weighing, checking his or her skin, and trying to immunize the child. The nurse had no knowledge of her client's culture and how culture influenced health and illness states.

There was a small hospital about 25 miles from the Gadsup village, but this service was seldom used by the villagers; they feared it was a "house of sorcery." Periodically, when I visited this hospital, I could see the fear of many natives who came there. Very infrequently, Akunans came there for an illness that did not respond to folk practices. While in the two Akunan villages I studied, I found no evidence of cancer, mental psychoses, or heart attacks. There were, however, sorcery conditions, pneumonia (during rainy season), and gastrointestinal disturbances (i.e., villagers with diarrhea). Skin lacerations, and broken bones or head injuries were other of the more common health conditions of the Akunans. The latter were often due to village fights within or at another village and usually appeared more commonly in men than women. Occasionally, however, I found women with head and body injuries due to women fighting over men or due to adulterous relationships. The women, however, seldom went to the hospital. Children and elderly died most frequently due to pneumonia during the rainy season. Parenthetically, when I made a return visit in 1978, the Akunans suffered new kinds of illnesses: drug dependency, broken bones due to car accidents (not fights), and severe malnutrition. The impact of Western contacts and a poor cash economy, plus other factors too numerous to discuss here, had markedly changed the Akunan caring and health status. Clearly, the health status of Akunans was more favorable in the early 1960s then in late 1978.

Cultural Value Influences

Thus far I have identified and discussed some of the major Gadsup Akunan cultural values as derived from grounded *emic* ethnonursing and ethnographic data. These values, extremely important to understand culture care fully, were embedded in the social structure and values of the Gadsup and can be summarized as follows:

1. *Patriarchialism* was a culture value evident in male authority decision making and authority in diverse aspects of the social structure as reflected in the daily lifeways of the people.

2. *Extended family ties and social relatedness* were important culture values which influenced Gadsup patterns of relationships to different groups, and in marriage, birth, festive, and death ceremonies. Kinship patterns and relationships influenced what was acceptable and non-acceptable behavior in the village and with non-Gadsups.

3. *Egalitarianism* was identified as a cultural value reflecting ways the villagers attempted to maintain and value equal peer relationships and to avoid "showy man or woman behaviors." "Big Men" in the village had to watch their behavior in political and economic affairs and not be too different from other village men.

4. *Acknowledging gender differences* was a cultural value held to be extremely important among the Gadsups. Males and females had different roles, material items, capabilities, and responsibilities. Female and male secrets were important in all ceremonies and rituals, and were viewed as complimentary attributes of humans. Separate material objects and symbols were valued, owned, and used by males and females.

5. *Maintaining communal relationships* was a value upheld by the Akunans who saw themselves as part of the largest social and cultural Gadsup community. They believed they came from "one vine" (symbol of continuity, growth, and unity) and should remain aligned. Hospitality and communal respect was expected among all Gadsups, but still silently acknowledging friendly and enemy villages. Communal care values within and outside the villages was an ideal to prevent unfavorable relationships, hostilities, open aggression, feuds, sorcery accusations, and remain a Gadsup. However, open feuds did occur in the larger Gadsup community despite efforts to suppress them. The care values of surveillance,

protection, and communal assistance among "Gadsup brothers" were expected.

6. *Experiential learning* was greatly valued because it was essential to help Akunans discover and know their ecology (immediate physical environments) including: trees and plants, animals, material culture, legends, and all aspects of current and past Gadsup life. Gadsups were expected to share whatever they had learned with other villagers and of their spiritual lessons from Gadsup ancestors. Concrete, practical, and mundane life experiences were important to know and to transmit to current and future generations. These cultural values and others (along with many beliefs) were confirmed and had meaning-in-context with recurrent patterning in the Akunan daily lifeways and as part of the enculturation process.

Thematic Data Analysis and Culture Care Theory

During the 18-month period I spent in two villages conducting this ethnonursing and ethnographic study, I gathered much new knowledge and experiences. Detailed observations and participatory experiences along with tape recordings and use of photos for stories brought forth meaningful data of Akuna care, health, and lifeways. The full account will be published in a forthcoming book, but here only major findings related to the theory of Culture Care Diversity and Universality will be presented.

Data analysis specific to the ethnonursing method was done in accord with Leininger's Ethnonursing Phases of Analysis for Qualitative Data Analysis already explained in Chapter 2. Data bearing on the theory were systematically examined using the five qualitative criteria discussed in Chapter 2. I systematically collected, recorded, and analyzed all raw or grounded field data beginning from the first day in the village. I also made nightly observations to obtain a full account of caring for a 24-hour period. The grounded *emic* (local people) data were a saturated and very rich source of data on which to identify themes and other findings related to the domain of inquiry. I analyzed all ethnonursing *emic* data from Phase 1 (raw data) to Phase 2 in which

I focused on specific descriptors and components as revealed in the Sunrise Model. In Phase 3, I studied these data further for recurrent patterns, specific contextual meanings, and credibility. Finally, in Phase 4, I abstracted themes and diverse or similar research findings from both raw *emic* and *etic* data.

In this next section, I will demonstrate how I arrived at themes from Phase 1, 2, 3, and 4 using one major theme. Space does not permit such an explication for the remaining themes. Before presenting one example of one theme and findings, however, I should discuss some culture care constructs to bring forth fuller meanings from the findings. These *culture care emic* constructs were largely embedded in data related to the worldview, social structure, language environment, and folk care system. They would be essential to help the transcultural nurse to focus on each care construct to provide congruent care to Gadsup Akunans. Below are presented *culture care meanings and action modes* in order of greatest importance to the villagers (established largely with the criteria of credibility, confirmability, recurrent patterning, and saturation) (Leininger 1987, 1990).

1. *Surveillance* (look out for, watching for as surveillance care). Two kinds of surveillance were identified namely, *surveillance nearby* and *surveillance-at-a-distance*. These modes of surveillance were held important for well being and health of all Akunan key and general informants. The commitment to be surveillant was seen repeatedly in practice in the village by all villagers but especially in the gardens by the women and in the forest by the men. Women were more surveillant than men; men were more watchful with protective care outside of the village.

2. *Protection* (protective care and caring). This construct was extremely important to the Akunans. It had two major features, namely, (1) *protecting Akunans inside and outside the village;* (2) *protective care of infants throughout the lifecycle.* Protective village care was manifested in daily observations and participatory activities by *obeying cultural taboos and sanctions.* Such protective care was critical to protect the villagers from sorcery, illnesses, death, and unfavorable cultural situations. Lifecycle protective care was maintained well

by women in early years of life (up to 15 years); whereas the men were more effective in protective village care.

3. *Nurturance* (nurturant care and caring). Nurturance was manifest primarily with women in ways they helped infants and adults grow, function, and survive in Gadsup land. Males learned how to nurture young boys and married men. Nurturance was an integral part of child and adolescent care. The women were resourceful in providing nurturance. Women key informants said, "We believe in nurturance for our survival . . . It helps children to grow and be good strong Gadsup." This concept of nurturance was the first concept identified in transcultural nursing research and it supports the epistemic roots of nursing being derived from nurturance with special meanings to the Gadsup. (This was an important discovery in the 1960s, and is still little studied in nursing.)

4. *Prevention* (preventive care and caring ways). This care construct was an integral part of daily and nightly living to avoid negative sanctions, harm to group, illnesses, disabilities, and sudden death. Preventive care also was manifested by caring actions such as avoiding intervillage conflicts, problems, and stresses which could lead to feuds, potential killing, or "crippling" of the villagers. Prevention as caring was demonstrated through cultural stories, legends, narratives, alarming events, and experiential informal education in daily contextual experiences. All villagers were active supporters for preventive caring modes, and if not, one was suspected to be a sorcerer or "too deviant a person."

5. *Respecting for sex differences.* Care meant respect for and observance of differences between males and females from birth to death. Role entailments, responsibilities, and activities by sexes was a feature of being a caring Gadsup and to facilitate village work and regulate village stresses and behaviors. All villagers upheld their longstanding beliefs in sex differences in work role, play, and other facets of Akuna life being a caring community.

6. *Touching* (touching as care and caring). Touching was expressed by bare body hugs, mainly between men, and by

women stroking, rubbing, and kissing infants. Women touched infants for growth and stimulation and to console. Intimate touching between sexes was only for married spouses, and if sexual intercourse occurred outside of marriage and was discovered, this led to fights and other serious repercussions. The firm shaking of a child for not obeying cultural taboos was used, but seldom severe physical punishment. Intensive touching in domestic quarrels or in male or female feuds also was identified. Wife and spouse abuse occurred and was viewed as a noncaring form of touching and protection.

MAJOR THEME FINDINGS

As one examines a major theme of the Akunans in light of the theory and Leininger's mode of data analysis, one will note special features and findings.

Major Theme One

Culture care means surveillance and protective action to ensure the health or well being of Gadsup Akunans.
This major theme was confirmed repeatedly as credible and important by all key and over 90 percent of all the village informants in Akuna village. Several said to me, "Now you speak true of us and know our lifeways . . . This is our lifeways and what we believe is important." Some verbatim statements with action patterns as an example to establish confirmability, credibility and meanings-in-context of theme one at each phase of Leininger's (1987, 1990) data analysis are as follows: (Code: FAKI = Female Adult Key Informant; MAKI = Male Adult Key Informant).

Phase 1: Documentation with Raw Emic (Local) Care Data
FAKI: "We watch over our infants, small boys and girls and others in the village so that no harm comes to them; We keep healthy and well because we protect our children from sorcery, illnesses, and outside threats to us."

MAKI: "Akuna men know how to watch at a distance . . . We watch over the grassland, our enemies and friends, and down the road to protect our villagers from strangers and sorcerers . . ." "It is a man's protective job to do this and not a woman's."

Phase 2: Care Descriptors and Components (only key phrases are identified from the raw data).

FAKI: *Watching over* is important for health and well being; Watching and *being there* and *over the person*; *Protecting* is done by *watching out for others* (demonstrated by many actions of *watching over* and *watching for* others).

MAKI: "Must *protect* our children and adults . . . *Watch out for the sorcerers* is essential . . . Our families, lineages, and villages need to be protected day and night . . . In the past we had surprise attacks and some did not watch well, we lost villagers."

Phase 3: Care Patterns and Meanings-in-Context Features (stated as patterns from above descriptors and components).

FAKI: *Female patterns:* (1) The researcher found that every morning for nine months the women and young girls went to the garden (universal); (2) Mothers placed their infants in net bags on a post which held the child in a pandanus mat to protect them (universal); (3) Mothers relied on young girls (7–12 years) to protect and watch over siblings to keep well; (4) Women watched over adolescent girls when delivering betel nut to strangers for their well being. (The meanings-in-context can be trailed to the raw data.)

MAKI: *Male patterns:* (1) Accompanied young boys with their bows and arrows into forest area to hunt animals, to eat, to be spiritually inspired, and to be healthy; (2) Men watched over villagers and protected the males and females from sorcery in order to keep them well; (3) Males conduct male initiation rights to "protect males who still have female blood in them."

Phase 4: Stating the Major Theme (this was the abstracted theme grounded in Phase 1 and could be trailed with detailed data in Phases 2 and 3): "*Culture care means surveillance and protective actions to ensure health and well being.*" This theme is grounded in Phase 1 and can be trailed in Phases 2 and 3.

There were, of course, other interesting findings related to this theme such as the following: (1) young children (5–19 years) could only walk down the road to a certain place and then turn around and come back to the village (this was a strong past culture value still alive); (2) watching meant to Akunans to be *attentive to* and *listen for sounds* across the lands of enemies several miles away; (3) Gadsup women were solely responsible for bearing healthy children to see that their children became adults, got married, and had children. Male and female roles were very different, and yet complimentary for watching and preventing care role activities.

Major Theme Two

Culture care means nurturance that helps people grow, perform roles, and survive throughout the lifecycle and is influenced by social structure factors and folk care practices.

This theme was firmly confirmed by 95 percent of key and village informants. The credibility and confirmability of this theme was trailed from *emic* verbal statements, to daily observations, and to participatory actions by the villagers at different phases of the lifecycle, i.e., from birth, young child, older child, young man, and finally adult married men and women. Essential to grasp the significance of the theme and to understand patterns, norms, symbols and ways that nurturance took on meaning to the Akunans was meaning-in-context. Mothers were central figures to nurture female infants (often on demand) and at birth ceremonies. Male kinsmen, especially the mother's brother, were involved in nurturance to help the child grow strong and healthy. Garden foods were the "best" nurturant food, and the people valued their homegrown foods as safe to eat. Men provided diversity of foods.

This theme had evidence of saturation and recurrent patterning criteria throughout the lifecycle accounts and in social structure factors (especially political, education, and economic factors). It was extremely important that I observed, with some regularity, the many *folk* and *generic* care practices on different occasions, in different contexts, and over an extended period of time.

Major Theme Three

Culture care (caring) means keeping "good" culture values and lifeways based on Gadsup ethnohistory, social structure, and worldview in order to prevent illnesses, keep well, healthy, and to avoid unnecessary intervillage conflicts and stresses.

Key and village Akunan informants established as credible and confirmed this theme. Saturation with recurrent patterning became evident in practically every aspect of Gadsup living, and with only slight variations or diversities. The culture history, political, kinship, and religious beliefs and practices greatly influenced direct and indirect caring patterns to remain well, become ill, or unhealthy. Women kinfolk who married into the village (newcomers) expressed the greatest differences in their ways of viewing care and health. Folk tales, village stories, and caring narratives reinforced recurrent patterns of well being, health, or illness. Non-caring ways of strangers who influenced or "caused" sorcery and illnesses, which often led to feuds and intervillage accusations, constituted the greatest areas of conflict related to this theme.

Major Theme Four

Care means respecting male and female sex differences in order to confirm role complimentarity, to maintain health, and to fulfill prescribed village role responsibilities.

Over 93 percent of key and village informants established as credible and confirmed this theme. I documented this theme via field journal notes by observing recurrent patterns of behavior regarding sex role attributes and action modes and with saturation data from the Observation-Participation-Reflection Guide. Male and female role differences prevailed in every aspect of the villager's lives. The social structure, worldview, past history, folk care, and many different life span data supported sex differences. Birth, marriage, and death ceremonies had sex role performance differences revealed in folk legends and language expressions of both sexes. Such sex differences were held as essential for a division of labor (role complimentarity) as serving as role modeling for children and young adults. Such gender differences had a definite impact on the quality of health or well being of individuals, families, and lineage members. When sex roles were culturally violated or daily roles not performed properly, cultural conflicts and potential harm to the "deviant" individual arose via village gossip and direct actions by the "Big Men" or other involved kinsmen. Ethical sanctions related to proper sex behavior was often buttressed by the ancestor's moral life essence principles and beliefs. The five criteria used for qualitative research (Leininger, 1990) supported this theme, especially *meaning-in-context* and *recurrent repatterning* in political, kinship, education, and human care expressions.

Although other qualitative findings from this study arose, the above themes were, from an ethnonursing perspective, the most dominant and prevailing. These findings were important indicators to substantiate the assumptions and tenets of Culture Care theory which have been presented throughout this chapter. From the above themes and other findings, the nurse would have knowledge to provide culturally congruent nursing care—the goal of the theory.

NURSING CARE ACTIONS AND DECISIONS FOR GADSUP AKUNAN

In light of findings from this study, the nurse is challenged to use worldview, social structure, language expressions, environment, and folk practices to study ways to provide culture-specific and culturally congruent care. Although many nursing care actions and decisions are evident from the thick and rich inductively derived ethnonursing study, several areas will be presented only. The reader will note that I prefer not to use the term *intervention*. All too frequently this term implies curtailing or changing the status of something or in imposing a different mode of acting in a culture. As the nurse functions in different cultures, it may be quite inappropriate to change or curtail something, and indeed, the nurse may need to preserve or maintain that which exists as beneficial to clients.

From this study, *generic folk care* knowledge would be essential for *professional nursing care* knowledge and practices. *Emic generic care* and *caring* that was largely embedded in the worldview, social structure, and other areas depicted in the Sunrise Model influenced Akunans' health and well being as well as illness patterns. Interestingly, *health* was frequently used interchangeably with *well being*, reflecting a comprehensive view of total functioning within a given environment; whereas *health* was a state of being that enabled a person to perform role functions within cultural expectations.

Turning to the three modes of decision and action, professional nurses need to use culture-specific care knowledges that *preserve* and *maintain* health. Among these expectations and of major focus would be to preserve most male and female role responsibilities that support their well being. It would be quite difficult to change male and female roles without serious cultural conflicts and major disruptions of social structure and lifeways of the people. Gender differences are strongly confirmed and embedded in the social structure. While a Western feminist nurse might be inclined to alter gender roles "to improve Akunan women lifeways," this could lead to major difficulties. Likewise, Akunan males generally value their role entailments as complimentary to the women. While males expressed protective care roles, they also envied female fertility and procreative abilities—females believing here that they were a key factor in bearing and nurturing healthy infants and children. (Future care repatterning of belief systems might be considered as role changes are desired by the villagers.) The nurse also might be tempted to provoke Gadsup women toward overt activity in political affairs. However, Akunan women, for one, believed they were quite effective in domestic political affairs as they were, and I found evidence to support some of their beliefs and action modes. Women did influence men's public decisions and actions. (This finding dispels a Western conceit that as "third world women" have virtually no power, men have all the power; hence, "empowerment" becomes a goal.)

Given the discovery of the knowledge and importance and use of the care constructs of *surveillance, protection, nurturance, prevention,* and *appropriate touching,* such care constructs with meanings and action modes would require preservation. These care constructs have been quite effective in maintaining health and well being for many years and through many generations. Knowledge of each care construct and how it could be used to preserve the ongoing health of the Gadsup for congruent care would be important.

The value of *egalitarianism* among extended family members was another major knowledge area discovered in this study. To preserve and maintain Gadsup relationships as *"true brothers"* and *equals in social and cultural relationships* would be essential to reduce sorcery accusations, conflicts, and maintain health.

Care knowledge discovered with regard to *nurturance* as a means to *preserve* the idea of helping Akunans to grow, survive, and stay healthy by many nurturant activities would be extremely important. In addition, some rituals, such as feeding of the infant by kinsmen as a symbol for growth, would be valuable to *preserve*. Nurturant care by female girls in the culture might be considered for *culture care negotiation* or *repatterning* with the free roaming young boys who had nothing to do. Care by elders who no longer worked in the gardens and who cared for children in the village was appropriate and protective of the children's health; hence, *care preservation* would be needed here. In a culture where sex differences predominate, the effect on health of women as *caregivers* and men as *curers* was curious. When women caregivers were in control, they maintained good health; when men curers were in control, they maintained poor health. Further study of how care and cure differ with women and men in generic care is needed.

Knowledge generated from this study regarding illness and prevention modalities also needs to be preserved for congruent Akunan care practices. In addition, the role of preventing conflicts and illness by preserving culture values needs to be considered by Western culture. For example, Western medications could be viewed as potential sorcery materials in the village unless the nurse had developed trust with the Akunans. The nurse also would need to keep in mind that as a woman is a potential sorceress, a male nurse (as a "doctor boi") might make Western emergency medications or treatments more acceptable to Akunans. In this regard, the nurse could use the Leininger Stranger-Friend Guide in assessing his or her relationship with strangers.

The professional nurse could consider repatterning and restructuring with the Akunans regarding their beliefs about menstrual blood as harmful or destructive to others by talking to the women and letting them reflect on other possible ideas. Helping the women realize (from the nurse's professional knowledge) that menstrual blood usually does not kill women in other cultures, again, is something for the women to reflect on and repattern if desired or chosen. In changing this belief, a trusting friend relationship would be necessary.

Knowledge of the many positive generic folk health practices with the use of cultural care constructs of *surveillance, protection, nurturance, prevention,* and *touching* in caring relationships with others would need to be preserved and used with professional generic care practices. Western professional values such as self-care, assertiveness, treating sexes alike, competition, and use of high technologies would encounter much difficulty in this culture.

The healthy foods in the Akunan culture, such as the fresh garden greens, fruits, seasonal nuts, sweet potatoes, bananas, and other fresh foods, should be preserved. Introduction of milk is inappropriate as Akunans had a lactose ingestion problem. Introducing some meat and fish was much desired and this could be done as culture care accommodation. Preventing mental illness, dreaded diseases, and obesity as known in our Western world should be given full thought and as lessons for the "why" of these transcultural differences. We have much to learn from this culture. A number of other nursing care decisions could be considered related to the three modes predicted in the theory of culture care. The nurse would need to complete this phase of examining the theory by systematically studying what transpired with the use of each of the three modes of care and its impact to provide culture congruent care.

CONCLUSION

In this chapter, I have examined the theory of Culture Care with the Gadsup (Akunans) of the Eastern Highlands of New Guinea with the ethnonursing research method. The method was extremely important in teasing out and obtaining in-depth data to confirm the theory. Studying the worldview, social structure, ethnohistory, language, and folk beliefs and practices were essential in discovering care and caring influences on Gadsup health and well being. For the Gadsup universals predominated over diversities related to human care. The embedded care form, expression, and values are extremely important to provide culturally congruent care that is meaningful, appropriate, and beneficial to the culture. This study reveals the importance of *generic* care that must be explicated to develop humanistic and scientific care for the discipline of nursing. Such knowledge will help us shift from the traditional medical model to a true nursing model with care as the essence of nursing. This first transcultural care study should encourage nurses to realize the significance of care and why care has been difficult to explicate because of its invisible features lodged in social structure and other areas as depicted in the Sunrise Model. Finally, this research had a profound influence on my professional life, for it gave me new confidence about discovering care knowledge and the diverse care expressions, meanings, and forms of care. This body of knowledge gives hope for future nurse researchers to become full participants in a culture to document the epistemic source of generic care and its potential relationship to advanced professional nursing knowledge. Although I took a certain personal risk in doing such nursing and anthropological research in a culture that views women as potential sorceresses, I learned much from the people who became my "true friend" and teacher.

NOTES

[1] It should be noted that a girl is not called a woman until she has married and had a child; likewise, a boy is not called a man until he has married and had a child. Hence, the terms of *girl* and *boy* were used until marriage. (Leininger, 1966b, 1978).

REFERENCES

Aamodt, A. (1978). Sociocultural dimensions of caring in the world of the Papago child and adolescent. In M. M. Leininger (Ed.), *Transcultural Nursing Theory and Practices*. New York: John Wiley & Sons.

Bohay, I. (1989). *Ethnonursing study: Lithuanian parent beliefs and experiences*. Unpublished master's dissertation. Detroit: Wayne State University Press.

Brown, E. L. (1948). *Nursing for the future*. New York: Russell Sage Foundation.

du Toit, B. M. (1975). *Akuna: A New Guinea Village Community*. Rotterdam: A. A. Balkema.

Dougherty, M., & T. Tripp-Reimer (1985). The interface of nursing and anthropology. *Annual Review of Anthropology, 14,* 219.

Gates, M. (1989). *Care and care meanings, experiences and orientations of persons dying in hospital and hospital settings*. Unpublished doctoral dissertation. Detroit: Wayne State University Press.

Horn, B. (1978). Transcultural nursing and child-rearing of Muckleshoot people. In M. M. Leininger (Ed.), *Transcultural nursing: Concepts, theories, and practices*, New York: John Wiley & Sons, 223–239.

Leininger, M. M. (1964). A Gadsup village experiences its first election. New Guinea's first national election: A symposium. *Journal of the Polynesian Society, 73*(2).

Leininger, M. M. (1966a). *Convergence and divergence of human behavior: An ethnopsychological comparative study of two Gadsup villages in the Eastern Highlands of New Guinea*. Doctoral dissertation. Seattle: University of Washington.

Leininger, M. M. (1966b). *New Guinea micro-evolution studies*. Department of Anthropology, University of Washington, Seattle, memorandum no. 18, 32–37.

Leininger, M. M. (1970). *Nursing and anthropology: Two worlds to blend*. New York: John Wiley & Sons.

Leininger, M. M. (1978a). *Transcultural nursing: Concept, theories, and practices*. New York: John Wiley & Sons.

Leininger, M. M. (1978b). The Gadsup of New Guinea and early child-caring behaviors with nursing care implications. In *Transcultural nursing: Concepts, theories, and practices*. New York: John Wiley & Sons, 375–397.

Leininger, M. M. (1979). *Transcultural nursing*. New York: Masson Publishing Co.

Leininger, M. M. (1985). *Qualitative research methods in nursing*. Orlando, FL: Grune and Stratton.

Leininger, M. M. (1987). *Care: Discovery and uses in clinical and community nursing*. Detroit: Wayne State University Press, 1–30.

Leininger, M. M. (1988). *Care: An essential human need*. Detroit: Wayne State University Press.

Leininger, M. M. (1990). The philosophic and epistemic bases to explicate transcultural nursing knowledge. *Journal of Transcultural Nursing*. Memphis, TN: University of Tennessee Press, 1(2), 40–51.

Littlewood, R. A. (1972). *Physical anthropology of the Eastern Highlands of New Guinea*. Anthropological studies in the Eastern Highlands of New Guinea. Seattle and London: University of Washington Press, 2.

McCabe, G. (1960). Cultural influences on patient behavior. *American Journal of Nursing, 60*(8), 1101.

McKaughan, H. (1973). *The languages of the eastern family of the East New Guinea Highland stock*. Anthropological studies in the Eastern Highlands of New Guinea. Seattle and London: University of Washington Press, 1.

Mead, M. (1956). Understanding cultural patterns. *Nursing Outlook, 4*(3), 260.

Orem, D. (1980). *Nursing: Concepts of practice*. McGraw-Hill.

Pataki, K. J. (1970). An environment through time: A comparison of precontact and post-contact habitats in the Eastern Highlands of New Guinea. Boulder, CO: Institute of Behavioral Science, University of Colorado.

Rosenbaum, J. (1990). Cultural care, culture health and grief phenomena related to older Greek-Canadian widows with Leininger's theory of culture care. Unpublished doctoral dissertation. Detroit: Wayne State University.

Saunders, L. (1954). Cultural differences and medical care. New York: Russell Sage Foundation.

Spangler, Z. (1990). Nursing care values and practices of Philippine-American and Anglo-American nurses. Unpublished doctoral dissertation. Detroit: Wayne State University.

Staziak, D. (1990). An ethnonursing study of folk care and health beliefs and practices with Mexican-Americans using Leininger's theory of cultural care. Unpublished master's thesis. Detroit: Wayne State University.

Watson, James B. (1963). A micro-evolution study in New Guinea. Journal of the Polynesian Society, 72(3), 188–192.

Watson, V. & J. D. Cole (1977). Prehistory of the Eastern Highlands of New Guinea. Anthropological studies in the Eastern Highlands of New Guinea. Seattle and London: University of Washington Press, 3.

Wenger, A. F., (1988). The phenomenon of care of the Old Order Amish: A high context culture. Unpublished doctoral dissertation. Detroit: Wayne State University.

8

Culture Care Theory for Study of Dying Patients in Hospital and Hospice Contexts

Marie F. Gates

Improving care for dying patients involves the study of meanings of care and cure of those patients. An important focus of this study also involves the effects of care providers and hospital and hospice settings on dying patients' experiences with and views toward care and cure. Leininger's theory of Cultural Care and her use of ethnonursing as a qualitative method to study the care of dying patients, for example, have all led me to conduct the investigation described here.

Initially, this study included discovery of the meanings, experiences, and orientations that dying patients gave to care and cure. Second, this study focused on discovery of the ways in which the culture of the hospital and hospice influenced the meanings, experiences, and orientations of care and cure for those dying persons who were chosen as the study informants.

Significant research questions guiding this study were:

1. What are the meanings of care and cure to persons who are dying?

2. What experiences do persons have with care and cure during
    the living-dying interval (Pattison, 1979)?
3. What are the characteristics of care and cure orientations as
    described by persons who are dying?
4. In what ways does the cultural context of hospital and hos-
    pice settings influence the care and cure meanings, experi-
    ences, and orientations as described by persons who are
    dying?

THEORETICAL CONCEPTUALIZATION

As foundation for this study, Leininger's theory of Cultural Care Diversity and Universality (1988) involves several major tenets: (1) there
is a link between the care and well being of persons who are dying
(Leininger, 1984, p. 5); (2) an explication of cultural care knowledge in
nursing will lead to improving care and providing culturally congruent
care for persons whether living or dying; and (3) there are different
forms, expressions, meanings, and experiences related to care in different cultures. These tenets guided my thinking.

Cure, of course, is the other important aspect of any consideration
of the phenomenon of dying. For Leininger (1981), however, cure is
not developed as a concept separate from care. In fact, "There can be
no curing without caring" (p. 11). The systematic study of care and
cure concepts, then, in two different contexts with people encounter-
ing the experience of dying was predicted to reveal new knowledge and
understanding of care and cure expressions and meanings. Exploration
of the relationship between cultural care and cure also was seen as a
way to give additional insights to these important concepts in nursing.

The orientation definition of care used in qualitative studies was
based on Leininger's (1988) definition of generic care. For the purposes of this study, *care* was defined as physical, psychological, spiritual, cultural, and other informant-identified acts or measures designed
to promote quality of living while dying. *Cure*, on the other hand, was
defined as surgery, medication, intravenous solutions, radiation, and
other informant-identified acts or measures designed to eradicate or
halt the progression of disease. Pattison's (1977) concept of the living-

dying interval was included within the conceptualization to specify a time frame for when "dying" begins. The definition of living-dying interval as the time when persons were aware that their illness was likely to lead to death and not recovery was critical in the selection of study subjects.

While nursing's essential focus is care, there is need to study cure in terms of nursing's additional function, of carrying out physicians's orders which normally have a curing intent. Several nursing authors have stated that cure is an important aspect of nursing as well. For example, there is Vredevoe's (1984) basic science of care as curology and Loomis and Wood's (1983) position that "nurses are capable of curing the actual or potential health problem." With the increase in chronic disease, and with the need to focus on those who no longer can be "cured," the attempt to look at cure and care together and to determine meanings and experiences patients held was an important consideration.

Leininger's (1978) theory also was important for studying institutional units of hospital and hospice as subcultures with their own values, norms, and practices. Comparing and contrasting of experiences of persons who were dying either in hospital or hospice was a major interest. Findings from the study would add new cultural care knowledge as institutional knowledge to guide nursing practice. In terms of nursing theory development as a whole, such refinement of caring knowledge is urgent (Leininger, 1981, 1984; Morse et al., 1990).

Ethnonursing was developed by Leininger (1985) specifically to study the theory of Culture Care. The care and cure meanings and experiences as expressed by persons who are dying represent a domain which fits within the ethnonursing qualitative research method. The goal of discovering nursing knowledge based on the experiences and perceptions of dying persons and their caregivers also is congruent with the use of ethnonursing.

LITERATURE REVIEW

Care theorists, among them Leininger (1970, 1978, 1981, 1984, 1988), Watson (1979, 1985), and Benner and Wrubel (1988), have studied and emphasized the essential nature of care within nursing both from philosophical and empirical viewpoints. Gaut (1981, 1984) identified three components essential to care: disposition or feeling in the one giving care, the enactment of activities, and the combination of affect and doing for the welfare of others. Leininger identified the universality of care but emphasized the importance of studying its diverse forms, patterns, expressions, and meanings as expressed transculturally (1970, 1978, 1981) in professional and cultural groups and institutions, to name a few. Watson (1979) identified the "carative" factors that enable a person to die a peaceful death. Ray (1984, 1987) identified the need to study care in clinical and institutional settings and emphasized the need to see how the culture of those settings influences care.

Qualitative inductive studies related to care include Riemen's (1986) identification of caring and noncaring behaviors of nurses as identified by patients. Mayer's (1986) examination of care concluded that cancer patients and their families valued both instrumental behaviors (physical action-oriented helping behaviors and cognitive-oriented helping behaviors) and expressive behaviors (behaviors establishing relationships based on trust, hope, sensitivity, genuineness, and support). Gardner and Wheeler (1981) studied support as a specific component of care from the viewpoint of nurses and patients in three speciality areas in one hospital: surgery, medicine, and psychiatry. Emotional support was strongly emphasized, social support was not.

Swanson-Kaufman (1986) studied 20 women who had miscarried and identified the following elements of caring: knowing or the desire to be understood for personal meaning of loss; being with or feeling with the women who miscarried; doing for or needing to have others do; enabling or facilitating capacity to grieve; and maintaining belief— having others believe in their capacity to get through the loss.

Brown (1986) found that patients who were in a non-life threatening condition emphasized their need, when being cared for, for professional knowledge and skill, surveillance, and reassuring presence when threat was present, or threatening reactions to conditions were present. Patients also emphasized recognition of individual qualities and needs, the promotion of autonomy, and time spent with clients when threat was not present as empowering. Larson (1984) found similarity in caring expectations with cancer patients.

These studies revealed persons in various kinds of health-illness situations are able and willing to discuss, describe and categorize meanings, experiences, and values regarding care. Such persons also consider care important, can differentiate essence and nuance regarding care, and value the opportunity to share their experiences.

While the above studies focused on patients' expressions of care from professional care providers and identified patients' willingness to participate in such investigations, no studies specifically identifying dying patients' views on cure were found. Nonetheless, the act of patients linking care with cure can be inferred, for example, from the popular literature of de Beauvoir (1966), Gunther (1949), Lear (1984), Radner (1989), and Ryan (1966). Kennison (1982), however, in her study on the clinical reality of sickness, did interview persons diagnosed with cancer—some were nurses, some were not. One of her findings indicated that nurses were surprised when patients hoped for a cure when medical status indicated otherwise.

To maintain the balance of care and cure as a primary ethical concern for nursing, Benoliel (1979) has suggested a reordering of priorities in health care delivery services. She encouraged nurses to conduct research related to care and cure with dying patients (1983, 1987–1988).

The questions regarding what constitutes cultural care and cure and why dying persons continue with cure activities even when a potential cure is not attainable remain. The present study was proposed to focus on these unexplored areas.

RESEARCH DESIGN

Ethnonursing (Leininger, 1985) is the systematic study of nursing and related phenomena bearing on nursing. This method was used to discover the meanings and expressions of care and cure as experienced by persons spending part of the living-dying interval (Pattison, 1977) within the hospital and hospice cultural settings. I used several enablers as part of the ethnonursing method. Observation-Participation-Reflection model (O-P-R) (Leininger, 1985) was a major guide for the study. I did in-depth interviews with key and general informants and used field journal documentation to record reviews along with other field information (i.e., newspaper articles, organization charts, memos, letters). Other features of the study followed the ethnonursing method as presented in Chapter 2.

Settings

Sites chosen for study were an oncology unit of a large community teaching hospital and a free-standing hospice unit. After approval by the institutions' review boards, and preliminary contact by the managers of each setting, I proceeded with the O-P-R process. (See Figure 1 for a summary of typical activities occurring within Leininger's O-P process model.)

I documented observations and experiences related to care and cure practices in brief and later expanded notes. I recorded reflection and hunches about what transpired during the course of the study in a personal journal. In addition, I included data from patient records to substantiate data from key informants and to provide care providers' responses to interviews, as well as helpful information related to patients' conditions.

Informants

I conducted unstructured interviews with 12 key and 12 general informants in each setting purposefully selected from each of the two settings. Key informants were patients who had an illness designated by the primary physician or nurse as likely to lead to death within the next year. Other criteria for selection included awareness of prognosis, ability and willingness to participate in the study, ability to speak English, and minimum age of 21 years. Key informants were chosen because they were held to be knowledgeable about care and cure related to death and dying. Interviews were conducted in informants' rooms or homes. Two to three interviews, averaging 45 minutes each with a total range of two to three hours were spent with each key informant.

As Table 1 shows there were a total of 24 key informants from the hospital and hospice ranging in age from 25–84 years. Only 7 of the 24 informants were male since fewer met the primary criterion particularly in the hospital setting. All had a diagnosis of cancer. Two-thirds were Anglo-American, one-third African-American, representing the Midwestern urban population of the area. The informants varied in marital status, but all had an identified family member or support person. All but two informants had an identified religion, but two of

Figure 1
Leininger's Observation-Participation-Reflection Phases with Researcher's Time Span

Phases	I Observation	II Observation and Participation	III Participation	IV Observation and Reflection
Types of Activities	Observe interactions events, activities, people, structure functions Identify key and general informants Record data	Focus on domains: care, cure, dying process, setting Continue observations Begin participation in activities, e.g., rounds, meeting, pt. conferences Begin interviews with key and general informants Construct similarities and differences in settings	Continue participation in events, activities, interactions Continue interviews with key and general informants Confirm analyses and impressions with informants, participants, experts	Examine effect researcher has on participants Confirm patterns, themes, conclusions with participants, practitioners, researchers, experts Ongoing writing of analyses and results
Relative Time Frame	*Hospital* Aug/Sept 1987 *Hospice* Dec 1987/Jan 1988	Oct 1987 Feb 1988	*Hospital* – Feb 1988 *Hospice* – May 1988	*Hospital* Feb 1988/Oct 1988 *Hospice* June 1988/Oct 1988

287

Table 1
Characteristics of Key Informants

Characteristic	Total	Hospital	Hospice
Number	24	12	12
Age (Range 25–84)			
21–39	1	0	1
40–49	5	2	3
50–59	6	4	2
60–69	5	4	1
70–79	6	2	4
80–89	1	0	1
Gender			
Female	17	10	7
Male	7	2	5
Cultural Background			
African-American	9	6	3
Anglo-American	15	6	9
Marital Status			
Married	13	9	4
Divorced	5	1	4
Widowed	2	0	2
Single	4	2	2
Religion			
Protestant	13	8	5
Catholic/Orthodox	6	2	1
Jewish	3	2	1
Agnostic	2	0	2

the Catholic/Orthodox group specified that they no longer practiced their religion.

The 12 general informants in each setting were interviewed to provide reflective viewpoints related to the settings and experiences key informants had shared, as well as to provide descriptive data regarding the settings themselves. General informants included nurses, other care providers, family members, volunteers, and visitors. Interviews averaged 45 minutes duration and took place in offices, the solarium, the cafeteria, conference room, visitor room, or wherever a quiet environment could be found.

Audiotaping of interviews with key and general informants took place when feasible and if permitted. Sixty percent of the total interviews were

Table 2
Sample of Coding Items
from Leininger's Sunrise Model

Code Number	Item
1	Worldview
5	Linguistic terms and meanings
13	Kinship
15	Religious, philosophical, ethical
23	Folk care/caring
24	Professional care
25	Professional nursing care
26	Non-care
36	Political factors of institution
38	Technological factors of institution
58	Life passages
71	Dialogue by interviewer
74	Informed consent factors

taped. Field notes were systematically recorded regardless of taping, and were transcribed within 48 hours. Comparison of field notes to transcribed notes revealed similarity of data and confirmed the use of field notes as a helpful way to document events and experiences.

The large volume of ethnonursing data from O-P-R, records, personal journals and interviews were entered into the computer using the Leininger, Templin, and Thompson (LTT) (1990) ethnoqualitative software package. The field research data were identified and coded within Leininger's theory, components of the Sunrise Model, and the domains of inquiry of the study. The computer package facilitated the sorting of data by single or multiple codes, words, and code/word combinations. (See Table 2 for an example of codes used in this study.)

ANALYSIS OF DATA

In keeping with the ethnonursing method to study Cultural Care Diversity and Universality, Leininger's Phases of Ethnonursing Analysis for Qualitative Data (1985, 1987) was used. In Phase I, detailed statements of interviews from informants and O-P-R experiences were studied in depth to become fully aware of the raw data within the diverse hospital and hospice contexts. Reviewing, coding, and classifying data to identify and compare descriptors constituted Phase II of data analysis. In Phase III analysis, patterns of care and cure were formulated from descriptors. In Phase IV, themes were abstracted from the identified patterns, descriptors, and raw data. Overall, such analysis permitted in-depth study at each phase as well as the ability to move back and forth between phases to confirm and establish credible and accurate findings.

Since the purposes and goals of the qualitative paradigm differ from those of the quantitative paradigm, only suitable criteria for analysis were used: credibility, dependability, recurrency, saturation, and confirmability as described by Leininger (1985) and Lincoln and Guba (1985). Of particular importance to this study was the criterion of *dependability*. To ensure dependability of data, use of a variety of approaches—establishing an audit trail so that another researcher could observe the raw data, computer print-outs, and organization of data into themes and patterns—was established. Certainly, researcher dependability was enhanced by fluency in the language of informants by practicing observation and listening skills, and by being open to a variety of stimuli (Lincoln & Guba, 1985). I found informants and others in the settings receptive, open, willing to talk, and willing to say they found me open, receptive, and nonjudgmental.

The criterion of *credibility*, determination of the accuracy or truth value evident in the research process and conclusions of the study (Leininger, 1985; Lincoln & Guba, 1985), also was critical. As observations and interviews were completed, I summarized, analyzed, and discussed emerging patterns and themes with key and general informants in the settings. Another technique, peer debriefing, in which the research mentor and other peers engaged in qualitative research by questioning me to clarify accuracy of data regarding emerging patterns and themes, helped to support the criterion of credibility.

Findings

In this section, I will present major themes related to cultural care and cure with their meanings and expressions. I have presented in detail a comparative description and analysis of the settings of hospital and hospice and the theme of *caring ambience present in the settings* is in another publication (Gates, 1991) as well as in the full investigation (Gates, 1988). This chapter, however, will focus on the themes related to care and cure and on the dying experience as described by the patients.[1]

Theme 1—Patient caring for others. A significant finding here was the expressed wish of patients to give care to others. Such *altruistic care*, patients giving care to others without receiving something in return, differed from *mutual care*, patients giving care with the expectation of receiving something in return. The theme of *patient caring for others* was apparent in both the hospital and hospice settings. Such care was directed toward family or significant others, roommates, and professional service providers. All key informants provided examples of giving care to others during this study.

Patient Caring for Family. Patients expressed in large and small ways how they cared for their family members, for example, teaching a husband how to shop and cook; sitting with a fiancee while she's fixing dinner because she liked company; dog-sitting for friends; arranging for a dinner tray for a wife who was visiting the hospital later that evening; or spending time discussing school problems with a teenage daughter. One woman kept a pink notebook in which she organized the bills and other finances for her husband and detailed what to do in preparation for her funeral arrangements. The following example from one key informant, a woman married over 50 years, exemplifies the pattern of caring for family:

> *I thank God for giving me this time. . . . I have seen so many people . . . written so many things. I have given cherished things away which I think if I didn't . . . you don't know what's going to happen later. I have also made the dresser . . . it was so very feminine with perfume, powder, etc. . . it's changed to his [husband's] way. So that transition won't be so bad. . . . I thought it would be easier. My clothes need to be out . . . that's another thing that has to happen quickly so his clothes will be in both closets. As I say, "I'm thinking of them."*

Whether it was with the intention of receiving something in return or not, patients wished to *give*, to *do*, to *be*, in some way, caring for their family or significant others. They saw it as a way to "care back" for all the caring they received, to find some meaning in their living during their difficult times, to make sense of their lives immediately, or to make up for what they did not do in the past. Patient desire to care for others was paramount—an extremely important and necessary aspect of their lives.

Patient Caring for Roommates.   The caring acts extended to their roommates as well and identified a second pattern. Measures they described and I observed included such activities as "showing each other the ropes," calling the nurse for one other, asking family members to bring in treats or perform something special for one another, feeding one another, writing letters or calling one another after discharge, and sharing experiences about treatment or personnel. Due to the greater likelihood of roommate interaction in the hospital, roommate caring was more apparent there than in the hospice setting. For example, there was the relationship between Jan and Nellie:

> Jan, a 57-year-old Irish-American woman, and Nellie, a 65-year-old African-American woman shared a room for a number of days. Nellie referred to Jan as "my friend." Jan talked about having a "sympatico" relationship with Nellie. Jan, upon receiving chemotherapy, experienced a decrease in her white blood cell count, necessitating a move to a private room. Staff delivered notes between the women. Upon Nellie's discharge home, she asked to be wheeled to the door of Jan's room to say good-bye. They continued phone calls until Jan's death.

Patient Caring for Staff or Care Providers.   Expressions of this pattern of caring for staff included bringing in treats for staff, telling jokes, or buoying a staff member's spirits. One critical example was the decision of patients to continue with cure treatments. Six of the key informants indicated they decided to continue with chemotherapy or radiation even though they knew it would not increase their life spans as a way to "care for" their physicians. General informants were universal in their confirmation of the third pattern. As one nurse general informant stated: "I learned a lot—not just about oncology, but about life—how by their perspective it's not gloomy—you keep living, even when dying, and that's helped me with living." Key informants did not always identify this behavior as caring, but staff and family members as general informants did. One experienced nurse stated she made it a point to tell patients when they were doing this so they were aware of *patient caring for others.*

The agreement to participate in studies, or to continue treatment even when no longer seen as helpful, exemplified caring not only for physicians or staff, but in a larger sense of caring for others who might benefit in the future from the patient's decision.

Theme 2—Patient receiving care from others. The second primary theme involved the expressions of care received from family members and professional care providers. In both hospital and hospice, patients placed greatest value on receiving care first from family or significant others than from professional staff, especially nurses and physicians.

In the hospital setting, care as *doing* was emphasized, while in the hospice care as *presence* of family was more strongly described. Receiving care from significant others was identified as crucial and essential by all key informants in hospital and hospice settings.

While all categories of staff were identified as important to key informants in terms of receiving care, both nurses and physicians were identified as most important to key informants in both settings. One hospital key informant stated, "The nurses care about whether or not I'm constipated, and about how I'm holding up emotionally." Another described how a nurse "cleaned me up when I experienced a sudden bout of diarrhea and left me with my dignity intact." In the hospice setting all staff other than physicians were identified as nursing staff. This may have occurred due to the blurring of roles in hospice.

In both hospital and hospice settings, patients stressed the importance of receiving care from their physicians. In the hospital, key informants generally had ongoing relationships with their physicians. Patients found physicians caring when physicians spent time talking with them, did not rush them, explained what the treatment was in detail, and treated them with respect. In hospice, the unit physician often became the patient's physician and was described as "loved" by patients. In each setting and with both nurses and physicians, the caring acts themselves and the manner in which they were extended were critical attributes of caring in the experiences of key informants.

Key informants described physical and psychological care as having priority, but there were differences in expressions between the two settings. Physical care acts in the hospital were referred to as dressings, pain control measures, central lines, chemotherapy, and intravenous therapy. Patients expected and found technological expertise essential to care received from physicians and nurses in the hospital. Hospice patients emphasized that personal care, such as bathing and feeding, and control of symptoms, especially pain management, respiratory distress, and nausea was more important. As Clara, a hospice patient, stated, "my pain was controlled with beauty and sensitivity."

In terms of psychological care, key informants in the hospital setting were *surprised* that staff were aware of their psychological needs. Mary exemplified a number of hospital key informants in commenting how nice it was to have someone "Know when I'm depressed and need to talk or don't need to talk but just need someone there." Hospice key informants, on the other hand, *expected* to receive psychological care. Typical statements included: "Talking about what was important to me"; "having someone there when I need to and being left alone when I need that."

In relation to care received by professional staff, hospital key informants valued expertise in terms of physical care and were surprised to receive psychological care. Hospice key informants were more appreciative of personal care acts and expected to receive psychological care.

Theme 3—Cure as hoped-for outcome. Both hospital and hospice patients viewed cure as eradication of disease. Hospital patients were more hopeful that cure was still possible and were more likely to be engaged in cure acts. Eleven of the twelve hospital patients were receiving chemotherapy or radiation therapy, which represented cure acts for them. Cure meant: "completeness"; "wonderful, terrific, everything that's good"; "coming back like you were before." Despite what they said regarding their hope for therapy, all the hospital informants also said that they knew their therapy would not cure them. Why, then, did they engage in the treatment? Some did it as a way of caring for their physicians: "Dr. A. thinks I should, so why not do it for him?" exemplifies a common response. Others, particularly those for whom religion was important, saw it as a way that God might choose to heal them.

Family members' requests to continue therapy, as a way to care for their family members, was another reason. A need to be doing something, a common symptom of American positivist mentality, an optimistic worldview, and having a positive attitude were still other reasons given to continue therapy. Another significant reason to continue therapy came into play here: the cure orientation of the hospital unit, in which participation in cure acts came as a matter of course. All these factors contributed to the idea of cure as a "hoped-for" outcome. In no case did a key informant say cure was just going to happen for them, "but you never know."

For hospice informants, cure meant: "hope"; "completely getting rid of the cancer"; "eradicating it totally." During the study none of the hospice patients were receiving treatment. Five had never received treatment and one discontinued treatment after only one session due to its deleterious effect on her quality of life. The hospice philosophy supported the patients' decisions to refrain from treatment. In fact, patients could not continue with hospice services if they chose to continue cure acts. A more realistic worldview also may have contributed to their decision. However, even with hospice patients, cure as a "hoped for" outcome was still a possibility. For example, one hospice patient noted he had "already exceeded the six-month limit and was going for another six months."

Theme 4—"Living while Dying." The fourth theme which emerged clearly from the data, "living while dying," was named for the title of a book based on a nurse researcher's experiences with dying patients (Martocchio, 1982). The phrase succinctly captured how patients asked to be seen. "Please see me as living while dying, with an emphasis on the living" was one patient's plea. Patterns which characterized this theme included: openness in talking about feelings, particularly about death and dying; support systems which promoted living; participation in daily tasks; and caring for others.

Openness in Talking about Feelings.   This pattern emerged early as each key informant engaged in life history and life review. All patients were candid in using such words as *death, dying, die, terminal* or *cancer* in describing their recent life experiences. They were clear in saying their time was limited, and also clear in sharing their feelings about that time. Communicating about feelings was an important feature of living while dying. Why? One hospital patient, a single woman who raised her sister's children, said:

> My sister died, and we all pussyfooted around, wouldn't talk about what was happening. My family vowed if anyone else came down with something like this, we'd talk, we'd be open.

Another key informant described a recent incident with the doctor coming in to tell her "grim news"—her fracture was the result of additional metastasis. When her family was left alone in the room with her, she reported that:

> My family was waiting for me to come out with words of good cheer—I couldn't give them the words but I sensed they were looking to me for that and I couldn't hack it; we cried together, we shared where we were; I owed them more than a false front.

Reliance on Support Systems. The second pattern focused first on a personal belief system. The presence of God, faith, or prayer in living the experience was spoken of by all but one of the hospital key informants and eight hospice informants. Even those not practicing a defined religion and those seeing themselves as agnostic identified the importance of "love," nature, and an examination of the meaning of life as ways which helped them live more fully. Reliance on a defined religious system was especially noted with the African-American key informants. Literature was cited as a second important pattern, especially the Bible. Simonton (1978), Siegel (1986), and Kübler-Ross (1969, 1976) were other frequently cited authors who were viewed as providing comfort and support to patients during the "living while dying" experience.

Participating in Daily Events. Patients wished to continue to participate in daily events as much as they could. They expressed a desire to talk about the baseball game or a staff nurse's vacation as well as their own experiences. For example, one key informant in hospice came home, was sitting in her living room chair while members of her family came in daily to care for her, clean house, and so forth. She said, "I'm going to die in this chair, bored to death. So I fired the lot of them and decided to do what I did before." Her schedule included getting her hair done, having visitors over, accompanying her husband on shopping trips designed to orient him to tasks he wasn't used to doing. In order to see her, I had to sandwich my visits within her busy schedule. She died two weeks later.

Patients talked about keeping diaries or writing letters. One young man was compiling a book of his thoughts, ideas, poems, and stories regarding his "living while dying" experiences which he hoped would be published after his death. His hope was realized.

Openness in sharing feelings about living and dying, reliance on support systems, participating in routine events, and caring as described in the *patient caring for others* theme were patterns which characterized the theme of *living while dying*.

Other Findings

Leininger's theory encourages the exploration of diverse and universal findings. Two such areas were described by several informants: euthanasia and setting limits. Although euthanasia was not part of my interviewing, several patients took it on themselves to initiate discussion on this topic. Selected comments included:

A person of reasonably sound mind should be able to decide his own future within limits—that includes turning off the power.

If I knew how to do it, I would, but I wouldn't put that guilt on anyone, the repercussions can be horrendous.

If I have a spell, I don't want anyone bringing me back, I just wanna go—no tubes or machine.

Setting limits was particularly identified by general informants. While it is necessary for care providers to encourage patients to exert control, it also is advantageous to help patients analyze behavior that might become detrimental to themselves or to others. One staff nurse at hospice raised the question of challenging patients, not permitting an "anything goes" attitude. She set limits with patients when it seemed appropriate and found patients thanked her for doing so.

Challenging patients who are dying when they are inappropriate allows me to see them and them to see themselves as living, as having a choice, as making a mistake.

Patients confirmed the importance of this challenge as a way of seeing them as living, as not "getting away with absurd behavior." These findings were shared by too few informants to extrapolate themes; however, the findings indicate areas for further study and analysis.

DISCUSSION

Patient Caring for Others

Key informants either directly expressed or were observed engaging in *patient caring for others. Patient caring for others* represented a great desire to do and to be for others, of being seen as living more fully during the dying experience. All persons who are dying may not be able to or willing to engage in caring behaviors, nor should they be expected to do so. However, those persons who choose to do so can be accommodated by staff and significant others. Leininger (1988) identified cultural care accommodation as a major mode of nursing practice in her theory. Ways in which staff and others may assist in cultural care accommodation include orienting family members to patients' wishes to become engaged in caring behaviors, fostering closer patient-patient, patient–family, and patient–staff relationships, and informing patients of the ways they *are* caring for others. Nurses must be careful, however, not to impose expectations of such caring on patients. Providing opportunities for patient caring and encouraging families to allow such caring are important avenues for some patients. Other patients, however, may not wish to do so.

Since patient caring for others seems closely related to appropriate living while dying, nursing can study that aspect of care more fully. Marck (1990) has developed a concept analysis in therapeutic reciprocity that explores the patient aspect of mutually experienced caring. Findings from this study provide data to support her premise.

The concept of *patient caring for others* supports Leininger's research (1978) of the many cultures that value caring for others. In this light, a pertinent research question comes to mind involving a study of the concept of *patient caring for others* with other persons facing other life crises (e.g., traumatic injuries) or diseases (e.g., AIDS), in other developmental levels (e.g., the old-old), in other settings (e.g., nursing homes). A second research question which comes to mind involves both patient and staff: Does the ability of patients to engage in caring for others contribute to the satisfaction of staff or the decision of staff to continue to serve in palliative care units, hospices, and home care?

Care Received from Others by Patients

The particular significance of care received from family/significant other is congruent with Mor & Kidder's (1985) finding that dying patients identified supportive others as their most important strength. Ways of fostering family care, preventing caregiver burden, and providing opportunities for family to support each other are important activities for nursing to promote. Leininger (1988) has proposed cultural care preservation as a mode of nursing action. Where families are attuned to caring for their loved ones, such caring can be seen as a means of cultural care preservation.

The finding that physicians as well as nurses provide significant care to patients may seem surprising. Physicians are beginning to appreciate the importance and value of care, particularly in situations where cure is no longer possible. Leininger's emphasis on care as essential for cure has influenced that growing appreciation. The popularity of Siegel's (1986, 1989) works may be viewed as a catalyst for continued physician interest in care as well. Nurses can support efforts of physicians to learn about and value care, especially when that care involves dying patients.

Concern of key informants for psychological care as well as physical care is consistent with findings from Brown (1986), Larson (1984), Mayer (1986), Riemen (1984), and Swanson-Kaufman (1986) in valuing both physical/facilitative and expressive aspects of caring. That technological expertise and attention to body needs would be paramount in the hospital was an expected finding. Nonetheless, the skill with which symptom control, particularly pain control, was handled in hospice indicates an area in which hospice can provide assistance to hospitals in facilitating care. Hospice personnel are noted for expertise in managing symptoms such as pain, respiratory distress, and nausea, as experienced by dying patients. Kastenbaum (1987–1988) has encouraged the broader dissemination and utilization of hospice research for symptom control to other settings where dying patients receive care. Dying patients gave much attention to physical and psychological care. Nurses need, however, to consider ways to increase patients' awareness of and sensitivity to social, cultural, and spiritual components of care.

Cure as "hoped for" outcome. Data did not support a predominant cure orientation with patients who were dying. Instead, patients valued cure and expressed a desire to have cure. While cure was not an expectation, cure continued to be a hope even in the final days.

In hospital settings, nurses may find it more congruent with patient needs to support treatment acts when that is the patient's choice. Such support exemplified Leininger's (1988) mode of cultural care accommodation. Furthermore, nurses need to encourage patient understanding and discussion of choices regarding cure acts. If care providers and family members understood the rationale for patients' continuation of cure acts, decision making would be more clearly outlined.

This study provided confirmation for Leininger's proposition that cure was a component of care. Findings revealed that cure was interdependent with care for persons who were dying. Furthermore, patients expressed willingness to continue with cure acts, which they openly discussed as futile, as a means of caring for others, particularly physicians and family members. Participation in cure acts was seen as an aspect of caring for others.

Living while dying. This theme has been found by a number of researchers working with those who are dying (e.g., Castles & Murray, 1979; Hurley, 1977; Martocchio, 1982; Paige, 1985). Kübler-Ross (1976) characterized death as the final stage of growth. Leininger's theory (1988) identified assisting patient to achieve a peaceful death as a goal for culturally congruent nursing care. Nursing can foster "living while dying" as a means of helping patients achieve their goals for peaceful or appropriate deaths through: (1) acknowledging and supporting opportunities for patients to engage in caring for others; (2) encouraging discussion related to sharing of life history, life experiences, and expression of feelings; and (3) including patients in the lifeways of the settings in which they're located. Such actions are examples of cultural care preservation.

CONCLUSION

This ethnonursing study conceptualized within Leininger's theory offers findings to link care with cure, particularly with persons who are dying. It was discovered that dying persons engage in caring behaviors with family, roommates, and care providers. Those caring behaviors are a primary means for dying persons to live more fully while they are dying. The examination of caring acts and processes which dying persons gave and received provide support for the richness of the phenomenon of caring and its importance to nursing.

NOTE

[1] The term *patient* is used interchangeably with *key informant*. Emic comments indicated that was an acceptable, even preferred term as expressed by key informants.

REFERENCES

Beauvoir, S. de (1966). *A very easy death*. New York: Putnam.

Benner, P. & Wrubel, J. (1988). *The primacy of caring—stress and coping in health and illness*. Redwood City, CA: Addison-Wesley.

Benoliel, J. Q. (1979). Dying in an institution. In H. Wass (Ed.), *Dying: Facing the facts*. Washington, DC: Hemisphere Publications.

Benoliel, J. Q. (1983). Nursing research on death, dying and terminal illness: Development, present state, and prospects. In H. H. Hurley & J. J. Fitzpatrick (Eds.), *Annual review of nursing research*, (pp. 101-130). Vol. 1. New York: Springer.

Benoliel, J. Q. (1987-1988). Health care providers and dying patients: Critical issues in terminal care. *Omega*, *18*, 341-363.

Brown, L. (1986). The experience of care: Patient perspectives. *Topics in Clinical Nursing, 8*(2), 56–62.

Castles, M. R., & Murray, R. B. (1979). *Dying in an institution: Nurse-patient perspectives.* New York: Appleton-Century-Crofts.

Gardner, K. G. & Wheeler, E. (1981). Patients' and staff nurses' perceptions of supportive nursing behaviors. A preliminary analysis. In M. M. Leininger (Ed.), *Caring: An essential human need* (pp. 109–114). Thorofare, NJ: Slack.

Gates, M. F. (1988). *Care and cure meanings, experiences, and orientations of persons who are dying in hospital and hospice settings.* Unpublished doctoral dissertation. Wayne State University, Detroit.

Gates, M. F. (1991). Transcultural comparison of hospital and hospice as caring environments for dying persons. *Journal of Transcultural Nursing, 2.*

Gaut, D. (1981). Conceptual analysis of caring: Research method. In M. M. Leininger (Ed.), *Caring: An essential human need.* Thorofare, NJ: Slack, 17–44.

Gaut, D. (1984). A theoretic description of caring as action. In M. M. Leininger (Ed.), *Care: The essence of nursing and health.* Thorofare, NJ: Slack, 27–44.

Gunther, J. (1949). *Death be not proud, a memoir.* New York: Harper.

Hurley, B. A. (1977). Problems of interaction between nurses and dying patients. In M. V. Batey, (Ed.), *Communicating nursing research,* Vol. 9, Boulder, CO: WICHE, 223–226.

Kastenbaum, R. J. (1987–1988). Theory, research, and applications. Some critical issues for thanatology. *Omega, 18,* 397–410.

Kennison, B. J. (1983). *Nurses and patients: The clinical reality of sickness.* Vol. I & II. Doctoral Dissertation. Ann Arbor: University of Michigan,.

Kübler-Ross, E. (1969). *On death and dying.* New York: Macmillan.

Kübler-Ross, E. (1976). *Death: The final stage of growth.* Englewood Cliffs, NJ: Prentice-Hall.

Larson, P. (1984). Important nurse caring behaviors perceived by patients with cancer. *Oncology Nursing Forum, 11,* (6), 46–50.

Lear, M. W. (1980). *Heartsounds.* New York: Simon & Schuster.

Leininger, M. M. (1970). *Nursing and anthropology: Two worlds to blend.* New York: John Wiley & Sons.

Leininger, M. M. (1978). *Transcultural nursing: Concepts, theories, and practice.* New York: John Wiley & Sons.

Leininger, M. M. (1981). The phenomenon of caring: Importance, research questions and theoretical considerations. In M. M. Leininger, (Ed.), *Caring. An essential human need.* Thorofare, NJ: Slack, 3–16.

Leininger, M. M. (1984). Care: The essence of nursing and health. In M. M. Leininger (Ed.), *Care: The essence of nursing and health*. Thorofare, NJ: Slack, 3–16.

Leininger, M. M. (1985). Ethnography and ethnonursing: Models and mods of qualitative data analysis. In M. M. Leininger (Ed.), *Qualitative research methods in nursing*. Orlando, FL: Grune & Stratton, 33–72.

Leininger, M. M. (1987). Importance and uses of ethnomethods: Ethnography and ethnonursing research. In M. Cahoon (Ed.), *Recent advances in nursing*. London: Churchill Livingston, 17, 23–25.

Leininger, M. M. (1988). Leininger's theory of nursing: Cultural care diversity and universality. *Nursing Science Quarterly 1*, 152–160.

Leininger, M. M., Templin, T., & Thompson, F. (1989). *Leininger-Templin-Thompson ethnoscript qualitative software program: Users handbook*. Detroit: Wayne State University College of Nursing.

Lincoln, Y. S., & Guba, E. G. (1985). *Naturalistic inquiry*. Beverly Hills, CA: Sage.

Loomis, M. E., & Wood, D. J. (1983). Cure: The potential outcome of care. *Image, 15*, 4–7.

Marck, P. (1990). Therapeutic reciprocity: A caring phenomenon. *Advances in Nursing Science, 13*, 49–59.

Martocchio, B. M. (1982). *Living while dying*. Bowie, MD: Robert J. Brady.

Mayer, D. K. (1986). Caring behaviors of cancer patients and their families. *Topics in Clinical Nursing, 8*(2), 63–89.

Mor, V. & Kidder, D. (1985). Cost savings in hospice: Final results of the National Hospice Study. *Health Services Research, 20*, 407–421.

Morse, J. M., Solberg, S. M., Neander, W. L., Bottorff, J. L., & Johnson, J. L. (1990). Concepts of caring and caring as concept. *Advances in Nursing Science, 13*, 1–14.

Paige, S. (1980). *Alone into the alone: A phenomenological study of the experience of the dying*. Unpublished doctoral dissertation. Boston: Boston University.

Pattison, E. M. (1977). *The experience of dying*. Englewood Cliffs, NJ: Prentice-Hall.

Radner, G. (1989). *It's always something*. New York: Simon & Schuster.

Ray, M. A. (1984). The development of a classification system of institutional caring. In M. M. Leininger (Ed.), *Care: The essence of nursing and health*. Thorofare, NJ: Slack, 95–112.

Ray, M. A. (1987). Health care economics and human caring in nursing: Why the moral conflict must be resolved. *Family and Community Health, 10*(1), 35–43.

Riemen, D. J. (1986). Noncaring and caring in the clinical setting. *Topics in clinical nursing, 8*(2), 30–36.

Ryan, C. (1966). *The last battle.* New York: Simon & Schuster.

Siegel, B. S. (1986). *Love, medicine & miracles. Lessons learned about self-healing from a surgeon's experiences with exceptional patients.* New York: Harper & Row.

Siegel, B. S. (1989). *Peace, love & healing.* New York: Harper & Row.

Simonton, O., Matthews-Simonton, S., & Creighton, J. (1978). *Getting well again.* Los Angeles: J. P. Tarcher.

Swanson-Kaufman, K. M. (1986). Caring in the instance of unexpected early pregnancy loss. *Topics in Clinical Nursing, 8*(2), 37–46.

Vredevoe, D. L. (1984). Curology: A basic science related to nursing. *Image, 16,* 89–92.

Watson, J. (1979). *The philosophy and science of caring.* Boston: Little, Brown.

Watson, J. (1985). *Nursing: Human science and human care.* Norwalk, CT: Appleton-Century-Crofts.

9

Culture Care Theory and Greek Canadian Widows

Janet Rosenbaum

The rich tapestry of Canadian life includes many cultures. Among widows of these cultures, clinical observations confirm diverse beliefs and expressions regarding care, health, and grief. Professional help, however, is infrequently incapable of understanding or appreciating the culturally specific expressions of widows' care values.

With the large number of Greek families now living in many Canadian cities, Greek Canadian widows form a unique cultural group. An appreciation of Greek contributions to civilization as a whole stimulated my interest in doing this study.

A growing body of care theory and research documents the importance of providing culturally relevant care (Leininger, 1981, 1984a, 1988; Gaut, 1983, 1984; Wenger, 1988; Gates, 1988; Luna, 1989; Rosenbaum, 1990). Although Anderson (1985) studied Greek Canadian women and Tripp-Reimer (1983, 1984) reported on health in the Greek American culture, no studies to date regarding care with Greek American or Greek Canadian widows have been reported.

PURPOSE AND DOMAINS OF INQUIRY

In this transcultural nursing study, I will describe and explain the meanings and experiences of older Greek Canadian widows in regard to their cultural care, cultural health, and grief phenomena. Worldview, general culture, and social structure will be viewed within the theory of Culture Care Diversity and Universality. Four research questions and five orientational definitions helped to form the study's scope.

Research Questions

1. What are the meanings of cultural care, cultural health, and grief phenomena to older Greek Canadian widows?

2. What cultural care values of Greek Canadian widows contribute to the meanings of their cultural care?

3. What are the meanings and experiences of the transition from wife to widow for Greek Canadian older women?

4. How does cultural care contribute to the cultural health of Greek Canadian older widows who are experiencing grief phenomena?

Orientational Definitions

Cultural care:
Those supportive or facilitative acts specific to a particular culture which assist individuals or groups to improve their human conditions or lifeways (derived from Leininger, 1985a, p. 209).

Cultural care continuity:
Culturally learned, sustained, patterned, and supportive acts to improve human conditions or lifeways, which are given and received by persons over an extended period of time while they are in transition to a different life cycle phase, involve the use of their cultural care values.

Cultural health:
A state of culturally defined well being which reflects the ability to perform daily role activities (derived from Leininger, 1988, p. 156).

Grief phenomena:
Culturally based beliefs, practices, emotional expressions, and sorrow follow the death of a significant person. Within this orientational definition the concepts of grief and mourning were included as follows:

Grief: The meanings and expressions of sorrow following the death of a significant person.

Mourning: The culturally based practices that are performed following the death of a significant person.

Greek Canadians:
Persons of Greek ancestry who were born in Canada or who immigrated to Canada, who identify themselves as Greek Canadians.

THEORETICAL CONCEPTUAL FRAMEWORK

The theoretical framework used in this study derived from Leininger's theory of Culture Care Diversity and Universality, as delineated in Chapter 1. Cultural care, cultural care continuity, cultural health, and grief phenomena was investigated by focusing on older Greek Canadian widows' descriptions, explanations, and meanings for these domains.

Cultural care was assumed to be essential to face a critical life event such as the death of a spouse (Leininger, 1985a). Cultural care expressions, meanings, and practices were predicted to influence the cultural health of the widows, congruent with Leininger's theory (1984a), which predicted that cultural values, as the preferred ways of guiding behavior, influence care. Accordingly, the discovery of the Greek Canadian widows' cultural care values assisted in determining how such values influenced cultural care, and, ultimately, cultural health. The Sunrise Model was used to study conceptual components of Leininger's Culture Care theory (see Chapter 1).

All of the social structure features and worldview were considered along with language and environmental contexts in order to discover the Greek Canadian widow's care and health patterns. Folk and nursing systems were the focus for cultural care nursing decisions and actions.

Cultural care was explored as it was given and received within the concept of cultural care continuity. That is, widows received care, but they also gave care to others. It was conceptualized that when widows gave forms of cultural care to others as a culturally learned and valued pattern, the widows themselves should benefit as well as the recipients of care. If cultural care positively influenced the cultural health of both the person giving and receiving care, then widows who experienced cultural care continuity were predicted to maintain their cultural health.

It was assumed that while their husbands were alive, there were meaningful patterns of giving and receiving generic care between spouses which would be missed upon death. Therefore, cultural care continuity would be beneficial to the cultural health or well-being of these older Greek Canadian women during their transition from wives to widows.

Van Gennep's (1960) analysis of rites of passage also assisted in understanding the meanings and experiences of the transition to widowhood. His discussion of cultural rituals as mechanisms for helping people pass from one life cycle stage to another focused on three phases: rites of separation, which removed the individual from the previous situation; rites of transition, which assisted movement to a new stage; and rites of incorporation which provided integration into the new stage. The transitional stage ended when mourning was completed and the survivors were integrated again into society.

Previously, Rosenbaum (1988) explored the theoretical ideas of van Gennep (1960) and Leininger (1984a, 1988) in a mini ethnonursing study that described and explained the experience of widowhood of Greek American women. In Rosenbaum's study, informants reported that their well being was increased when they received care and gave care which had been culturally learned as they made transition from being married to being widows. This helped to provide a culturally healthy lifeway after the death of their spouses.

REVIEW OF THE LITERATURE

Cultural Care

Leininger (1967, 1970, 1978, 1979, 1984b) spearheaded the cultural movement in nursing to study care as the essence of nursing. She developed ideas on care from an inductive (emic) nursing perspective in the mid 1960s through ethnonursing field research of such diverse cultures as the Afro-American and Gadsup of New Guinea in an effort to describe the meanings and expressions of their cultural care.

Other nurses followed Leininger's leadership to contribute to the body of care theory and research. Aamodt (1979) studied children and adolescents in the Papago Indian culture of Arizona finding that care practices were altered during lifecycle changes. Boyle (1984) investigated care and health in a Guatemala community learning how those people promoted health and prevented illness. Gaut (1981, 1983, 1984) used philosophical analysis to explicate caring as a series of actions. Although she did not identify care meanings for specific cultures, her approach did help to clarify the philosophical basis for the study of care.

Ray (1981) identified themes of caring such as mutual self-actualization, love, and copresence within the social structure of a general hospital. Using philosophical analysis, phenomenological and ethnonursing research, she discovered that patients were assisted to maintain their health through caring. Watson (1979, 1985) stressed that caring is a moral ideal in nursing and identified ten carative factors derived from psychiatry to promote transpersonal caring relationships between nurses and clients.

Wenger (1988) discussed the meanings and expressions of care in the Old Order Amish culture. She found care had the same meanings over generations related to the high context of the culture. Luna (1989) contributed an understanding of care and cultural context for Lebanese Muslims in a U.S. community. She identified a theme of care as equal but different for men and women. Men were expected to protect and provide for the family while women were expected to nurture and comfort their children and husbands. Gates (1988) studied care and cure meanings of dying people in hospital and hospice settings. She found these people benefited from giving as well as receiving care, enabling them to sustain a better quality of life through the dying experience.

From these examples and others not mentioned here, cultural care literature has demonstrated that cultural care as given and received has multiple dimensions, expressions, and meanings which must be discovered. Additional issues in need of exploration include influence of generation of immigration and life cycle stages on cultural care.

Cultural Health

Although most nursing theorists defined health per se (King, 1981; Newman, 1979; Neuman, 1989; Orem, 1985; Watson, 1985; Roy, 1984), only Leininger (1988) has focused on cultural health. According to Leininger (1978), as health and illness are culturally defined, they must be studied within the context of particular cultures. In 1988, Leininger defined health as "a state of well-being which is culturally defined" (p. 156) and involves performance of role activities. In fact, and as she found, many cultures use health and well being interchangeably. Because health for Leininger is a fundamental aspect of culture, it must be defined within the context of specific cultures.

The research literature confirms the multiplicity of beliefs and practices for cultural health. Tripp-Reimer (1984, 1985), who developed an emic-etic grid to conceptualize health, identified disease as etic and illness as emic, using Greek American immigrants as study informants. In her study of beliefs regarding the *evil eye* among several generations of Greek Americans, she identified protective practices which included the use of charms to ward off harm. Tripp-Reimer found Greek Americans retained folk health and illness practices along with the use of professional care.

Using the ethnographic method, Ragucci (1979) studied the health beliefs and practices of three generations of Italian American women, who defined health in terms of well being which diminished with age. She also found that folk practices were more prevalent in older women. Ragucci urged nurses to provide care appropriate for their clients' cultural needs.

Anderson (1985) compared Greek Canadian immigrant women to South Asian Canadian immigrant women. Using a case study method to learn about health concerns and help-seeking behavior, Anderson found differences between the two groups. For example, South Asian Canadian women did not discuss their feelings while Greek Canadian women shared their feelings in regard to states of loneliness and depression.

Other studies, such as those done by Wiggins (1983) and Louie (1976), illustrated the diverse beliefs and practices of cultural health. This literature also confirmed Leininger's (1984a) position that cultural groups have diverse patterns of health expressions.

Grief Phenomena

The nursing literature to date reveals only limited conceptualization and research studies of grief phenomena among widows, especially widows of specific cultures. With several exceptions (Saunders, 1981; Carter, 1989; Dimond, 1981), nursing studies have been conducted within the more restrictive paradigm of quantitative measures (Brock, 1984; Vachon et al., 1976; Vachon & Stylianos, 1988; Lund et al., 1985-1986; Gass, 1987).

Dimond (1981) conceptualized adjustment to bereavement by developing a model which included support networks, concurrent losses, and coping skills as intervening factors for adaptation. Unfortunately, she did not identify the culture which is integral to support networks and coping skills.

Carter (1989), in a thematic analysis of reports by adults who were bereaved, identified five core themes: being stopped, hurting, missing, holding, and seeking. She concluded that reappearance of grief after many years of loss can be expected.

In the psychiatric literature grief was conceptualized as an intrapsychic emotional pain which resolved with orderly stages in time, or it became pathological. Freud (1917) described melancholia resulting from pathological grief. Lindemann (1944) depicted grief as a six-week crisis. Engel (1964), who described three stages of grief necessary for healing—shock and disbelief, developing awareness, and restitution—also described cultural grief practices (e.g., funeral ceremonies) as helpful to the bereaved.

In response to Lindemann's (1944) position that recovery from grief might be achieved in six weeks, Glick, Weiss, and Parkes (1974), in their study of the first year of widowhood, found that resolution of grief might require many years and multiple crises. Other studies confirm that grief can pose illness and even death risks for widows following the loss of their spouses (Parkes, 1975; Bornstein et al., 1973; Ball, 1976-1977; Shneidman, 1980; Rigdon, Clayton, & Dimond, 1987).

The anthropological literature offers numerous rich descriptions of cultural influences on grief. Rosenblatt, Walsh, and Jackson (1976), in their study of grief in 78 cultures, reported that, while people in all cultures react with emotional distress to the loss of loved ones, specific cultural practices exist to assist people to work through their losses. Danforth and Tsiaras (1982), for example, described death rituals of rural Greece, where memorial services and the eating of specific foods assisted grieving persons to resolve their loss.

These anthropological researchers and others (Gorer, 1965; Kalish & Reynolds, 1976; Kalish, 1985) described grief phenomena in a variety of situations. Mathison (1970) discussed institutional controls such as wearing special clothing to mark widowhood. Matchett (1972) related the hallucinatory experiences of Hopi Indian women during grieving. Yamamoto et al. (1969) reported that Japanese widows are comforted by offering their dead husbands gifts and food.

In summary, the literature demonstrated that expressions of care, health, and grief exist in cultures expressed by diverse patterns. However, little is known about the meanings and experiences of Greek Canadian widows. Hence, the linkage between culture and care, health, and grief needed further systematic documentation in this investigation.

RESEARCH METHODS

To discern the Greek Canadian widows' lifeways, beliefs, and values, and answer the research questions, the ethnonursing, ethnographic, and life health-care history methods were selected. Ethnonursing is discussed in detail in Chapter 2.

Ethnography was used in conjunction with ethnonursing to systematically observe, detail, describe, document, and analyze the lifeways of the Greek Canadian widows in their environment (Leininger, 1985d). In contrast with ethnonursing (focused on nursing phenomena), ethnography documented the broader general lifeways. Additionally, the life health care history method gave a sequenced account of cultural care, cultural health, and grief phenomena experienced by informants. Leininger developed this method based on the anthropological life history method (Leininger, 1985e).

Selection of Informants

Through the assistance of church and Greek Canadian community leaders, entrance was gained into three Greek Canadian communities in order to select informants and collect data.

The most effective informants were those who were knowledgeable about their own culture, currently involved in the culture, and were willing to teach the investigator (Spradley, 1979; Leininger, 1985b). Twelve key informants and 30 general informants were purposefully selected during observation-participation in churches, the community, and at senior citizen functions, where the appropriateness of potential informants were appraised (Pelto & Pelto, 1978).

Key informants were selected who met the following criteria: widows who identified with the Greek culture, widowed for six months or more, able to speak and understand English, willing to participate in the study, and were 50 years of age or older. Older widows were chosen because research suggested that experiences of widows whose families were grown were different than that of younger widows (Vachon et al., 1976). They ranged in age from 50 to 81 years, and were widowed from 6 months to 24 years. They were Canadian residents born in a variety of countries: two in Canada, two in the United States, six in Greece, and two in Turkey.

During less intensive interviews than those given key informants, general informants were selected to reflect on the meanings expressed by the key informants. General informants, who included Greek community leaders, family and friends of widows, ethnohistorians, and 15 widows, confirmed the patterns which emerged from key informants.

DATA COLLECTION

Observation-Participation-Reflection
Ethnonursing Model

Leininger's (1990) Observation-Participation-Reflection phases were used to guide systematically the study of key and general informants in their cultural contexts at family gatherings, senior citizen activities, church services, and a funeral service. Beginning by observing, then observing with some participation, the investigator moved to primarily participating. Finally, observation-participation culminated in reflective observations to confirm findings by rechecking key informants.

Ethnographic/Ethnonursing Interviewing

Interviews were conducted in naturalistic environments such as informants' homes or churches. Interviewing guides consisting of semistructured and open-ended statements were developed specifically for this study. Observations and meanings were regularly checked with informants to strengthen credibility of the findings.

Inquiry Enabling Guides

Several enabling guides were used in addition to the interviewing guides. A field journal recorded investigator observations and reactions, as well as informants' linguistic expressions. The Leininger (1985e) Life History Health Care Protocol recorded six key informants' health care histories. The acculturation of each first and second generation key informant was contrasted using the Leininger's (1991) Acculturation Rating and Profile Scale of Traditional and Nontraditional Lifeways. These ethnocare enablers are discussed fully in Chapter 2.

Data Recording

The Leininger-Templin-Thompson Ethnoscript Qualitative Software program (1984) was used with a personal computer in combination with Data Base III Plus for data management and retrieval by code and text.

Data Analysis and Evaluation Criteria

Data analysis progressed through incremental higher levels of abstraction by using Leininger's (1990) Phases of Ethnonursing Analysis for Qualitative Data. The analysis moved from collection of rich qualitative raw data, identification of descriptors, pattern analysis, and to eventual theme formulation.

Criteria for ongoing systematic evaluation included credibility, confirmability, meanings-in-context, recurrent patterning, saturation, and transferability (Leininger, 1990). These evaluation criteria are discussed in depth in Chapter 2.

FINDINGS

Seven major themes and research findings were abstracted from the raw data, descriptors, and patterns. Six themes reflected commonalities among the Greek Canadian widows, and one reflected differences among the widows based on generation of immigration. Major themes are presented with supporting descriptors and patterns using Leininger's (1990a, p. 50) Phases of Ethnonursing Analysis for Qualitative Data.

Theme 1

For Greek Canadian widows, cultural care meant responsibility for, reciprocation, concern, love, companionship, family protection, hospitality, and helping, derived from their kinship, religious, and cultural beliefs, and values.

Family and church were focal in the cultural care of older Greek Canadian widows. Grown children took responsibility for assisting with decision making, handling finances, and activities of daily living. They also assisted their mothers in deciding where to live, with most widows choosing to remain in their own homes, and protected them from additional sorrow.

Cultural care meant that widows and their families reciprocated concern, love, hospitality, and companionship. It also meant comfort from prayer and support from the Greek Orthodox Church. Verbatim descriptors confirmed that cultural care, derived from the widows' cultural beliefs and values, had numerous meanings. A key informant emphasized the importance of family and religion:

My children take care of me, bringing things to me, visit. They remember me on Mother's day, bring me fresh fish. I lived with one of my children when I first came to Canada. . . . I would say (advise) . . . get religious support.

General informants who were the grown children of widows, said they respected their elderly mothers for their wisdom, and included them in their family and social activities. Observations confirmed caring interactions between widows and their daughters, sons, and grandchildren. Grandchildren interacted affectionately with the widows, calling them "*Yaiyai*," a Greek word meaning grandmother.

Family members reciprocated care, illustrated by a key informant who said, "At first I don't care for my hair and make-up. I say, 'you better change yourself.' I say [to daughter], 'You need me and I need you. I make me to have a life again'." Community care was evident with neighbors and members of the church rendering care by visiting, bringing food, and inviting widows to their homes.

From the descriptors, the following patterns were derived:

1. Grown children assisted their mothers with decision making, transportation, paying bills, and interacting with the larger community.

2. Widows continued the pattern of remaining in their marital homes after their husbands died.

3. Regular visiting was evident between widows and their families.

4. Widows were part of a social network that spanned several generations.

5. Family and community members were concerned about and protected the widows from additional sorrow.

6. Members of the Greek community reflected respect for the elderly.

7. Grown children reciprocated their mothers' loving care.

8. Family, friends, and members of the Greek community provided food, hospitality, and companionship for the widows.

9. Widows sought care from God and the Greek Orthodox Church as they prayed.

Theme 2

Greek Canadian meanings and expressions of grief focused on beliefs about the endurance of the husbands' life spirit as an integral part of the widows' cultural care lifeways.

Grief care practices assisted in the transition to the status of widow-hood. The black symbols, designated time periods, and memorial services honored the deceased as symbolic care. A key informant confirmed what others reported:

> *Believe me, the memorial services helped. . . . People came who we hadn't seen in years. . . . Forty days afterwards we had another memorial service. We brought* koliva *[sweetened wheat] to the church to give to the parishioners, and we said special prayers. At 60 days and one year we also had special prayers. I also go to the cemetery. It really helped when all the friends and people came around me.*

All widow informants related that in the early days after their husbands' death their family and friends brought food, visited, and gave encouragement to go on with life. *Trisayio* prayers services were conducted at the funeral home and at the church. *Mnimosina* memorial services to honor and protect the souls of their husbands were conducted on the fortieth day and recurrent times over three years. Thereafter, the major prayers for the dead occurred on *Soul Saturdays.* Informants reported they visited and cared for their husbands' graves to continue to honor them.

Key informants, who wore black for varying time periods, said black symbolized the sadness they felt. Most widows wore black for one year and then dark colors for several years after, although one discontinued black immediately after the funeral.

Attachment to their husbands was evidenced by the comfort care which many widows received from their husbands' presence after death as continuation of care within spiritual dimensions. A key informant said, "He's directing my life. He tell me things to do. The spirit is right in my life now."

At the same time that widows participated in attachment rituals to their deceased husbands such as prayers, wearing their wedding rings, and avoiding remarriage, they engaged in tie-breaking expressions such as giving away their husbands' clothes. A key informant said, "My mother packed all my husband's clothes and put them in the garage. . . ."

The following patterns were derived from the emic data to support this theme:

1. Family, friends, neighbors, and members of the Greek community gave grief care to the widows by giving comfort, providing food, visiting, and giving encouragement to carry on with life.

2. Prayer by informants maintained family honor by showing respect to their deceased husbands.

3. Widows wore black for one year and dark colors for several years after their husbands' death.

4. Caring for their husbands' graves meant care as honor to their husbands' memories.

5. A pattern of giving away their husbands' clothes and possessions after they died prevailed.

6. Widows received comfort from the belief in their deceased husbands' presence was evident.

Theme 3

For Greek Canadian widows, transition from wives to widows meant resignation to their husbands' death based upon the belief that "life goes on," with active remembrances of the husbands' care values and lifeways.

Emotional expressions of grief diminished over time but the grief and remembrances of the husbands continued; transition to widowhood meant resignation rather than acceptance. Life continued for the widows as they carried on their husbands' care values and lifeways.

A key informant expressed the sentiments of many informants when she said, "I never forget him." Grief came and went over the years expressed by crying and yearning for their husbands. A key informant said:

I never get used to it. I am happy for a few hours—then I feel so empty. I got my kids, I'm proud of them. Kids can't make you feel happy. Can be happy, but different than if I have my husband.

Another key informant confirmed similar feelings by saying, "It's not as severe as it is in the beginning, you know, you don't cry every time you think of your man, your person, your partner in life. Many times you do though."

Even though all the informants said they cried, especially immediately following their husbands' death and at the funeral, most stated that crying was not helpful. A typical belief about crying was expressed by a key informant who said, "You try to control yourself and you learn how to control, and eventually you face the fact of life and say life is like that, beginning and end."

All widows said they experienced disbelief when their spouses died, some saying this continued for many years. One widow of several years said, "I still can't believe my husband's dead . . . I feel like I'll lose my mind." Except for one widow who expressed anger about her husband, most widows overlooked negative remembrances to maintain their husbands' honor.

Informants stressed that their families and religion provided them with care to "go on with life." Religious memorial services gave the informants opportunities to express their grief as well as to honor their husbands. Many of the informants verbalized gratitude that their husbands had a "peaceful death" which reflected a good life. They also prayed for such a death for themselves to avoid burdening their children. A key informant expressed this poignantly:

Yes, he passed out, but didn't have the agony, he passed out like a good Christian, like a good man he was. . . . If I was in Greece people would sit at my table and they would say "and I wish you Cala Esterna," a good ending. . . . a peaceful death . . . the end of your life will be peaceful and without any struggle.

The following recurrent patterning supported this theme:

1. Widows continued with their lives by attempting to maintain stability of lifeways and care values.

2. Expressions of disbelief, crying, and sorrow abated but did not terminate in the widows' daily lives.

3. A recurrent belief held by widows was that crying was not helpful.

4. Widows honored their dead husbands and expressed their grief at religious memorial services.

5. A pattern of gratitude for husbands who died peacefully was reflected by the widows.
6. Widows prayed for their own peaceful death to decrease the burden on their families.

Theme 4

Differences in gender roles for Greek Canadian spouses revealed distinct care meanings and expectations.

All key informants said the major role responsibility of their husbands was to maintain authority, be strong, and function as head of the patriarchal household. Husbands were to provide financially for the families' everyday needs as well as the children's education. However, some key informants said they had financial power within the household as explained by one key informant, "I was boss in house, he was boss in business."

If the wife worked outside the home, it was often done with reluctance and out of necessity to augment the family income. One key informant who worked indicated that her employment reduced her husband's self-concept as provider. She said, "I didn't tell my husband when I went to get the job because he would be embarrassed. . . . My husband was a proud man".

Many informants said their husbands had worked long hours in family businesses or as laborers resulting in long absences from home. When they returned from work their wives tried to please them by making their homes as harmonious and tranquil as possible.

Most key informants said they were expected to administer their homes, have meals ready to serve their husbands, bear children, and discipline and teach the children Greek values. A key informant explained the importance of child rearing:

Life begins with childhood and what the child is exposed to from the very beginning has such a great value for the rest of growing up. . . . You take an oak tree. You plant a little seed and up comes the seedling. And if that seedling is crooked and nobody puts a stick

beside it to straighten it up—that oak tree, the proud oak tree will
be crooked.

Despite the expectation that the husbands would be the sole bread-winners, 9 of the 12 key informants held jobs while they were married. Those who worked in the family businesses assisted their husbands rather than being major decision makers. This data confirmed the pattern of the wives working despite the value for women to be housewives, suggesting a hierarchy of values, whereby the value for families to avoid government assistance was stronger than the value for wives to remain at home.

Most informants reported that care by the husbands and wives to each other was based on mutual commitment to family life. They provided care to each other during illness, performing roles which were not usual gender activities. For instance, many informants said their husbands cooked, cleaned, and took care of the children when they were ill. The widows described caring activities which they performed when their spouses were dying. A key informant said, "I learned how to give him nasal feeding because he wanted to come home (from the hospital)." Care between husbands and wives did not usually take the form of public shows of affection. Together, the husbands and wives were responsible to protect family honor, cherishing the "good family name."

Despite a few unhappy marriages related to alcohol abuse, most widow informants spoke about great spousal mutual respect and shared love. They talked about the different contributions which the husbands and wives made to family life and care.

The following patterns substantiated this theme:

1. In Greek Canadian homes husbands provided financially for their families' everyday needs and the children's education.

2. Greek Canadian husbands exhibited care by maintaining final authority over decisions which reflected protection of the family.

3. Husbands preferred that their wives did not work outside their homes, but if wives did work it was to augment the families' income.

4. Women who worked outside their homes while married were expected to fulfil their female role activities.

5. The pattern of care by Greek Canadian wives included child-bearing, child rearing, cultural food preparation, and maintaining a peaceful home atmosphere for their hard working husbands.

6. Women who worked in their husband's businesses were assistants to their husbands rather than major decision makers.

7. Spousal care was based upon love, companionship, helping, fulfilment of gender role expectations, and mutual obligation to family life.

Theme 5

Cultural health of Greek Canadian widows meant a state of well being, ability to perform daily role activities, and avoidance of pain and illness.

Good health, highly valued, was commonly expressed by informants in this proviso: "Health and family are the most important things in life." Three major meanings of health were identified: well being, ability to perform daily role activities, and avoidance of pain and illness.

The health of the widows was an extended family concern. Grown children took responsibility to drive their mothers to doctors' appointments, assist them with daily role activities such as housework, and provide them with companionship to increase their well being.

Well being as health was expressed by a widow holistically in this way: "The body, spirit, and mind can't be separated." Verbatim expressions such as "happy," "feeling good about myself," "vigor," "having my mind to make judgements," expressed well being as health. A key informant said, "I think health is feeling good, enjoying the things available in life, for instance, going to movies and having good friends."

Many informants identified the importance of performing culturally defined daily role activities as health, exemplified by, "Health means being able to get out of bed each morning, do my functions, be free, be independent." Role activities included caring for their husbands' graves, providing hospitality, taking care of their grandchildren, cooking and baking for themselves and family, cleaning, attending church, going on family outings, and doing volunteer work. Maintenance of independence was viewed as important to performance of role activities.

Health also meant avoidance of pain and illness. A key informant related, "I want health because I'm afraid if I get sick I don't know what will happen to me. I worry about getting sick." Many key informants said they sought physician services to treat illnesses. Pain was viewed as a sign of poor health. A key informant summed up several concepts of health when she said:

Health means a lot. I don't want to see myself in an old age home . . . Health means happy. I not afraid, I don't [want] to be dependent, can do the things I want. If I want to go to Windsor, I go . . . If I sick, [I] don't want to say take me for a bath or washroom.

The following patterns, which were derived from the verbatim descriptors, reflected recurrent meanings and expression in support of this theme:

1. There was a belief that the state of the widows' health affected the extended family.

2. Health as well being reflected "feeling good," "happiness," "vigor," "enjoying life," having cognitive ability, and high self-esteem.

3. Health meant performing daily role activities reflecting the culturally expected behaviors for their many statuses of widows, mothers, grandmothers, friends, volunteers, and employees.

4. Widows visited physicians and took medications to avoid illness and pain.

Theme 6

Cultural care continuity diminished the spousal care void and contributed to the cultural health of Greek Canadian widows.

When their husbands were alive, Greek Canadian wives and husbands reciprocated care to each other. This spousal care was expressed

by love, companionship, assistance, fulfilment of gender role expectations, sick care, and protection.

The husbands' death meant that widows lost important givers and
recipients of care. The widows missed this reciprocity of care, experiencing *a spousal care void*. A key informant said, "Losing a partner
changes your life. Life is made up of many details. Suddenly all is gone.
You have to work out everything without a husband." Considerable
data supported the pattern of giving and receiving care during the
transition to widowhood, *cultural care continuity*, as reducing the
spousal care void.

Verbatim data from key and general informants confirmed that
care received by the widows positively influenced their health. One
widow said, "Oh yes, when they show they care about me, I feel
happy and healthy." Another widow said, "Before I don't feel good.
They [family] take care of me even before I miss something to make
me better."

In addition to being the recipients of care, widows who gave care to
others improved their well being. A key informant who received culturally learned care from her grown children and grandchildren told of
her satisfaction from also giving care:

> *I have full days. I'm busy with the children, help my daughter, cook
> supper. I help my daughter from the time I lost my husband. [Before
> I came] she had a babysitter. I do something good. I raise two little
> kids with no worries. I am very happy about this. I have my own
> apartment. I go there Friday night and come back here on Sunday
> night.*

Many widows reported they improved their health when they "kept
busy" by giving care to other people within the cultural contexts of
family, community, and church. A key informant said, "I believe that
giving care helps me stay healthy. It helps me and it helps them . . . I
don't expect them to care for me, I give because I want it. I don't
expect [care] back." Another key informant said, "If you are caring, and
are cared for, you feel good mentally. I guess that's health."

Patterns which supported cultural care continuity as diminishing
the spousal care void and contributing to the health of the widows
were as follows:

1. Love, companionship, protection, and helping as care was reciprocated between wives and their husbands as patterned relationships.
2. Husbands and wives provided illness care for each other.
3. "Keeping busy" with activities which reflected Greek Canadian cultural care values enhanced the widows' well being as a pattern of behavior.
4. Giving and receiving care was viewed by key informants as attenuating the spousal care void that was created by their husbands' death.
5. Improvement in widows' health occurred when they gave and received care.

Theme 7

Cultural care and grief had different patterns, beliefs, and expressions for Greek Canadian widows born in Greece and Turkey, and those born in Canada and the United States.

Cultural care differences between informants born in Greece and Turkey, and informants born in Canada and the United States, was evident from prominent indicators such as mourning clothes, social interaction, household symbols of religion, and maintenance of composure.

All eight first generation key informants said they wore black for a minimum of 40 days. Some said they wore black for one year, others for three years. A key informant from Greece said:

I wear black for three years. I wear a kerchief, then prints with dark. Now I put everything on. Inside I feel like black [depressed]. My kids say "no like" wearing dark clothes. My kids bring back light colored clothes [for me] when they go away.

The four second generation key informants were all observed wearing lighter clothes. Two said they wore black for 40 days, while the remaining two said they did not wear black as mourning attire after the funeral. A key informant summed up why she discarded black mourning attire by saying "I tried to have life continue as it was."

Diversities between the two groups of key informants extended to the action pattern of social interaction. First generation informants interacted primarily in the Greek language with other Greek and Turkish born ladies in activities which revolved around the church. A key informant born in a small city in the United States commented about the cohesiveness and ethnocentrism of the first generation Greeks in large cities: "The Greeks [in large cities] are backward. They stay together. If there is only a handful, they would have to mix." Many of the first generation key informants verbalized their difficulty mastering the English language, learning English gradually from their children. All first generation key informants confirmed that they spoke Greek at home, and with their friends and relatives. Second generation key informants spoke English to their children, could understand and speak Greek, and encouraged their children to learn Greek. A second generation key informant illustrated the social interaction differences by saying, "We're more aware of what goes on outside our home in politics and the world around us, as compared to, for instance, my mother who wouldn't understand as much."

There was substantial credibility and confirmability, however, that second generation key informants also were deeply involved in Greek communal life in Canada. While they each said they had a circle of Greek friends born in many countries, they also had many non-Greek friends. Most of these women said they felt "different" than Greek-born women.

Another contrast between the groups was the pattern of household symbols of religion. Each of the first generation widows displayed vigil lights and icons. Only one second generation informant had a vigil light, but several reminisced about religious symbols from their childhood days.

A final difference was the meaning of composure. Many first generation key informants expressed the need to "keep a happy face" for their children. While they said their "hearts were sad," they believed their Canadian born children expected them to "keep their feelings inside" and make the best of life. In contrast, second generation informants said they did not feel pressured to suppress expressions of grief, suggesting their emotional expressions were viewed as appropriate by their children. Several informants commented that first generation widows were more expressive of emotions.

To further establish credibility regarding the diversity between first and second generation key informants, the two groups were compared using Leininger's Acculturation Rating and Profile Scale of Traditional and Nontraditional Lifeways to determine differences in acculturation. The overall median scores (Figure 1) demonstrated a greater traditional profile for key informants born in Greece and Turkey than those born in Canada and the United States, the differences related to acculturation. The major commonalities between generations of immigration occurred with similar traditional family, educational lifeways, cultural values, and nontraditional use of technology.

The following patterns represented meanings-in-context reflective of differences between first generation and second generation informants:

1. First generation widows remained in dark mourning clothes longer than widows born in Canada and the United States.

2. Widows born in Canada and the United States expressed the daily lifestyle pattern of social interaction beyond the Greek community into the larger community.

3. Household symbols of religion such as vigil lights and icons were evident with first generation widows.

4. First generation widows stifled their expression of grief to appease their acculturated children.

DISCUSSION

The major findings are discussed in relation to Leininger's theory of Culture Care Diversity and Universality with reflections on van Gennep's rites of passage as the conceptual framework.

Cultural care was confirmed to be essential for persons to face a critical life event such as the death of a husband (Leininger, 1985a). The care constructs of responsibility for, reciprocation, concern, love, companionship, family protection, hospitality, and helping were abstracted from the emic data. These enabling behaviors were embedded in the worldview and social structure features within language and

Figure 1
Median Acculturation Rating and Profile Scale of Traditional and Nontraditional Lifeways of First and Second Generation Key Informants (*n* = 12)

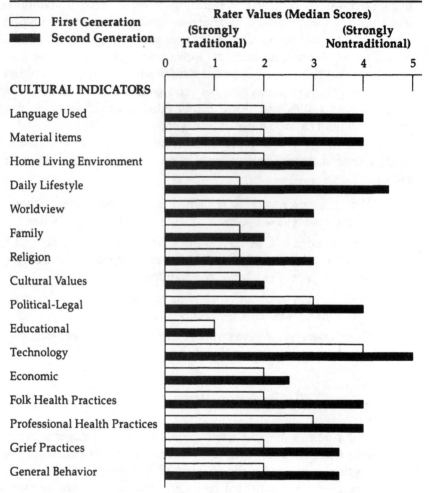

environmental context in the Greek Canadian culture. The meanings and practices of kinship, religion, and cultural beliefs and values were major influencers on the care patterns of the older widows which led to their health. This is in accord with Leininger's theory about social structure and other features influencing care and in turn health.

Grief care practices such as visiting and bringing food comforted the new widows. Practices such as praying and wearing mourning clothes gave posthumous spiritual care by honoring the memories of the deceased. This also is congruent with Leininger's theory which holds that human care patterns are based upon cultural care values, practices, and beliefs (1985a).

Grief practices assisted the transition to widowhood, substantiating van Gennep's conceptualization (1960). During the mourning period, when the widows were in a transitional stage, memorial prayers were said at specific intervals until the conclusion of the three-year period which marked the widows' reintegration into society. In rural Greece, the transition period is clearly completed when the deceased are exhumed and their bones placed in the village ossuary (Danforth & Tsiaras, 1982). Since the cultural practice of secondary burial is not performed in Canada, it may be speculated that the incorporation phase for Greek widows in Canada might be delayed, particularly for first generation immigrants who were enculturated into this exhumation practice.

The widows performed several grief practices which accomplished paradoxical functions of tie-breaking and attachment to their deceased husbands. Van Gennep (1960) stated the transition period is complex, with ongoing processes for the deceased and for the mourners. Hence, the complexity of the transitional period was marked by the tie-breaking ritual of giving away the deceased husbands' clothes concurrently with the attachment rituals of prayers and remembrances. The finding that widows received comfort care from the belief in their deceased husbands' presence was confirmed by the Greek Orthodox Christian spiritual literature (Carlson & Soroka, 1954) but conflicted with the psychiatric literature which tended to categorize this as pathological (Clayton, Desmarais, & Winokur, 1968).

The findings give credibility to cultural diversities of grief expressions and raise questions about categorizing grief as "pathological" without knowing cultural care beliefs, values, and practices. The process of grief did not follow linear stages as the literature suggested (Engel, 1964; Lindemann, 1944). Instead, grief expressions ebbed and flowed as waves of sorrow which abated but did not terminate, as Carter found in her study (1989). The women did not accept their husbands' death. They surrendered to widowhood with resignation.

The finding that crying was not considered helpful beyond the early days of bereavement conflicted with the psychiatric and psychiatric nursing literature (Freud, 1917; Stuart & Sundeen, 1987) which purports that crying is cathartic. Even though crying may be a universal expression of grief (Rosenblatt, Walsh, & Jackson, 1976), the findings confirm there are diverse cultural beliefs about the value and appropriateness of crying.

Greek Canadian husbands and wives performed different gender roles and made unique care contributions to each other and to family life. These gender roles were learned from their parents through enculturation in a patriarchal family structure (Leininger, 1978). Both the husbands and wives valued their roles, saw them as equal but different, and expected role performance from themselves and their spouses.

Spousal care patterns supported Leininger's prediction that "Humans are caring beings capable of being concerned about, holding interest in, or having regard for other people's needs, well being, and survival" (1985a, p. 210). The complementarity of gender roles supported Luna's (1989) similar finding among Lebanese Muslims living in the U.S. The findings from this investigation and Luna's study emphasize the importance of viewing gender roles within the total context of care and culture.

The orientational definition of cultural health referred to "well being expressions" and "ability to perform daily role activities." However, Leininger (1988) said orientational definitions may be changed to fit the people's perspective. The findings substantiated avoidance of pain and illness as an additional meaning of health. Therefore, the definition of *cultural health* has been altered in keeping with the mission of ethnonursing research to develop emic meanings of nursing phenomena:

Cultural health of Greek Canadian widows meant a state of well being, ability to perform daily role activities, and avoidance of pain and illness.

Credibility, recurrent patterning, confirmability, meanings-in-context, and saturation were established regarding the essential nature and benefits of cultural care continuity, the giving as well as receiving of care during the transition to a different lifecycle phase such as widowhood. A growing body of care literature documented the rewards of receiving care, but only Gates (1988) explicated the advantages gained by the givers of care. The provision of cultural care continuity was found to facilitate promotion of health for Greek Canadian widows, demonstrating the comprehensiveness and richness of care.

While first and second generation Greek Canadian widows had similar values for family, religion, and education, they expressed several diverse patterns regarding cultural care and grief. Leininger's (1991) Acculturation Health Care Assessment Tool for Cultural Patterns in Traditional and Nontraditional Lifeways confirmed the finding that first generation widows were more traditional than second generation widows, a difference explained by acculturation. The second generation widows were socialized into a Greek Canadian culture which blended both Greek and Canadian cultural features. Leininger (1978, p. 104) stated, "acculturation refers to the process by which a given culture is adapting to or learning how to take on the behavior of another cultural group." They learned to be Greek from their parents and their Greek Orthodox church; they learned to be Canadian from the public schools, their neighbors, and their non-Greek friends.

CULTURAL CARE NURSING DECISIONS AND ACTIONS

Leininger (1985a, 1988) predicted that cultures know care in diverse ways. Therefore, nurses must be guided by knowledge of clients' social structure and worldview within language and environmental contexts to provide culturally relevant care. Clients' values, beliefs, and practices must be integrated into their nursing care. Culturally congruent care, the ultimate goal of nursing, can be provided through three modes of supportive or enabling professional actions and decisions: cultural care preservation or maintenance, cultural care accommodation or negotiation, and cultural care repatterning or restructuring.

Cultural Care Preservation/Maintenance

In this study, cultural care preservation/maintenance refers to professional actions which perpetuate cultural resources to maintain health
and caring lifeways of grieving Greek Canadian widows. The widows
were sustained by cultural care from their loving families, faith in their
religion, and the Greek community. Cultural care preservation could
be used by nurses to encourage and strengthen those resources already
available to the widows.

The church, binding people to the Greek language and Greek Orthodox religion and culture, is an important element in cultural care
preservation. The wives of priests, known in Greek as *Presvytera*, are
often available for advice and counsel to Greek people in need of care.
Widows who participate in church activities and who talk to priests'
wives do seem to benefit from such interaction. When widows pray at
memorial services, for example, they fulfill a culturally created need
to provide symbolic care to their deceased husbands.

Because kinship is a central social structure feature in the Greek
Canadian culture, focus on the entire family rather than on individual
widows seems an appropriate perspective. Particularly for first generation informants, grown children are expected to be active in decision
making for their mothers. While family members can usually be
counted on to provide care activities when their mothers are ill or in
need, it is important to work with the delegated family leaders such as
grown sons and daughters who will orchestrate the care.

Hospitality, a cultural care activity which is embedded in the culture, is another available element of giving. Widows who isolate themselves in their sorrow, for whatever personal reasons, also will miss the
solace of hosting family and friends in their homes, can be encouraged
to invite family and friends to their homes. Visiting and sharing Greek
food has been shown to promote care activities as well as support good
nutrition.

The widows' spiritual belief in the presence of their husbands can be
understood to be culturally appropriate as comfort care and fostered by
the nurse. Encouraging the widows to reminisce about their husbands'
contributions to the family and community is another method to perpetuate family honor and bring comfort.

Finally, nurses who support cultural care continuity in promoting
the health of Greek Canadian widows also can reawaken the widows'

interest in caring for others. Data shows that, for these study subjects, assisting their grown children, participating in the charitable activities of the *Philoptochos Society*, the women's group of the Greek Orthodox church, and visiting the ill are examples of activities for provision of care to others congruent with cultural care values under discussion here. Nurses need to be mindful that widows gain benefits from giving as well as receiving care.

Cultural Care Accommodation/Negotiation

Findings from this study give direction for adaptive actions to promote the health of Greek Canadian widows through cultural care accommodation/negotiation.

Nursing assessment information about ways the widows and their husbands gave care to each is beneficial. If their husbands provided authority and total family income, inquiry could be made about plans to assist the widows. The nurse needs to assess the family, church, and community involvement to determine deficiencies in care. For example, the nurse might involve Greek community resources, if they are available, to strengthen families' ability to give care when grown children's jobs or young children keep them from providing all the required care. Even in a culture which maintains strong family values, family members may be troubled by their own grief and obligations, and adaptation may be necessary.

It is helpful to avoid imposing nursing's value for self-disclosure on widows of cultural groups who are hesitant to share negative feelings about their husbands for fear of dishonouring them. This reluctance to disclose these feelings should be respected. Nurses can adapt their approach by empathetic listening without prodding; if the widows wish to share negative feelings, they should be counselled over several sessions to diminish guilt.

When community health nurses visit the homes of Greek Canadian widows, they need to take time to establish trust. This may mean sitting down for coffee and Greek cultural food, because refusing the hospitality of a first generation immigrant may be taken as an insult. Learning about religious patterns, discovering family relationships, and learning folk care and health practices assist the nurse to adapt health teaching to provide culturally relevant care.

Cultural Care Repatterning/Restructuring

Cultural care repatterning/restructuring refers to altering behavior of either the client or the nurse to promote health.

Group counselling is a common mode in modern nursing. However, it would be culturally incongruent for most first generation immigrants to ventilate their feelings in a group of strangers, especially if they could not speak English well and had little formal education. Cultural care repatterning would result, however, if nurses assisted in individual discussion with widows of their widowhood lifeways with a trusted Greek Orthodox priest, for example, or with staff at a Greek community social service agency.

Nurses must repattern their attitudes if they believe that widowhood is a crisis which terminates in a few weeks or months. The practice of diagnosing dysfunctional grieving in Greek Canadian widows who continue to experience sorrow needs restructuring since the findings confirm grief diminished rather than terminated. Concluding that these widows were experiencing prolonged pathological grieving may be ethnocentric conclusions based on the nurses' own cultural beliefs and values.

Finally, nurses will avoid stereotyping when they understand there is cultural variability as well as similarities among people of cultural groups. The finding that important differences exist between first and second generation Greek Canadian widows illustrates the need for nurses to examine their belief that patterns are automatically shared by all people within a culture.

CONCLUSION

This investigation was conceptualized within Leininger's theory of Culture Care Diversity and Universality, a comprehensive theory which assisted discovery of cultural care, cultural health, and grief meanings and expressions for Greek Canadian widows. The use of Leininger's theory enabled holistic understanding of the widows' lifeways by exploring social structure, worldview, language, and environmental contexts.

The research findings reported here contributed to Leininger's theory by building and substantiating a body of nursing care and cultural health knowledge which identified, described, explained, and interpreted culturally specific care as a therapeutic mode. It is the hope of this author that such findings will aid nurses in providing culturally congruent nursing care.

REFERENCES

Aamodt, A. (1979). Social-cultural dimensions of caring in the world of the Papago child and adolescent. In M. M. Leininger (Ed.), *Transcultural nursing* (pp. 47–56). New York: Masson Publishing.

Anderson, J. (1985). Perspectives on the health of immigrant women: A feminist analysis. *Advances in Nursing Science, 8*(1), 61–76.

Ball, J. (1976–77). Widow's grief: The impact of age and mode of death. *Omega, 7*(4), 303–333.

Bornstein, P., Clayton, P., Halikas, J., Maurice, W., & Robins, E. (1973). The depression of widowhood after thirteen months. *British Journal of Psychiatry, 122,* 561–566.

Boyle, J. (1984). Indigenous caring practices in a Guatemalan Colonia. In M. M. Leininger (Ed.), *Care: The essence of nursing and health.* Thorofare, NJ: Slack, 123–132.

Brock, A. (1984). From wife to widow: A changing lifestyle. *Journal of Gerontological Nursing, 10*(4), 8–15.

Carlson, S., & Soroka, L. (1954). *Faith of our fathers: The eastern orthodox religion.* Minneapolis: Olympic Press.

Carter, S. (1989). Themes of grief. *Nursing Research, 38*(6), 354–358.

Danforth, L., & Tsiaras, A. (1982). *The death rituals of rural Greece.* Princeton: Princeton University Press.

Dimond, M. (1981). Bereavement and the elderly: A critical review with implications for nursing practice and research. *Journal of Advanced Nursing, 6*(6), 461–470.

Engel, G. (1964). Grief and grieving. *American Journal of Nursing, 64*(9), 93–98.

Freud, S. (1917). Mourning and melancholia, in *The complete psychological works of Sigmund Freud,* Vol XIV. London: Hogarth Press, 1957, 243–258.

Gass, K. (1987). The health of conjugally bereaved older widows: The role of appraisal, coping and resources. *Research in Nursing & Health, 10,* 39–47.

Gates, M. (1988). *Care and cure meanings, experiences and orientations of persons who are dying in hospital and hospice settings.* Unpublished doctoral dissertation. Detroit: Wayne State University.

Gaut, D. (1981). Conceptual analysis of caring: Research method. In M. M. Leininger (Ed.), Caring: An essential human need. Thorofare, NJ: Slack, 17-24.

Gaut, D. (1983). Development of a theoretically adequate description of caring. Western Journal of Nursing Research, 5(4), 312-324.

Gaut, D. (1984). A philosophical orientation to caring research. In M. M. Leininger (Ed.), Care: The essence of nursing and health. Thorofare, NJ: Slack, 27-44.

Glick, I., Weiss, R., & Parkes, C. M. (1974). The first year of bereavement. New York: John Wiley & Sons.

Gorer, G. (1965). Death, grief, and mourning. Garden City: Doubleday & Co.

Kalish, R. (1985). Death, grief, and caring relationships. Monterey: Brooks/ Cole Publishing.

Kalish, R., & Reynolds, D. (1976). Death and ethnicity: A psychocultural study. Los Angeles: University of Southern California Press.

King, I. (1981). A theory for nursing. New York: Wiley.

Leininger, M. M. (1967). The culture concept and its relevance to nursing. Journal of Nursing Education, 6(2), 27-39.

Leininger, M. M. (1970). Nursing and anthropology: Two worlds to blend. New York: John Wiley & Sons.

Leininger, M. M. (1978). Transcultural nursing: Concepts, theories, and pratices. New York: John Wiley & Sons.

Leininger, M. M. (1979). The Gadsup of New Guinea and early child-caring behaviors with nursing care implications. In M. M. Leininger (Ed.), Transcultural nursing. New York: Masson Publishing, 167-185.

Leininger, M. M. (1981). The Phenomenon of caring: Importance, research questions and theoretical considerations. In M. M. Leininger (Ed.), Caring: An Essential human need. Thorofare, NJ: Slack, 3-16.

Leininger, M. M. (1984a). Care: The essence of nursing and health. In M. M. Leininger (Ed.), Care: The essence of nursing and health. Thorofare, NJ: Slack, 3-15.

Leininger, M. M. (1984b). Southern rural Black and White American lifeways with focus on care and health phenomena. In M. M. Leininger (Ed.), Care: The essence of nursing and health. Thorofare, NJ: Slack, 133-159.

Leininger, M. M. (1985a). Transcultural care diversity and universality: A theory of nursing. Nursing and Health Care, 6(4), 209-212.

Leininger, M. M. (1985b). Qualitative research methods in nursing. Orlando, FL: Grune & Stratton.

Leininger, M. M. (1985c). Nature, rationale, and importance of qualitative research methods in nursing. In M. M. Leininger (Ed.), Qualitative research methods in nursing. Orlando, FL: Grune & Stratton, 1-25.

Leininger, M. M. (1985d). Ethnography and ethnonursing: Models and modes of qualitative data analysis. In M. M. Leininger (Ed.), *Qualitative research methods in nursing*. Orlando, FL: Grune & Stratton, 33-71.

Leininger, M. M. (1985e). Life health-care history: Purposes, methods, and techniques. In M. M. Leininger (Ed.), *Qualitative Research Methods in Nursing*. Orlando, FL: Grune & Stratton, 119-132.

Leininger, M. M. (1988). Leininger's theory of nursing: Cultural care diversity and universality. *Nursing Science Quarterly, 1*(4), 152-160.

Leininger, M. M. (1990a). Ethnomethods: The philosophic and epistemic bases to explicate transcultural nursing knowledge. *Journal of Transcultural Nursing, 1*(2), 40-51.

Leininger, M. M., Templin, T., & Thompson, F. (1990b). *Leininger-Templin-Thompson ethnoscript qualitative software program: User's handbook*. Detroit: Wayne State University Press.

Leininger, M. M. (1991). Leininger's acculturation health care assessment guide for cultural patterns in traditional and non-traditional lifeways. *Journal of Transcultural Nursing, 2*(2), 40-42.

Lindemann, E. (1944). Symptomatology and management of acute grief. *American Journal of Psychiatry, 101*(1), 141-148.

Louie, T. (1976). Explanatory thinking in Chinese Americans. In P. Brink (Ed.), *Transcultural nursing: A book of readings* (pp. 240-246). Englewood Cliffs, NJ: Prentice-Hall.

Luna, L. (1989). *Care and cultural context of Lebanese Muslims in an urban U.S. community: an ethnographic/ethnonursing study conceptualized within Leininger's theory*. Unpublished doctoral dissertation. Detroit: Wayne State University.

Lund, D., Dimond, M., Caserta, M., Johnson, R., Poulton, J., & Connelly, J. (1985-86). Identifying elderly with coping difficulties after two years of bereavement, *Omega, 16*(3), 213-225.

Matchett, W. (1972). Repeated hallucinatory experiences as a part of the mourning process among Hopi Indian women. *Psychiatry, 35*, 185-194.

Mathison, J. (1970). A cross-cultural view of widowhood, *Omega, 1*(3), 201-218.

Neuman, B. (1989). *The Neuman systems model*. Norwalk, CT: Appleton and Lange.

Newman, M. (1979). *Theory development in nursing*. Philadelphia: F. A. Davis.

Orem, D. (1985). *Nursing: Concepts of practice*. New York: McGraw-Hill.

Parkes, C. M. (1975). Determinants of outcome following bereavement. *Omega, 6*(4), 303-323.

Pelto, P., & Pelto, G. (1978). *Anthropological research: The structure of inquiry*. Cambridge: Cambridge University Press.

Ragucci, A. (1979). The urban context of health beliefs and curing practices of elderly women in an Italian American enclave. In M. M. Leininger (Ed.), *Transcultural nursing*. New York: Masson Publishing, 222–242.

Ray, M. (1981). A philosophical analysis of caring within nursing. In M. M. Leininger (Ed.), *Caring: An essential human need* (pp. 25–36). Thorofare, NJ: Slack.

Rigdon, I., Clayton, B., & Dimond, M. (1987). Toward a theory of helpfulness for the elderly bereaved: An invitation to a new life. *Advances in Nursing Science, 9*(2), 32–43.

Rosenbaum, J. (1986). Relationship between ethnocaring value continuity and perceived health of Greek American widows: A mini ethnography. Unpublished manuscript.

Rosenbaum, J. (1990). *Cultural care, cultural health, and grief phenomena related to older Greek Canadian widows within Leininger's theory of culture care*. Doctoral dissertation. Detroit: Wayne State University.

Rosenblatt, P., Walsh, R., & Jackson, D. (1976). *Grief and mourning in cross-cultural perspective*. New Haven: HRAF Press.

Roy, C. (1984). *Introduction to nursing: An adaptation model*. Englewood Cliffs, NJ: Prentice-Hall.

Saunders, J. (1981). A process of bereavement resolution: Uncoupled identity, *Western Journal of Nursing Research, 3*(4), 319–336.

Shneidman, E. (1980). *Voices of death*. Cambridge: Harper & Row.

Spradley, J. (1979). *The ethnographic interview*. New York: Holt, Rinehart and Winston.

Stuart, G., & Sundeen, S. (1987). *Principles and practice of psychiatric nursing*. St. Louis: C.V. Mosby.

Tripp-Reimer, T. (1983). Retention of a folk-healing practice (Matiasma) among four generations of urban Greek immigrants. *Nursing Research, 32*(2), 97–101.

Tripp-Reimer, T. (1984). Reconceptualizing the construct of health. *Research in Nursing and Health, 7*(2), 101–109.

Tripp-Reimer, T. (1985). Expanding four essential concepts in nursing theory: The contribution of anthropology. In J. McCloskey & H. Grace (Eds.), *Current issues in nursing*. Boston: Blackwell, 91–103.

Vachon, M., & Stylianos, S. (1988). The role of social support in bereavement. *Journal of Social Issues, 44*(3), 175–190.

Vachon, M., Forms, A., Freedman, K., Lyall, W., Rogers, J., & Freeman, S. (1976). Stress reactions to bereavement. *Essence, 1*(1), 15–21.

van Gennep, A. (1960). *The rites of passage*. London: Routledge & Kegan Paul.

Watson, J. (1979). *Nursing: The philosophy and science of caring*. Boston: Little, Brown & Co.

Watson, J. (1985). *Nursing: Human science and human care: A Theory of nursing*. Norwalk, CT: Appleton-Century-Crofts.

Wenger, F. (1988). *The phenomenon of care in a high context culture: The Old Order Amish*. Doctoral dissertation. Wayne State University, Detroit.

Wiggins, L. (1983). Health and illness beliefs and practices among the Old Order Amish. *Health Values: Achieving High Level Wellness, 7*(6), 24–29.

Yamamoto, J., Okanogi, K., Iwasaki, T., & Yoshimura, S. (1969). Mourning in Japan. *American Journal of Psychiatry, 125*(12), 74–79.

RESEARCH FINDINGS FROM DIVERSE CULTURES WITH USE OF LEININGER'S CULTURE CARE THEORY AND ETHNOMETHODS

In this section, sample research findings from 23 out of 54 Western and non-Western cultures are presented. Dominant culture values with care meanings and action modes obtained directly from culture informants (*emic* based data) define the knowledge base. These findings are shared to serve as a general guide to the nurse in clinical or community practices. In addition, a list of 172 care constructs from the 54 cultures studied are presented to show considerable diversity in the linguistic terms or phrases used by informants. Another chapter is focused on the potential uses of Culture Care theory in nursing administration, education (including curriculum), and clinical practices within hospitals and other institutions, or in community based home care.

In the last chapter, I look to the future and reflect on ways Culture Care theory and the use of ethnonursing and other qualitative paradigmatic methods can facilitate the generation of a new body of humanistic and scientific nursing care knowledge to move nursing into the twenty-first century. This section should awaken nurses to see the rich and still largely untapped care knowledge yet to be discovered, refined, and applied to nursing. Culture Care theory has been invaluable in opening doors to a hitherto untapped fund of epistemic and ontologic knowledge. The section closes with a list of nurse researchers using Leininger's Culture Care Theory and a selection of available publications on the theory, its meaning, and uses.

10

Selected Culture Care Findings of Diverse Cultures Using Culture Care Theory and Ethnomethods

Madeleine M. Leininger

During the past three decades, I have worked with a number of graduate students and colleagues studying Western and non-Western cultures using the theory of Culture Care with the ethnonursing and other qualitative research methods. Presented here are sample research findings of different cultures derived from the study of worldview, social structure, environmental context, ethnohistory, and other dimensions of the theory. Unfortunately, space does not permit a full report on all cultures studied. Instead, dominant cultural care values, care meanings, and action modes will be presented to assist nurses, in part, to consider using these findings to guide their nursing practices with clients from 23 different cultures studied. These data are being shared because of frequent requests from many nurses who have heard about or seen several of these research findings, and are eager to improve the quality of care to clients from the cultures studied.

345

To use the findings reported in this chapter, the reader needs to keep in mind several facts and realities when reporting only partial but important findings from the cultures studied. Some of these realities are briefly summarized below.

First, the reader needs to realize that full ethnonursing systematic studies were done with each culture often over an extended period of time (usually one to several years) by the author or another transcultural nurse researcher who was knowledgeable about the theory, the ethnonursing method, my enablers, and my data modes of analysis. Second, the primary focus of the research was on the people's *emic* knowledge (the inside culture) views, and not on the nurse's *etic* (or outsider's) views, meanings, and practices related to culture care or caring. Third, the data presented are focused on cultural values and care meanings and actions. The findings represent only the "tip of the iceberg"—there is a wealth of ethnonursing data below the tip that could not be presented here. Nonetheless, the findings offer important data to understand the culture with its *patterned* care meanings and action modes as an initial basis for nursing care.

Fourth, since each culture was studied indepth by transcultural nurses who knew the theory of Culture Care, ethnonursing, and related qualitative methods, the findings reflect credible and accurate data for the cultures studied during the past 15 years. As researchers studied these cultures, approximately 13–18 *key* informants and usually twice that number of *general* informants (20–40) were participants in each study. Each researcher of a culture spent about three to five sessions (often 10–20 hours) with each key informant in their natural or familiar living environments (i.e., homes and communities). In keeping with the ethnonursing method, key informants were selected because they were held to be most knowledgeable about the culture and volunteered to share their lived-through insights about cultural care meanings, values, beliefs, and practices (Leininger, 1985a). The *general* informants participate as reflectors of the culture to help confirm some key informants' ideas, and to limit highly idiosyncratic or nonrepresentative culture data. In addition, the transcultural nurse made extensive observations, interviews, and direct-participant observations of the culture and of people's lifeways. Some ethnographic data were used with the ethnonursing method. The data were analyzed with Leininger's rigorous *Four Phase Data Analysis of Ethnonursing Data*. Of course, some methodological variables occurred via each researcher's procedure of study but this is expected with qualitative investigation.

Fifth, in presenting the data on the 23 cultures, only major, recurrent, and patterned culture values and care meanings and actions are included here. Thus, the reader gets the final analysis of the care *meanings* and *modes of action*. However, there is a wealth of rich detailed backup data to substantiate each of the care findings. These culture values and care meanings and actions can serve as a beginning guide or approach to the nursing care of clients or groups of these specific cultures to provide culturally congruent care. Users always must realize there were some cultural variations with clients due to acculturation and other factors. The reader also will note that, in keeping with the purposes of a qualitative paradigmatic study, no statistical data are presented. Instead, the goal is to understand the meanings and cultural experiences with culture care. These findings constitute the "gold nuggets" of nursing about care and caring, as they have been largely invisible or embedded in social structure factors, worldview, and other aspects of Culture Care theory dimensions awaiting ethnonursing studies. These care values, meanings, and modes of action can be considered the *epistemics* or root sources of people-centered care knowledge, and what nurses need to focus on in human caring.

Sixth, the reader needs to keep in mind that the findings revealed here were influenced significantly by the informants' ethnohistory, worldview, social structure, and environmental context. Although these dimensions were packed with information about care, they were embedded in areas which took much skill, time, and patience to explicate from informants. It seemed that the richest insights of informants were covert and deeply hidden in their thinking and experiences. Once trust was established, informants shared their very rich data with researchers.

The nurse learns to use such culture care findings of the 23 cultures as the beginning core or the "heart and soul of nursing," or what culture representatives tend to expect of nurses if care were provided. Most importantly, these findings should not be used rigidly or as fixed absolutes to stereotype people. Instead, care themes reflect *patterns of* care that can be considered to promote positive health to individuals or groups of a particular culture.

As nurses are taught how to do holistic culturalogical assessments using the Sunrise Model to assess an individual, group, or family in order to identify care variations, they will discover the sources of these findings (Leininger, 1978, 1981). In general, these findings can be used to provide specific care that *fits with* client's culture norms and lifeways, or they can be used as ways to change unfavorable or detrimental culture practices to clients. It is of interest that culture care values and action modes tend to remain with people over a period of time, and so these findings, which other nurses have used, remain extremely useful to understand clients and guide their care. These findings also revealed that culture values gave much meaning to the care actions in all cultures studied thus far. In using these findings, however, it is often well to consider them as "holding knowledge" to guide nursing care practices until the nurse has worked with and done his or her own assessment of an individual, family, or group. One can *anticipate* some variabilities among clients of a culture, but also some commonalities. To provide nursing care that is culturally based, nurses do require "holding knowledge"—that is, care values and beliefs similar to the way a physician uses medical science to handle cardiac clients. Most encouragingly, these care data are now becoming the new approach to nursing as nursing shifts from a *medical symptom-disease model* to a *nursing-centered care (caring) model.*

Finally, findings generated from the Culture Care theory can be used to help the nurse reflect on his or her *own* cultural care values and lifeways to consider what is different or similar in values and expectations as the nurse works with the client from a designated culture. Self-awareness of one's own culture is one of the "first principles" to master in transcultural nursing. Without self-awareness, the nurse may experience culture shock and be unable to help clients. Nurses may hold very different cultural care values and practices than clients. Recognizing such differences can help the nurse to understand and explain culturally based conflicts, frustration, and imposition practices. It also will help the nurse to understand why some nurses avoid clients because they are "true strangers." The nurse's professional values and practices often may be incongruent with those of the client, but awareness of such differences is essential in guiding the nurse's behavior. If the culture values of the nurse obstruct or hinder the recovery, cooperation, and progress of clients, this must be recognized and worked through with mentors in different counseling ways. Some nurses might be threatened with legal suits if they break cultural care taboos and reflect cultural care negligence or offensive behavior to some clients and families. With the rise in multiculturalism worldwide, legal cultural suits will markedly increase in the twenty-first century and beyond. Knowledge of culture care values and their constructs, thus, are helpful in preventing such undesirable legal potentials.

PRESENTATION OF CULTURE VALUES AND CARE MEANINGS WITH ACTION MODES OF SELECTED CULTURES

As one studies the findings from the 23 cultures, one will note that most cultures are from the United States of America, with some from Europe, Scandinavia, and other non-Western cultures. Some intergenerational and gender differences in each culture care were documented, but these still represent dominant findings within the culture. Only the *dominant emic* culture values, care meanings, and action modes are presented which were ranked by key informants of the culture. Thus, the first care construct listed was held most important by the informants and from the researcher's observations over a period of time. In the figure, however, not all the care meanings are reported as expressed in the native language; such linguistic terms or phrases, however, will be reported in a future publication. The informants were the translators of the terms into English. In some cultures, *care* as a native term did not translate readily into English, and so these linguistic phrases are the closest to the meanings and action modes of care. It is extremely important to keep in mind that the linguistic terms or phrases are the culture's. They may constitute stems of a sentence, or a partial sentence. Nonetheless, they are the care or essence of the value or action mode. It also is important to keep in mind that manifested care requires not only repeated verbal comments but daily or nightly care meanings and actions.

Finally, the orientational definition of culture values and culture care may help the reader as stated below:

Culture Values refer to the powerful, persistent, and directive forces that give meaning, order, and direction to the individual or group's thinking, actions, decisions, and lifeways, and usually over a span of time (Leininger, 1978).

Culture Care refers to those assistive, supportive, facilitative, and enabling acts for or toward another individual or group to ease or ameliorate a human condition, or lifeway in order to promote or maintain well being (or health), or to help clients face disabilities or death in given cultures or subcultures (Leininger, 1981, 1984).

REFLECTIONS ON RESEARCH: CULTURE CARE RESEARCH FINDINGS

Having seen the research findings from the above 23 Western and non-Western cultures as illustrative of approximately one-half of the cultures studied with the theory of Culture Care, a few reflections are in order. In reflecting on the findings, the reader begins to realize the diversity among cultures as well as some similarities in culture values and care meanings. These epistemic emic findings from culture informants are some of the "gold nuggets" and the "holding knowledge" to consider as the nurse assesses the client, family, and/or specific cultures wherever functioning. The nurse reflects further on these findings with professional nurses who may have had no preparation in transcultural nursing and who are expected to give quality care.

Most importantly, these culture care findings become a guide to help make decisions and actions with the three theoretical modes of decision making as previously discussed in Chapter 1: culture care preservation and maintenance, culture care accommodation or negotiation, and culture care repatterning or restructuring. These three modalities become important to consider in providing culturally congruent care to clients of the different cultures just presented. The nurse would creatively use the culture values and care meanings and action patterns to design nursing care for the client or family of a particular culture. For example, the Greek client will value daily exercise as a care preservation mode to promote health. At the same time, the Greek client expects the nurse to provide culture care accommodation or negotiation to let his or her Greek kin family be with him or her for satisfying and congruent care while in the hospital.

The challenge for the nurse is to provide care from the client's values and care meanings, using what may be relevant or helpful from professional knowledge with the client's generic care perspectives in order to design and arrive at congruent care practices. The nurse would study the effects of such care from both client and nurse viewpoints.

In using these culture care research findings, the nurse is keenly aware not to treat everyone exactly alike, but to use *culture-specific* care values and practices as a powerful directive for nursing practices. Such an approach differs from current emphasis on using NANDA nursing diagnosis—NANDA reflecting the use of another analogous linguistic label for nursing from the medical disease model. Focusing on "alterations," "deficits," and other diagnostic terms may seriously fail to provide for the cultural care needs of clients from a specific culture. Moreover, many of the NANDA labels are culture-bound and reflect dominant Anglo-American culture and nursing's values (Leininger, 1990). Thus, using Culture Care theory findings provides for an entirely new and different way to serve people.

To date, specific cultural care values, meanings, and actions of clients and nurses would remain unknown were it not for the transcultural research program launched in the 1960s. Whether clients want their care to be culturally congruent for more traditional values or new cultural values they are adopting, such research is more than timely. Some clients, for example, may want to adopt a new set of values permanently, but this is less frequently practiced—most humans do retain some or most of their traditional values. Nonetheless, it is very encouraging to see clients respond so formally to culture-specific care designed for them rather than having to accommodate themselves to professional or largely imposed professional practices. Indeed, it is virtually impossible for a nurse to care for people effectively and successfully without the use of transcultural care values and specific care knowledge of the cultures involved.

As the nurse becomes skilled in using cultural care knowledge, he or she will discover that professional skills take on new meanings. As the nurse's worldview greatly expands, a deep appreciation emerges for human diversities and similarities. The nurse becomes aware of the subtleties that make a difference in culturally based quality care practices, and especially that clients like cultural amenities, symbols, and actions to fit their cultural ways. As nurse's creative and professional skills grow, tailor-made care similar to giving a "perfect injection" may occur in using culture care practices. Exquisite, more assured, or confident care practices will occur as the nurse knows and understands the client of a particular culture. As the nurse uses specific care values and meanings, he or she does so with open communication with the client and often with the client's family. Sometimes remaining with the client and family can be a powerful caring mode to accommodate the client's needs. *Presence* often is deeply valued as well as promoting therapeutic outcomes. As the nurse uses such culture care knowledge, he or she also assesses client feedback and may alter care due to slight or major culture variations. The care constructs from the 23 cultures presented here are now being used in some clinical nurse settings, but will be used more as nurses learn about and try them. Such care constructs, however, need to be taught and studied further in nursing as the nursing knowledge base for the future.

In general, the research findings from the 23 cultures and the additional ethnonursing data reflect a lifelong research program of culture care studies by myself, other care scholars, students, clinicians, and faculty. The findings, with so much more still to be shared on every culture, also reflect the interest of key and general informants to share their *emic* (and often *etic*) experiences with nurses. Thus, it is fortunate that I have focused primarily on people-centered or *emic* ethnonursing findings for it provides a major breakthrough with some of "the best kept secrets about human care" of different cultures. This discovery must continue and will need to be updated with changing times. In the meantime, using the knowledge gained, the nurse has some insight of what can be used with clients. While the study of culture care is tedious and requires attention to a people's world, it is a most rewarding experience. Through it one discovers some of the most meaningful ways to know, help, and understand people.

LIST OF TRANSCULTURAL CARE CONSTRUCTS

During the three decades of discovering human care values, beliefs, meanings, expressions, patterns, and experiences, I found that with sensitive probing informants were able to identify, give meaning to, and prioritize their care values and meanings. The first care constructs were discovered with two Gadsup village peoples of New Guinea (see Chapter 1). This experience gave me courage to pursue the study in other cultures. Graduate students and others under my mentorship helped to keep this discovery process alive for nearly four decades. Accordingly, there are now 173 care constructs from 54 cultures, plus additional ethnonursing data to support the findings. In the beginning (in the 1960s), I had discovered 10 care constructs; in 1980 almost 37; in 1988, almost 100; in 1990, 175 constructs. Care constructs, therefore, have tended to remain largely invisible until nurse researchers probe, reflect on, and study them in depth in their embedded "homes" of social structure, worldview, and cultural values.

The findings presented in Figure 24 were obtained by the same method (ethnonursing) and with similar focus to that of discovering the care values and meanings with participants from ages 20 to 85 years of age. While there were some slight intergenerational and gender differences, these dominant care constructs prevailed. It was of interest that most informants were able to identify from four to eight care constructs *dominant* or *central* to them, and that no culture revealed *all* care constructs. Some informants, as they talked about the construct, wanted nurses to "be sure and know that they assess nurses as to whether they know these terms with the people's meanings and viewpoints." This was always encouraging to hear from informants. The criteria used to obtain these constructs and their meanings and actions (as presented also for the 23 cultures) were:

1. The informant(s) spoke English or a translator was available to help with the meanings in own native language.

2. The informant(s) identified themselves as belonging to and practicing the culture being studied about care and caring.

3. The informant(s) had been born and lived in the United States at least 15 years (the average had lived in the United States 35 years) or in their native non-U.S.A. country most of their lives (over 15 years).

4. The informant(s) volunteered and were usually interviewed in their homes or in a natural context so the researcher could also observe care practices in the natural home or work environment.

5. Culture care expressions, meanings, and patterns were studied by researchers using the Culture Care theory with the Sunrise Model over a considerable time span (often one year).

The purpose of sharing this list of constructs is mainly to alert the reader to be aware of the great diversity of constructs used and known by the people about human care and caring. Providing this list should help the nurse realize that care has different expressions, meanings and referents. All of these care constructs can be found in the 23 cultures presented earlier in this chapter and 31 additional cultures. The constructs also are offered to encourage nurses to do further work with these constructs with the cultures as we continue to discover the epistemic roots of care and health phenomena in many subcultures and cultures yet to be studied for care meanings and patterns within a nursing perspective.

My original question in the mid-1950s, *What is universal and diverse about human care/caring?* has been only partially answered with the care constructs listed in Figure 24. These care constructs and concomitant ethnonursing research data over three decades reflects the first systematization of the epistemic and ontologic transcultural care knowledge for the discipline of nursing. It reflects the ongoing work yet to be done to discover fully the meanings, functions, and structure of care knowledge transculturally.

Currently, I am in process of doing a comparative synthesis of the care knowledge drawing on data from the care constructs of different cultures in light of the tenets of my theory. Hopefully, this synthesis will lead to the identification of universal and diverse care meanings, practices, and structure of care so that this knowledge can ultimately be used both for clinical practices and for curricular and teaching purposes. In time, this care knowledge will be the substantive base of nursing knowledge in schools of nursing as well as in clinical settings in the next century. When this occurs, it will provide a very rich and sound knowledge base for the discipline and profession of nursing.

Finally, in presenting these culture care values, linguistic meanings, and action modes, keep in mind that there was no ethical or moral judgment made of what was "good," "bad," or "unethical." The findings are shared to reveal the human care expressions and patterns of cultures without moral judgements, and should be understood and used with this purpose and goal in mind.

Figure 1
Anglo-American Culture (Mainly U.S.A. Middle and Upper Class)

Cultural Values are:	*Culture Care Meanings and Action Modes are:*
1. Individualism—focus on a self-reliant person	1. Stress alleviation by: —physical means —emotional means
2. Independence and freedom	2. Personalized acts
3. Competition and achievement	—Doing special things
4. Materialism (things and money)	—Giving individual attention
5. Technology dependent	3. Self-reliance (individualism) by:
6. Instant time and actions	—Reliance on self
7. Youth and beauty	—Reliance on self (self-care)
8. Equal sex rights	—Becoming as independent as
9. Leisure time highly valued possible	—Reliance on technology
10. Reliance on scientific facts and numbers	4. Health instruction
11. Less respect for authority and the elderly	—Teach us how "to do" this care for self
12. Generosity in time of crisis	—Give us the "medical" facts

Figure 2
Mexican-American Culture*

Cultural Values are:	Culture Care Meanings and Action Modes are:
1. Extended family valued	1. Succorance (direct family aid)
2. Interdependence with kin and social activities	2. Involvement with extended family ("other care")
3. Patriarchal (machismo)	3. Filial love/loving
4. Exact time less valued	4. Respect for authority
5. High respect for authority and the elderly	5. Mother as care decision maker
6. Religion valued (many Roman Catholics)	6. Protective (external) male care
	7. Acceptance of God's will
7. Native foods for well being	8. Use of folk-care practices
8. Traditional folk-care healers for folk illnesses	9. Healing with foods
9. Belief in hot-cold theory	10. Touching

* These findings were from the author's transcultural nurse studies (1970, 1984) and other transcultural nurse studies in the United States during the past two decades.

Figure 3
Haitian-American Culture*

Cultural Values are:	Culture Care Meanings and Action Modes are:
1. Extended family as support system	1. Involve family for support (other care)
2. Religion—God's will must prevail	2. Respect (respecto)
3. Reliance on folk foods and treatments	3. Trust
4. Belief in hot-cold theory	4. Succorance
5. Male decision maker and direct caregivers	5. Touching (body closeness)
6. Reliance on native language	6. Reassurance
	7. Spiritual healing
	8. Use of folk food, care rituals
	9. Avoid evil eye (mal de ojo) and witches (bruja(o))
	10. Speak the language

* These data were from Haitians living in the United States during the past decade (1981–1991).

Figure 4
African-American Culture*

Cultural Values are:	Culture Care Meanings and Action Modes are:
1. Extended family networks	1. Concern for my "brothers and sisters"
2. Religion valued (many are Baptists)	
3. Interdependence with "Blacks"	2. Being involved with
4. Daily survival	3. Giving presence (physical)
5. Technology valued, e.g., radio, car, etc.	4. Family support and "get togethers"
6. Folk (soul) foods	5. Touching appropriately
7. Folk healing modes	6. Reliance on folk home remedies
8. Music and physical activities	7. Rely on "Jesus to save us" with prayers and songs

* These findings were from the author's study of two southern USA villages (1980–1981) and from a study of one large northern urban city (1982–1991) along with other studies by transcultural nurses.

Figure 5
North-American Indian Culture*

Cultural Values are:	Culture Care Meanings and Action Modes are:
1. Harmony between land, people, and environment	1. Establishing harmony between people and environment with reciprocity
2. Reciprocity with "Mother Earth"	
3. Spiritual inspiration (spirit guidance)	2. Actively listening
4. Folk healers (Shamans) (The Circle & Four Directions)	3. Using periods of silence ("Great Spirit" guidance)
5. Practice culture rituals and taboos	4. Rhythmic timing (nature, land and people) in harmony
6. Rhythmicity of life with nature	5. Respect for native folk healers, carers, and curers (Use of Circle)
7. Authority of tribal elders	
8. Pride in cultural heritage and "Nations"	6. Maintaining reciprocity (replenish what is taken from Mother Earth)
9. Respect and value for children	7. Preserving cultural rituals and taboos
	8. Respect for elders and children

* These findings were collected by the author and other contributors in the United States and Canada during the past three decades. Cultural variations among all nations exist, and so these data are some general commonalities about values, care meanings, and actions.

Figure 6
Gadsup Akuna of the Eastern
Highlands of New Guinea*

Cultural Values are:	Culture Care Meanings and Action Modes are:
1. Egalitarianism 2. Marked sex role differences 3. Patriarchal descent recognized 4. Communal unity ("one vine"/"line") 5. Prevent social accusations (sorcery) 6. Maintain ancestor "life-essence" and obligations 7. Have "good women, children, pigs, and gardens"	1. Surveillance (to prevent sorcery) —nearby surveillance —watch at a distance 2. Protection (protective male caring) —of Gadsups through lifecycle —obeying cultural taboos and rules 3. Nurturance —ways to help people grow and survive —know what they need (anticipate needs) through lifecycle —eat safe foods 4. Prevention (avoid breaking cultural taboos) to: —prevent illness and death —prevent intervillage fights and conflicts . 5. Touching

* This was the first transcultural care study done by the author in two villages in the early 1960s, with subsequent visits made in later years. (See Chapter 7 for a full account of these people.)

Figure 7
Philippine-American Culture*

Cultural Values are:	Culture Care Meanings and Action Modes are:
1. Family unity and closeness 2. Respect for elder/authority 3. "Leave one-self to God" (*Bahala na*) 4. Obligations to sociocultural ties 5. Hot-cold beliefs 6. Use of folk foods and practices 7. Religion valued (mainly Roman Catholic)	1. Maintain smooth relationships (*Pakikisama*) 2. Save face and self-esteem (*Amor propio*); (*Hiya*–avoid shame) 3. Respect for and deference to authority 4. Being quiet; privacy 5. Mutual reciprocity (*Utang Na Loob*) "the give and take" in relationships 6. Giving comfort to others 7. Tenderness 8. Being pleasant as possible

* These findings were from Philippines living in the United States for at least two decades and collected by the author Z. Spangler and other transcultural nurse researchers.

Figure 8
Japanese-American Culture*

Cultural Values are:	Culture Care Meanings and Action Modes are:
1. Duty and obligation to kin and work group	1. Respect for family, authority, and corporate groups; family included in caring
2. Honor and national pride	
3. Patriarchal obligations and respect	2. Obligations to kin and work groups
4. Systematic group work goals	3. Concern for group with protection
5. Ambitiousness with achievements	
6. Honor and pride toward elders	4. Prolonged nurturance "care for others overtime"
7. Politeness and ritual	
8. Group compliance	5. Control emotions and actions to "save face and prevent shame"
9. Maintain high educational standards	6. Look to others for affection (*Amaeru*) "save face and prevent shame"
10. Futurists with worldwide and plans	7. Indulgence from caregivers (young and old)
	8. Endurance to support pain and stress
	9. Respect for and attention to physical complaints
	10. Personal cleanliness
	11. Use of folk therapies (*Kanpo* medicine)
	12. Quietness and passivity

* These findings were from Japanese living and working in the United States the past two decades (1971–1991). Similar patterned findings were documented by informants in Japan, but with some recent intergenerational changes.

Figure 9
Vietnamese-American Culture*

Cultural Values are:	Culture Care Meanings and Action Modes are:
1. Harmony and balance in universe 2. Extended kinship family ties (centrality of extended family) 3. Religious and spiritual values (Buddhism and Catholicism) 4. Respect for elderly and authority 5. Folk-care practices 6. Food and environment	1. Harmony and balanced caring ways 2. Respect for elderly, family ties, cultural taboos 3. Using natural folk-care practices and food (hot-cold theory) 4. Spirituality in caring 5. Enabling others to do daily functions (other-care) 6. Family-centered carings 7. Touching to heal 8. Hopefulness

* These findings are mainly from Vietnamese refugees living in the United States and studied by authors and other transcultural nurses (1974–1990).

Figure 10
Southeast Indian American Culture*

Culture Care Meanings and Action Modes are:

1. Respect extended family members
2. Involve family as responsible caregivers
3. Use of folk treatment modes
4. Avoid cultural taboos with foods and culture lifeways
5. Use spiritual caring modes
6. Males responsible for public care decisions; females for domestic (home) care
7. Respect general role differences in care and curing
8. Use limit setting with children to discipline
9. Request religious beliefs and practices

* These findings were obtained from Southeast Indian men and women living in the United States the past decade and collected by transcultural nurses.

Figure 11
Chinese-American Culture*

Culture Care Meanings and Action Modes are:

1. Serving others (not self-care)
2. Compliance with authority and elders
3. Obedience to authority, elders, and government officials (discipline children)
4. Surveillance: watching near and at distances
5. Dependence on generic folk herbs, treatment modes (acupuncture, etc.)
6. Group communal assistance to others
7. Work hard and give to the society

* These findings are from Chinese living in the United States over five years. The data were collected by author and other transcultural nurse researchers (1983–1991). The author also documented similar findings in the People's Republic of China (1983).

Figure 12
Arab-American Muslim Culture*

Culture Care Meanings and Action Modes are:

1. Providing family care and support—a responsibility
2. Offering respect and privacy time for religious beliefs and prayers (five times each day)
3. Respecting and protecting gender culturally role differences
4. Knowing cultural taboos and norms (i.e., no pork, alcohol, smoking, etc.)
5. Recognize honor with obligation
6. Helping to "save face" and preserve cultural values
7. Obligation and responsibility to visit the sick
8. Following the teaching of the Koran
9. Helping especially children and elderly when ill

* These care meanings reflect several Arab-Muslims in Detroit (the largest Arab groups outside of the Middle East) and need to be viewed as common patterned expressions. While cultural variation existed among all Arab-Muslim groups, these were dominant themes supported by L. Luna's research (1989) and my work with the Arabs for nearly a decade (1982–1991). Many of these findings were also observed in Saudi Arabia by the author and L. Luna (1987).

Figure 13
Old-Order Amish-Americans*

Cultural Values are:	Culture Care Meanings and Action Modes are:
1. "Being Amish" (in dress, frugality, and lifeways)	1. Being aware of others: needs and actions
2. Community care action	2. Ministering to others: being present in thought and action
3. Family and community care for well being	3. Giving help generously: obligation and privilege
4. Non-materialism and limited technology	4. Receiving care with expectations and humility
5. Reliance on folk practices and God	5. Anticipatory care: (other-care)
6. Principled pragmatism	6. Obedience to God and elders
7. Non-government help	7. Community caring for well being
	8. Using folk-care ways
	9. Limiting use of technologies in caring

*The author drew from A.F. Wenger's (1988) research and other researchers who studied the Old-Order Amish (1984–1990).

Figure 14
Appalachian Culture*

Cultural Values are:	Culture Care Meanings and Action Modes are:
1. Keep ties with kin from the "hollows"	1. Knowing and trusting "true friends"
2. Personalized religion	2. Being kind to others
3. Folk practices as "the best lifeways"	3. Being watchful of strangers or outsiders
4. Guard against "strangers"	4. Do for others; less for self
5. Be frugal: always use home remedies	5. Keep with kin and local folks
6. Stay near home for protection	6. Use of home remedies "first and last"
7. Mother is decision maker	7. Help from kin as needed (primary care)
8. Community interdependency	8. Help people stay away from hospitals—"the place where people die"

* These findings were from a study in an urban community by the author and P. Shinkel (plus other transcultural nurses) as part of a larger urban Culture Care theory study (1984–1987).

Figure 15
Polish-American Culture*

Cultural Values are:	Culture Care Meanings and Action Modes are:
1. Upholding Christian religious beliefs and practices ("pray")	1. Giving to others in need
2. Family and cultural solidarity (other-care)	2. Self-sacrificing for others and God
3. Frugality as way of life	3. Being actively concerned about
4. Political activity for justice	4. Working hard whatever one does
5. Hardwork: "Don't complain"	5. Christian love of others
6. Persistence "Don't give up"	6. Family concern for others
7. Maintain religious and special days	7. Eating Polish foods and folk care to stay well or recover from illness (including home remedies)
8. Value folk practices	

* These findings are from transcultural nursing studies with midwest Polish-Americans (primarily in Detroit and Chicago—two of the largest Polish settlements in the United States) by several transcultural nurses over the past decade.

Figure 16
German-American Culture*

Cultural Values are:	Culture Care Meanings and Action Modes are:
1. Industriousness and being hard workers	1. Being orderly (orderliness) —things in "proper places" —right performance —being well organized
2. Maintain order and organization	
3. Maintain religious beliefs	
4. Stoicism	2. Being clean and neat
5. Keep environment and self clean	3. Direct helping to others —give explicit assistance —get into action
6. Cautiousness	
7. Knowledge is power	
8. Controlling self and others	4. Watch details —follow rules —be punctual
9. Maintain rules and norms	
10. Scientism with logic valued	
	5. Protecting others against harm and outsiders
	6. Controlling self and others
	7. Eating proper foods and getting rest and fresh air
	8. Do not complain, "grin and bear it"

* These findings are from urban and rural United States over the past three decades by author and other transcultural nurses. Similar values and care patterns also were observed and confirmed in Western Germany in past decades (1970–1980).

Figure 17
Italian-American Culture*

Cultural Values are:	Culture Care Meanings and Action Modes are:
1. Extended and close family ties	1. Well being of our families
2. Patriarchialism	—"best for the family good"
3. Strong religious practices (Roman Catholic)	—keeping family active and well
4. Being socially and politically active with extended family and wider community	2. Promoting family integrity —sharing among family —protecting family name and ways
5. Generosity and charitableness	3. Involvement with family and other Italians (being active and dealing with family affairs)
6. Expressive in music, art, and community service	
7. Responsible for Italians	4. Closeness with presence
8. Openly express feelings	—being there; "touching alot and hugs"
	5. Expressing oneself freely
	6. Eating fresh Italian market foods with some wine
	7. Family support (stay close to home)

* These findings were confirmed and substantiated by key and general informants living in a large Italian urban mid-central community in the United States by the author and several transcultural nursing researchers. Author worked in community project for ten years (1982–1992). While variability among Italians from the homeland was evident, the above commonalities prevailed.

Figure 18
Greek-American Culture*

Cultural Values are:	Culture Care Meanings and Action Modes are:
1. Maintain Greek family ties	1. Being responsible for other Greeks as religious and social obligation
2. Preserve religious beliefs and practices	
3. Be responsible for Greek families	2. Assisting others as soon as possible to prevent illnesses
4. Strong respect for cultural heritage	3. Actively involved with Greek families
5. Sacrificing for good of others and kin	4. Prevent illnesses with proper exercise; using family folk practices; avoiding hospitals; and eating "good healthy" Greek foods
6. Generosity to Greek kin, the arts, and other community groups	
7. Work with youth to help them become good adult Greeks	5. Hospitality (Greeks and strangers)
	6. Keeping active with family and church
	7. Reflecting on goodness of others
	8. Keeping clean and properly dressed
	9. Exercise daily
	10. Family tells kin of serious illness

* These care findings are from Greek families in urban United States by author's research team (1984–1988). Similar findings with other nurse researchers, and with Greeks in Australia and Greece (1978–1990).

Figure 19
Jewish-American Culture*

Cultural Values are:	Culture Care Meanings and Action Modes are:
1. Maintain respect for religious beliefs and practices (Judaism)	1. Express feelings openly
2. Keep centrality of family with patriarchal rule and mothercare	2. Get most direct and best help
	3. Accept shared sufferings
3. Support education and intellectual achievements	4. Maternal nurturance, i.e., overfeeding, permissiveness, and overprotection
4. Maintain continuity of Jewish heritage	5. Giving and helping others as social justice (tsdokeh)
5. Be generous and charitable to arts, music, and community service	6. Performing lifecycle (birth, marriage, and death)
6. Achieve success (financial and education)	7. Attentiveness to others
7. Be persistent and persuasive	8. Caring for own people
8. Enjoyment of art, music, and religious rituals	9. Teaching Jewish values

* These findings are from Jewish groups living in several urban communities in the United States (1975–1991). Pattern variations were evident with orthodox, conservative, and reformed Jewish-Americans and with intergenerational differences. Several transcultural nurses contributed to findings.

Figure 20
Lithuanian-American Culture*

Cultural Values are:	Culture Care Meanings and Action Modes are:
1. Extended family closeness	1. Presence (being there)
2. Religious beliefs and prayers (Roman Catholic)	2. Helping in times of need
	3. Hospitality to others
3. Education important	4. Sharing with others (other-care)
4. Hard work and industriousness	5. Flexibility to adapt
5. Thriftiness and good use of material resources	6. Cooperation with others
6. Endurance, persistence, and suffering with economic hardships	7. Praying with others
	8. Using subtle humor
7. Charity to others	

* These findings were from a large urban community in the United States. Rauda Galazis, doctoral student at Wayne State University, shared her findings from two studies in the United States and from a field study in Lithuania, her parent's homeland (1986–1991).

Figure 21
Swedish-American Culture*

Culture Care Meanings and Action Modes are:

1. Attention to detail
2. Self-responsibility
3. Maintaining privacy
4. Being hospitable
5. Showing orderly responsibility
6. Cleanliness: self and environment

* These findings were from Swedish informants in the urban midwest collected by author and research team (1984–1991). Many of these findings also were substantiated by key and general native informants in Sweden in the 1980s.

Figure 22
Finnish-American Culture*

Cultural Values are:	*Culture Care Meanings and Action Modes are:*
1. Enduring hardships	1. Being responsible for others (*Hetios*); charity and love (Caritas)
2. Being frugal and watchful	
3. Being productive	
4. Maintaining neutrality	2. Folk healing (Saunas)
5. Being nonpunitive	3. Listening attentively to others
6. Keeping beliefs (mainly religious)	4. Being quiet and contemplative
7. Maintaining national pride and traditionalism	5. Being able to suffer and obtain meaning with contemplation
8. Quiet action	6. Being non-assertive
9. Maintaining proper rituals and decorum	7. Loving others
	8. Protecting the vulnerable
10. Belief in folk and modern healing modes	9. Getting sick people well
	10. Taking care of self and others in the environment
	11. Communion with others

* These findings were from the United States, but with support from key and general informants from Northern and Southern Finland with help from Anita von Smitten, Dr. Pirkko Merilainen, Dr. Katie Eriksson, and authors research associates (1989–1991).

Figure 23
Danish-American Culture*

Cultural Values are:	*Culture Care Meanings and Action Modes are:*
1. Egalitarianism: "All alike;" "One as good as another"	1. Treating people alike
2. Society more important than family	2. Being quiet (leave alone at times)
3. Social obligations and responsibilities	3. Giving or sharing to others
4. Nongregariousness	4. Accommodating other (ideas and needs)
5. Consensus building	5. Avoiding conflicts
6. Cultural pride in heritage	6. Maintaining societal care responsibilities
	7. Eating proper foods
	8. Daily exercise

* These findings were from key and general informants in Denmark and the United States with limited variability.

Figure 24
List of Care/Caring (*Emic*) Constructs Derived from Leininger's Culture Care Theory Research (1960–91)

These *emic* (within the culture) care/caring constructs were identified in approximately 54 cultures through ethnonursing qualitative research methods(s) from 1960–1991. The cultural informants identified four or five dominant care constructs with their key meanings and action modes. None of the cultures identified more than eight major constructs. The professional nurses *etic* (or outsider's views) of care are not included in this list. The findings reveal a wide diversity in the *emic* culture care meanings and action modes. All foreign care/caring terms were documented and translated into English. This is only a small glimpse of the total care research findings.

Care and/or Caring Meanings and Action Modes:

1. Acceptance	14. Being authentic (real)
2. Accommodating	15. Being clean
3. Accountability	16. Being genuine
4. Action (ing) for/about/with	17. Being involved
5. Adapting to	18. Being kind/pleasant
6. Affection for	19. Being orderly
7. Alleviation (pain/suffering)	20. Being present
8. Anticipation (ing)	21. Being watchful
9. Assist (ing) others	22. Bribing
10. Attention to/toward	23. Care (caring)
11. Attitude toward	24. *Caritas* (charity)
12. Being nonassertive	25. Cleanliness
13. Being aware of others	26. Closeness to

Care and/or Caring Meanings and Action Modes:

27. Cognitively knowing
28. Comfort (ing)
29. Commitment to/for
30. Communication (ing)
31. Community awareness
32. Compassion (ate)
33. Compliance with
34. Concern for/about/with
35. Congruence with
36. Connectedness
37. Consideration of
38. Consultation (ing)
39. Controlling
40. Communion with another
41. Cooperation
42. Coordination (ing)
43. Coping with/for
44. Creative thinking/acts
45. Cultural care (ing)
46. Cure (ing)
47. Dependence
48. Direct help to others
49. Discernment
50. Doing for/with
51. Eating right foods
52. Enduring
53. Embodiment
54. Emotional support
55. Empathy
56. Enabling
57. Engrossment in/about
58. Establishing harmony
59. Engrossment in/about
60. Experiencing with
61. Expressing feelings
62. Faith (in others)
63. Family involvement
64. Family support
65. Feeling for/about
66. Filial love
67. Generosity toward others
68. Gentle (ness) & firmness
69. Giving to others in need
70. Giving comfort to
71. Group assistance
72. Group awareness
73. Growth promoting

74. Hands on
75. Harmony with
76. Healing
77. Health instruction
78. Health (well being)
79. Health maintenance
80. Helping self/others
81. Helping kin/group
82. Honor (ing)
83. Hope (fullness)
84. Hospitality
85. Improving conditions
86. Inclined toward
87. Indulgence from
88. Instruction (ing)
89. Integrity
90. Interest in/about
91. Intimacy/intimate
92. Involvement with/for
93. Kindness (being kind)
94. Knowing of culture
95. Knowing (another's reality)
96. Know cultural values/taboos
97. Limiting (set limits)
98. Listening to/about
99. Loving (love others)
    —Christian love
100. Maintaining harmony
101. Maintaining reciprocity
102. Maintaining privacy
103. Ministering to others
    —filial love
104. Need fulfillment
105. Nurturance (nurture)
106. Obedience to
107. Obligation to
108. Orderliness
109. Other-care (ing) non self-care
110. Patience
111. Performing rituals
112. Permitting expressions
113. Personalized acts
114. Physical acts
115. Praying with
116. Presence (being with)
117. Preserving (preservation)
118. Prevention (ing)

Care and/or Caring Meanings and Action Modes:

119. Promoting
120. Promoting independence
121. Protecting (other/self)
122. Purging
123. Quietness
124. Reassurance
125. Receiving
126. Reciprocity
127. Reflecting goodness
128. Reflecting with/about
129. Rehabilitate
130. Regard for
131. Relatedness to
132. Respecting
133. Respect for/about lifeways
134. Respecting privacy/wishes
135. Respecting sex differences
136. Responding appropriately
137. Responding to context
138. Responsible for others
139. Restoration (ing)
140. Sacrificing
141. Saving face
142. Self-reliant (reliance)
143. Self-responsibility
144. Sensitivity to others needs
145. Serving others (caritas)
146. Sharing with others
147. Silence (use of)

148. Speaking the language
149. Spiritual healing
150. Spiritual relatedness
151. Stimulation (ing)
152. Stress alleviation
153. Succorance
154. Suffering with/for
155. Support (ing)
156. Surveillance (watch for)
157. Symbols (ing)
158. Sympathy
159. Taking care of environment
160. Technical skills
161. Techniques
162. Tenderness
163. Timing actions/decisions
164. Touch (ing)
165. Trust (ing)
166. Understanding
167. Use of folk foods/practices
168. Use of limit setting
169. Using nursing knowledge
170. Valuing another's ways
171. Watchfulness
172. Well being (health)
173. Well being (family)
174. Wholeness approach
175. Working hard

REFERENCES

Leininger, M. M. (1978). *Transcultural nursing: Concepts, theories and practices*. New York: John Wiley & Sons.

Leininger, M. M. (1982-1990). *African-American and culture care theory in urban context*. Unpublished study. Detroit: Wayne State University Press.

Leininger, M. M. (1984). Southern rural black and white American lifeways with focus on care and health phenomenon. In *Care: The essence of nursing and health*. Detroit: Wayne State University Press.

Leininger, M. M. (1988). *Care: An essential human need*. Detroit: Wayne State University Press.

Leininger, M. M. (1988). *Care: The essence of nursing and health*. Detroit: Wayne State University Press.

Leininger, M. M. (1988). *Care: Discovery and uses in clinical and community nursing*. Detroit: Wayne State University Press.

Leininger, M. M. (1990, Summer). Issues, questions, and concerns related to the nursing diagnosis cultural movement from a transcultural nursing perspective. *Journal of Transcultural Nursing*, 23-32.

Leininger, M. M. (1991). *Culture care diversity and universality: A theory of nursing*. New York: National League for Nursing.

11

Culture Care Theory and Uses in Nursing Administration*

Madeleine M. Leininger

During the past three decades, several theorists, researchers, and scholars in the field of nursing have actively developed and systematically examined nursing's distinct domains of knowledge. A number of conceptual and theoretical perspectives have become evident with different research paradigms to explicate the phenomena of nursing. These developments have been encouraging as nursing delineates what constitutes its distinct focus to guide nursing education and practice. It has been a challenge to explicate nursing knowledge because of the complex and embedded ideas that characterize it, but also because of different theoretical interests and positions taken by nurses of what constitutes nursing's unique perspective as a discipline and profession.

* This chapter is a revised and shortened version of the chapter, "Cultural Care Theory and Nursing Administration," as published in *Dimensions of Nursing Administration: Theory, Research, Education, Practice*, by Henry B., Arndt, C., Di Vincenti, M., and Marriner-Tomey, A. (Eds.), St. Louis: Mosby Publication, 1988, pp. 19-34.
** In this chapter, *nursing administration* refers both to academic education and nursing service administration unless specified otherwise.

Unquestionably, there is no right or wrong theory of nursing; rather, there are theories that have a lesser or greater potential to explain, describe, interpret, and predict nursing from a local to a worldwide perspective. It is academically and theoretically healthy to see nurses deliberate about different theories and concepts and not close the door on theories that may show some of the greatest potential to explain the universality of nursing and its unique features. It is, therefore, encouraging to see different theories being systematically examined or tested to determine what characterizes the nature and essence of nursing.

It is interesting that some nurses have already been "fixed on" a few concepts, such as *man* (or person), *health, environment,* and *nursing* as the central concepts of the metaparadigm of nursing (Fawcett 1984). But as I have stated in other earlier writings, these four concepts must be reconsidered because of their questionable limitations as central, distinct, or unique to nursing (Leininger, 1981, 1984), and for several reasons. First, *man* as a generic concept is not distinct to nursing for most humanistic and scientific fields focus on generic man. Moreover, some disciplines such as anthropology have been intensively and extensively involved in studying generic man as culture groups through time and place for more than a century. Second, it is a logical contradiction to declare *nursing* as a distinct concept and then attempt to *explain* the same phenomenon by the same term. Third, while *environment* and *health* are possibilities to help explain nursing, further refinements and more specificity are needed to show nursing's unique focus in relation to many other disciplines that claim these concepts as central to their field. To date, very few nurses have been doctorally prepared in the environmental sciences such as ecology, geography, human environments, and other closely related fields, to ensure establishing environment as totally distinct to nursing. Unquestionably, health has been of historical interest to nurses since the Nightingale era, but only recently have nurses focused in-depth on health *per se.* Health as central to nursing will need more transcultural research to establish it as an epistemological base unique to nursing. Today, as in the past, many disciplines make firm claims to health as their unique discipline perspective so it may not be a major distinct phenomenon to nursing.

From an ethnohistorical and transcultural nursing perspective, *care* has remained central to nursing, but it has not been studied in-depth and from an epistemic, historical, and ontologic stance until the last three decades (Leininger 1976, 1981, 1984, 1990a). Since the 1940s, I have held that human care and caring is the distinct and unifying feature of nursing, and that this perspective will remain well into the future if nurses are committed to the full discovery and use of care knowledge. It is of interest that many consumers and society as a collective institution have long viewed nursing as a caring profession, but as one can see in the above metaparadigm (Fawcett 1984), care is omitted or not even mentioned by some nurse leaders. As I have stated in several of my writings, human care and caring acts are, indeed, the essence and the most promising construct to explain and predict nursing (Leininger 1970, 1974a, 1974b, 1978, 1981, 1984, 1988, 1990a). Care is *the unique, dominant, and unifying focus of nursing.* Moreover, care is a powerful concept with which to describe, explain, interpret, and predict nursing outcomes. Care as a noun is the phenomenon to be explained; caring as a gerund implies the action component of care. And care as a central phenomenon to transcultural nursing has been a major focus since this field was conceived in the mid-1950s (Leininger 1967, 1970, 1978).

In this chapter, the theory of Culture Care Diversity and Universality will be discussed for its importance and usefulness to academic and clinical nursing administrators. The rationale for nurse administrators to use Culture Care theory to promote and advance care is presented. To make humanistic and scientific care an integral and visible part of nursing requires support from nursing administrators. A transcultural comparative cultural perspective is essential, and a relatively new area of study and practice for most nurse administrators. It is a major focus for the future of nursing as our world of nursing becomes intensely multicultural. In addition, several research questions will be presented to stimulate nursing administrators to study and use findings generated from the theory of Culture Care.

RATIONALE FOR CULTURE CARE THEORY IN NURSING ADMINISTRATION

There are a number of reasons for focusing on the theory of Culture Care Diversity and Universality in nursing administration. First, the world of nursing administration with its norms, values, and practices is slowly beginning to shift from largely a unicultural to a multicultural focus. Nursing administration needs to change to a multicultural position to meet diverse consumer needs of clients, students, faculty, and others. Nurse administrators who are culturally alert to transcultural education and service practices realize the importance of understanding and working with people of many different cultures in the management processes, in decision making, and to obtain appropriate institutional goals. Accordingly, administrators in their organizational structures, functions, and processes need to reflect these societal and worldwide changes to accommodate cultural diversity factors in their work. For without such knowledge, practices, and commitments a host of cultural conflicts, stresses, and problems will undoubtedly occur.

Nursing administrators as leaders need to make their practices congruent with changing cultural values, beliefs, and lifeways in their local workplace, but they also must reasonably fit with societal and worldwide trends. Health care administrators with a unicultural view are challenged by consumers and employees today to make their services responsive to many diverse cultural, individual, and group needs and not treat all consumers alike. Moreover, nursing service and education leaders need to become proactive to meet the needs of clients, students, faculty, and staff of diverse cultures. Indeed, far more attention needs to be given to the cultural care diversity and universal administrative practices that reflect new and different ways to provide human services. Most importantly, nurse administrators need a broad, comprehensive, and culturally based theory in order to expand their worldview and to be sensitive to a global or transcultural view of administrative activities, action modes, and decisions. The theory of Culture Care Diversity and Universality is one of the broadest and most comprehensive theories in nursing to meet some of the major expectations cited above, related to accommodating similarities and differences in educational and service settings. Culture Care theory can provide a guideline for designing administrative practices based on specific modes of action and decision from a worldwide perspective (Leininger 1985a, 1988, 1990a).

A second major reason for using Culture Care theory is that diverse cultural groups expect or demand that their values and practices be respected as a culture and as individuals. This requires that nurse administrators consider multicultural perspectives and understand different cultures as clients enter and leave administrative systems. Currently, there is an increasing number of clients, staff, faculty, and students from many different cultures in the world and they expect that nursing administrators and staff will make decisions and judgments that meet or at least consider their cultural needs as human rights. Currently, cultural minorities in the United States and in foreign countries are not always represented in nursing care services and in nursing schools, and this must change with more minorities having rights to use health and educational services. In several schools of nursing in the United States, most students are predominantly Anglo-Americans and there are only a few cultural minorities (Leininger 1989). Much more visible administrative efforts are needed to recruit, attract, and retain nursing students from many diverse cultures and subcultures. Nursing administrators need to reexamine their organizational philosophies, structures, values, and recruitment-retention processes to support and nurture multiculturalism.

In nursing care services, it is interesting to observe that service values and practices tend to be focused on one dominant culture, and cultural minority needs, values, and viewpoints may be recognized and addressed in limited fashion only. When the latter occurs, signs often appear of misunderstanding, ineffective communication, cultural shock, cultural imposition and many kinds of problems or conditions related to cultural negligence or avoidance with minority consumers. The theory of Culture Care can serve as a broad conscious awareness framework to identify and develop nursing administration goals and programs, and as an action theory that will accommodate diverse cultural groups. At the same time, cultural care diversity practices can greatly enrich administrative cultural practices and experiences of any environment.

A third reason that nurse administrators need to consider the theory of Culture Care is to develop organizational structures and functions that reflect different cultural values and gender differences in nursing. These dimensions are essential to develop relevant cultural norms and practices in program development, implementation, and evaluation in clinical and educational settings. In clinical settings, for example, one can envision for the immediate future many nurses from diverse and foreign cultures in the world seeking staff positions for client care. Nursing service administrators need to plan now to accommodate and maximize nurses' abilities in many different cultures. Administrators need to develop cultural orientation programs and ways to use the talents and assets of nurses from many different cultures in the world. These nurses from other countries should be respected and understood for the ways they can provide effective, safe, and beneficial care to clients as well as for how they work with multidisciplinary staff. Nurses from diverse cultures have something to contribute to nursing education and service while learning about a new culture. Transcultural nursing is a two-way process and not a one-way system. As nurses from Egypt, Iraq, Philippines, Mexico, China, Japan, Korea, Eastern Europe, and virtually every place in the world are employed in different clinical settings and schools of nursing, their cultural value differences in gender, role expectations, and life experiences need to be identified and understood. How nursing administrators plan for and respond to these multicultural changes is important, for it is these nurses who will influence nursing care practices and educational systems. Cultural stresses and conflicts between nursing staff and clients will increase unless transcultural nursing education and services prevail that have been grounded in research findings generated from culturally based theory. Thus, nurse administrators need to anticipate worldwide changes and plan now to meet multicultural education and service needs in this rapidly changing nursing world. Most importantly, nursing administrators need to maximize and use the knowledge and skills which nurses bring with them, rather than discredit, demean, or misuse nursing talents (Leininger, 1986, 1989).

It also is important to realize that nursing education administrators as deans, associate and assistant deans, and other staff managers will play a major role in facilitating students and faculty from multicultures. Nursing educators will learn to support different teaching and learning methods and different ways to help students succeed and function in their career roles within different cultural orientations. Discovering and developing different teaching and learning methods for a new generation of multicultural students will be imperative, for students need to succeed and be successful in their career roles in diverse countries. Different teaching methods and a culturally based theory and guide administrators and faculty toward that goal. Currently, faculty and student problems and goals related to multicultural value differences are a major factor in student learning, in the recruitment and retention of students, and in educational goal attainment in schools of nursing. Educational administrative structures and policies should be sufficiently flexible and reflect philosophies and practices that help students and faculty use and learn about multicultural variabilities.

To date, very few studies exist in nursing service and education that are focused on transcultural organizational structures to support cultural value differences or to establish multicultural human service programs. Nor have the institutional cultures of nursing education and service been studied to identify and understand current practices that influence values, decision making, and normative practices. In the late 1960s and early 1970s, I described the culture of nursing along with cultural imposition practices, leadership styles, and some changing values and practices in both education and service in the United States (Leininger 1967, 1970, 1974a, 1978, 1987). A future publication will present a current portrait of the new or changed culture of nursing (1991a). The theory of Culture Care Diversity and Universality is a highly appropriate framework to study the culture of nursing and appropriate organizational structures in nursing education and clinical services for the future, especially since the theory includes the worldview, social structure factors, cultural values, environmental context, linguistic aspects, and ethnohistorical considerations. These dimensions are important to design administrative organizations for tomorrow's nursing service and education systems.

Fourth, the theory of Culture Care has great possibilities to examine different types of professional and academic administrative organizations and their effectiveness or limitations. Currently, there is a cultural movement to develop new types of organizations, other than those of the traditional bureaucratic structures, to meet societal and worldwide changes. Since Culture Care theory requires a systematic study of worldview, social structures, and cultural values, this would help identify potential patterns for differentiated administrative services. Comparative differences or similarities with nursing service and education with respect to their purposes, goals, and functions also is important to render quality nursing services. What types of organizational structures would be most effective or provide a better linkage between nursing education and service? What criteria should be used to support transcultural programs in nursing education and service? What kinds of nursing organizations would support multiculturalism? What would be the strengths or limitations of different prototypes of nursing organizations for worldwide transcultural nursing education and service? These questions could be explored with Culture Care theory.

In the United States, nursing faculty generally favor a *collegial type of academic administrative organization* in contrast to the traditional *rational-legal bureaucratic organization* (Henry et al., 1988; Leininger 1984). *Collegial* type refers to participatory management decisions and actions made in a spirit of collegial respect with participants who are informed on the subject; whereas *rational legal bureaucratic* type refers to decisions and actions that tend to be coercive, and are mandated from legal or rational stances (Rothschild & Russell, 1986). Some hospitals and clinics tend to espouse bureaucratic-like structures for efficiency and to support the dominant medical-authoritative organizational structure. With democratization growing in the world, one can expect more democratic cultural values and norms being used in a demonstration. This will be especially evident in nursing schools and clinical settings as nurses move between academic and clinical settings today and experience non-democratic structures. Most nurses become quite dissatisfied with autocratic structures. Moreover, "progressive" nursing administrators are eager to change existing structures for democratic participatory organizations, and especially in democratized countries or institutions.

Professional nurses worldwide are seeking more autonomy and freedom to attain nursing's goals as a discipline and profession. Nurses want to regulate, maintain, and control their professional affairs without undue external pressures and oppressive controls. Tightly controlled bureaucratic organizations and administrative practices in education or service have historically limited nurses to achieve their professional goals. Thus, more collegial rather than legal-bureaucratic organizations are much desired for the new culture of nursing administration, and with a strong caring ethos. Since most Western nursing education schools have moved into institutions of higher learning, several new types of democratization cultures in nursing administration undoubtedly will be developed. However, there will be some nursing education and service administrative organizations that will value what I call the "cult of efficiency," the "cult of compliance," and the "cult of pleasing others," and may, at times, function as highly rational-legal bureaucratic structures. These structures will limit the full development of nursing, reduce multicultural accommodations, and fail to nurture a caring philosophy of administration. These structures tend to show signs of staff dissatisfactions, frustrations, and staff problems. In general, oppressive, controlling, and rigid organizations seldom are supported by nurses because of past oppressive and limiting opportunities with patriarchal systems (Leininger 1974a). Thus organizational structures that anticipate and accommodate cultural care differences in management, human relationships, decision making, and respect female gender contributions will be in great demand. In addition, nursing education and service organizations will need to interface their organizations closely with local community and multicultural interest groups as well as with the larger society in which nursing functions. Being aware of local and societal perspectives with all their differences and similarities (including folk and professional group systems) will be important for nursing administrators.

An interesting area that merits study today is the growing trend toward the *corporatization of nursing education and health care services*. What are the actual or potential benefits and differences between corporate and non-corporate cultural care nursing systems? How will nursing systems interface and function within large corporate organizations? Comparative studies of corporate nursing systems as independent or interfacing cultures could well lead to some valuable insights about management and their effectiveness. In the future, it is reasonable to predict that corporate structures in institutions of higher educations will prevail. Most of these corporate structures will be cloned after business management models rather than transcultural academic and nursing care models. What effect will these business-driven focused corporate structures have on the quality of nursing education and service that values human caring services and from a multicultural viewpoint? How might nursing develop their own organizational or corporate care structure to fit with its distinct discipline and professional perspectives? Most assuredly, nursing organizational structures should be culturally congruent structures with its major discipline, theoretical, and service perspectives.

In general, nursing is entering a new and challenging era, with Western and non-Western nurses coming together. Worldwide administrative organizational structures or models that support culturally congruent care and multiculturalism will be valued and in demand by the year 2010. Nurse administrators are being challenged to establish organizational structures that reflect these philosophic aspects, but especially for a global humanistic care agenda. The theory of Culture Care is an appropriate theory to develop futuristic administrative organizations that can provide culturally congruent care in education and service (Leininger 1981, 1984, 1988). Most importantly, nursing administrators need futuristic plans that will accommodate rapid value changes and working with nurses from practically everywhere in the world. These administrators will need to support different configurations of different types of cultural and multidiscipline administration. Working with nurses who are highly mobile and for short time periods will be difficult but possible. The theory of Culture Care provides one means to design future administrative education and service programs with the above goals and trends in mind.

RESEARCH AREAS OF INQUIRY RELATED TO CULTURE CARE THEORY FOR NURSING ADMINISTRATORS

Since the theory of Culture Care is presented in this book and with transcultural care research studies, only research questions for nursing service and education administrators will be discussed in this last section. These areas of inquiry are offered to stimulate nurse administrators to explore what is universal or diverse about nursing administration worldwide, and to consider ways to get to new knowledge in order to develop new administrative organizations and practices. A comparative ethnoadministrative theoretical and research focus is needed to achieve this goal and to obtain fresh perspectives about nursing education and service (Leininger 1985b, 1990b). Culture Care theory with the ethnonursing research method is recommended to study ethnoadministrative practices. Other ethnomethods, however, such as ethnography, ethnoscience, life histories, audio-visuals, metaphors, and phenomenology could be used to discover the often invisible, covert and little known administrative aspects of human care and other nursing phenomena. The qualitative paradigm offers one of the best means to explicate cultural care with the ethnonursing method as the latter is a method designed specifically for Culture Care theory (Leininger 1985). The need for in-depth meanings and comparative cultural data bearing upon a human care and nursing administration within naturalistic and familiar context is important.

A. Research Questions for Nursing Service Administrators Using Culture Care Theory

1. What are the comparative meanings and interpretive expressions of cultural care to nurse administrators locally and in different countries?

2. In what ways can nurse administrators make human care a clearly visible, coherent, and central focus of nursing services?

3. What attributes and characteristics constitute universal and diverse features of nursing care administration in Western and non-Western cultures?

4. What alternative types or models of nursing service organization and management practices show the greatest potential to serve people of different cultures?

5. What are the strengths and limitations of a *collegial* type of organizational structure versus a *legalistic-bureaucratic* organization for Western and non-Western nursing service administration?

6. What cultural care stresses and conflicts do clients of diverse cultural backgrounds experience with administrators and staff who espouse cultural values that are clearly different from those of clients or staff nurses?

7. What innovative approaches can nursing service administrators use to accommodate cultural care differences in nursing care practices, and provide congruent care practices for clients?

8. In what ways do the worldview, social structure, cultural values, language, history, and environmental context influence nursing education and service practices?

9. What strategies could be used to help nursing administrators shift from the present emphasis on resource reallocation, technological efficiency, and "bottom line" cost effectiveness to that of quality nursing *care* services for specific clients of diverse or similar cultures?

10. Given the fact that a number of cultural groups, especially minority cultures, do not utilize or seek professional nursing and other health care services for many cultural reasons, what creative approaches or strategies could be used to attract

these cultural groups to use hospital or community-based nursing services when necessary?

11. What are some diverse or universal ethical and clinical problems of nurses in providing care to clients of different cultures, especially those whose values, beliefs, and practices differ considerably from the philosophy, norms and values of nursing service administration?

12. In what ways could nursing service administrators establish care as the central focus of nursing and with a highly favorable public image of nursing worldwide?

13. How could nursing service managers market quality of cultural care in a cost effective caring way to clients of diverse or similar cultures?

14. Since Western nursing care values and practices tend to contrast sharply with many non-Western cultural care values, how could nursing service administrators prepare nurses worldwide or locally to deal with such differences in order to reduce client stresses, conflicts, non-compliances, and non-therapeutic care practices?

15. Since cultural imposition practices are a serious and prevailing clinical problem (Leininger 1991a), how might nursing service administrators reduce or change cultural imposition tendencies?

16. In what ways does the theory of Culture Care contribute to differentiated nursing practices?

17. How can nursing service administrators and staff discover, document, and evaluate culturally congruent care?

18. What are some of the major reasons or factors preventing nurse administrators from focusing on comparative cultural care?

19. What research methods offer the greatest promise to accurately and credibly describe and interpret care phenomena of diverse cultures and their nursing care needs?

20. Given the litigious nature of human beings, what could nurse administrators do today to prevent serious legal suits with multicultural groups and of cultural care negligence?

21. With the future trend for community based home care services, what kinds of nursing service organizations need to be developed to accommodate lifecycle needs and provide culturally congruent home care?

B. Research Questions for Nursing Education Administrators Using Culture Care Theory

1. What are the universal and diverse meanings and interpretations of cultural care among nursing administrators and faculty in schools of nursing?

2. What universal and diverse administrative care approaches could be used to recruit and retain nursing faculty and students of diverse cultures, and especially cultural minorities that are under-represented in schools of nursing?

3. What types of organizational structures show the best promise to establish and promote a philosophy of cultural care and concomitant educational practices in schools of nursing?

4. How does the worldview, social structure, cultural values, linguistic expressions, history, and environmental factors influence cultural care education practices in nursing schools?

5. How might nurse administrators and faculty facilitate use of the theory of Culture Care to guide changes in philosophy, organizational structure, and curricula in schools of nursing to accommodate students, faculty, and staff from diverse cultures locally and transnationally?

6. Since so few nurse administrators and faculty have had formal preparation in transcultural nursing and human care, how might the theory of Culture Care help stimulate changes to meet this future emphasis in nursing?

7. In light of the rapid changes and demands for multicultural and transcultural nursing education, what could nurse administrators and nursing service leaders do together to prepare a new generation of nurses to care to be culturally sensitive, knowledgeable, and skilled in transcultural nursing?

8. What innovative administrative strategies could nursing deans use to support faculty to use a multicultural care approach to teaching, research and practice?

9. How could Culture Care theory be used in a collaborative way with nursing service staff in research projects to reinforce and build upon the goal of providing culture congruent care services?

10. How could Culture Care theory be used to help academic nurse administrators reduce cultural imposition practices with faculty and between nursing service and education?

11. Since cultural conflicts and stresses are anticipated to markedly increase in schools of nursing due to heightened multiculturalism, how might the three modes in Leininger's (1985, 1988) theory of cultural care actions and decisions be used to reduce multicultural conflicts and legal suits?

12. What incentives could be used to help nurse educators move from largely a unicultural to a multicultural perspective in administrative services?

13. What accounts for the diverse or similar administrative practices of deans in schools of nursing worldwide?

14. How might the theory of Culture Care be used to generate public policies in transcultural nursing and in administrative management practices on university campuses, in local communities, and in public sectors?

15. What is the potential consequence of having corporate cultures in schools of nursing? Will they support humanistic caring ethos with favorable benefits?

16. What might be the predicted outcome if nursing administrators were actively committed to and implemented culturally based humanistic care teaching and administrative practices?

17. What are the universal and non-universal ethical care problems that nursing administrators and faculty face when non-sensitive cultural care practices exist?

18. What universal cultural care concepts, principles, and research-based content needs to be taught to students in

baccalaureate, master's, doctoral, and postdoctoral nursing degree programs to increase transcultural care knowledge and practices?

19. What are the multicultural public images and interpretation problems related to the current public tagline: "If caring were enough anyone could be a nurse"? How might this tagline be improved or changed in the future for a more accurate and positive view of nursing?

From the above questions, one can note there are many studies which merit investigation to advance transcultural nursing administration with a care focus. The theory of Culture Care offers good possibilities for its use by nurse administrators in academic and service settings.

Administrators are truly faced today with a growing number of diverse cultural and social forces that are influencing nursing education and practice. Many of these critical administrative problems are bearing directly on our rapidly changing society and culture norms. With future demands from clients, nursing students, and faculty to have transcultural care knowledge an integral part of nursing and a specialization area, nursing administrators must be prepared to meet this need. No longer can they remain uniculturally oriented or use nursing theories and practices that are ethnocentric or culture-bound. Successful nurse administrators are challenged to be knowledgeable and open to accommodate consumers of multicultural orientations and backgrounds. An open and comprehensive theory such as Culture Care offers a means to discover new insights about administrative practices, and especially since it is not culture-bound nor a narrow theoretical view.

Currently, a number of nursing service and education administrators are using non-nursing theories, ideologies, or philosophies to guide their judgments and actions. Some of these nursing service administrators tend to rely heavily on biomedical disease and symptom alleviation ideologies and practices to guide their administrative decisions rather than nursing care theories and practices. There are some nursing service administrators who borrow, almost wholesale, specific theories and models from economics, public administration, and business to study and guide their administrative practices. In nursing education, there are deans and associate deans who rely on general education theories and practices. Still too few administrators have learned how to use and value our own theories to generate administrative decisions and actions. It seems ironic to find so many of our nursing administrators in education and service using only some of our 18 or more major nursing theories to guide their deliberations and for differentiated practices. This is a serious cultural lag and a problem that needs to be recognized if nurses are to advance nursing as a discipline and profession with its distinct perspectives. For without a nursing theoretical perspective, nurse administrators and those they serve may be offering questionable services.

As nursing moves into the future, I contend that nurse administrators in education and service can benefit from the use of Culture Care theory or from other similar care theories to help them move them soundly into the twenty-first century. These care theories are needed to provide a worldwide focus to nursing education and services because of future mobility and changing nurses practices. They need a broad holistic theory but also an action-oriented specific care theory. Therefore, it is time to prepare nurse administrators for top- and middle-level multicultural administrative care practices. These nursing administrators need to reflect nursing's distinct contribution to nursing through the use of current and future transcultural human care knowledge and practices. Nursing administrators are our leaders in nursing who can make a great difference in changing health care systems, in developing new policies and visible public care practices.

Although the future of nursing is promising, nursing administrators, as a key leadership group, must begin to shift from largely a unicultural to a multicultural perspective and use appropriate care theories to guide their judgments and decisions. Nurse administrators will find that the theory of cultural care with three modes of nursing actions (i.e. cultural care preservation or maintenance, cultural care accommodation or negotiation, and cultural care repatterning and restructuring) should be most helpful to develop new administrative practices in education and service. Unquestionably, the theory is a highly relevant and readily available for nurse administrators to use in our rapidly changing multicultural administrative and practice world.

REFERENCES

Fawcett, J., (1984). The metaparadigm to nursing: Present status and future refinements. *Image: Nurse Scholarship, 16*(3), 84–86.

Henry, B. et al. (1988). *Dimensions of nursing administration: Theory, research, education, practice.* St. Louis: Mosby Publication, 19–34.

Leininger, M. M. (1967). The culture concept and its relevance to nursing. *The Journal of Nursing Education. 6*(2), 27–39.

Leininger, M. M. (1970). The cultural concept and American culture values in nursing. *Nursing and anthropology: Two worlds to blend.* New York: John Wiley & Sons, 45–52.

Leininger, M. M. (1974a). The leadership crises in nursing: A critical problem and challenge. *The Journal of Nursing Administration, 4*(2), 28–34.

Leininger, M. M. (1974b). Towards conceptualization of transcultural health care systems: Concepts and a model. *Human care issues, transcultural health care issues and conditions.* Philadelphia: F.A. Davis, 3–23.

Leininger, M. M. (1976). Caring: The essence and central focus of nursing. American Nurses Foundation. *Nursing Research Report, 12*(1), 2, 14.

Leininger, M. M. (1978). *Transcultural nursing: Concepts, theories, and practices.* New York: John Wiley & Sons.

Leininger, M. M. (1981). *Care: An essential human need.* Thorofare, NJ: Slack.

Leininger, M. M. (1984). Care: The essence of nursing and health. In M. M. Leininger (Ed.), *Care: The essence of nursing and health.* Thorofare, NJ: Slack, 3–15.

Leininger, M. M. (1985a). Transcultural care diversity and universality: A theory of nursing. *Nursing and Health Care, 6*(4), 209–212.

Leininger, M. M. (1985b). *Qualitative research methods in nursing.* Orlando, FL: Grune & Stratton, 33–73.

Leininger, M. M. (1986). Care facilitation and resistance factors. In Z. Wolf (Ed.), *Clinical care in nursing.* Gaithersburg, MD: Aspen Publication, 1–24.

Leininger, M. M. (1987). *Care: Discovery and uses in clinical and community nursing.* Detroit: Wayne State University Press, 1–30.

Leininger, M. M. (1988). Leininger's theory of nursing: Cultural care diversity and universality. *Nursing Science Quarterly, 2*(4), 11–20.

Leininger, M. M. (1989). Transcultural nursing: A worldwide necessity to advance nursing knowledge and practice. In J. McCloskey & H. Grace (Eds.), *Nursing issues.* Boston: Little, Brown & Co.

Leininger, M. M. (1990a). Historic and epistemologic dimensions of care and caring with future directions. In J. Stevenson (Ed.), *Knowledge about care* and caring: State of the art and future developments. Kansas City, MO: American Nurses Association Press, 19–31.

Leininger, M. M. (1990b, Winter). Ethnomethods: The philosophic and epistemic basis to explicate transcultural nursing knowledge. Journal of Transcultural Nursing, 1(2), 40–51.

Leininger, M. M. (1991a). Becoming aware of types of health practitioners and cultural imposition. Journal of Transcultural Nursing, 3(1).

Leininger, M. M. (1991b). Current view of the culture of nursing. (in preparation).

Rothschild, J., & Russell, R. (1986). Alternatives to bureaucracy: Democratic participation in economy. In R. Turner & J. Short Jr. (Eds.), Annual review of sociology. Palo Alto: Annual Reviews, 12, 307–345.

12

Looking to the Future of Nursing and the Relevancy of Culture Care Theory

Madeleine M. Leininger

Theories help nurses to discover the future, and research findings guide nurses into future actions and practices.

Nursing is and will always be a transcultural adventure into the future with a challenge to care for people in a rapidly changing and uncertain world. Nurses will always be challenged by people of diverse cultures whose daily living experiences may bring them joyous occasions but also unexpected human tragedies or unfavorable life conditions. Nurses who are stimulated by nursing theories, and the use of transcultural research care findings will find many new and rewarding ways to care for or with people of different cultural backgrounds. Human caring also becomes a moral challenge and imperative as nurses realize the tremendous influence and positive consequences of skilled nursing care. This reality becomes even more important as nurses become highly knowledgeable and skilled to work with many different cultures in the world.

In the nursing profession and discipline, expert human caring will remain the hallmark and essence of nursing through time and place. Thus, it is important to look into the future and to anticipate the nature and direction of nursing in the twenty-first century. Indeed, futuristic nursing leaders must keep an open mind and remain alert to vague "cures," past historical trends, and be willing to envision what may not exist today.

The above thoughts and philosophy have guided my work to create new directions and beginnings in nursing. Indeed, during the past 40 years, it has been a great and stimulating challenge to use my nursing, anthropological, and general life experiences to look ahead at least three or four decades to imagine what nursing's possible future would be like. It also has been a challenge to carve new pathways and encourage nursing students and faculty to follow me down these paths to child psychiatric nursing, doctoral nursing education, transcultural nursing, human caring, use of qualitative research methods, and other new and important directions. But one of my greatest challenges has been to advance human care and transcultural nursing knowledge as central to nursing's discipline and profession. Discovering ways to guide nurses to learn about different lifeways of people in daily living, crises events, health struggles, and sickness episodes from a transcultural perspective remains a difficult challenge. However, the gradual discovery of culturally based care by nurses has greatly broadened and provided many new and different ways to help people and to discover themselves. Nurses have discovered new and important roles in the future of nursing with transcultural nursing knowledge and practices. Culture care knowledge has expanded the nurse's worldview and given a very different view of nursing. Culture Care theory has been an important means to discover such new insights about nursing, and challenges nurses to use a transcultural care focus in nursing education, research, and practice. The theory also has helped nurses to look into the future with many great challenges as nursing becomes a transcultural profession.

In this last chapter, I will discuss some of the major worldwide forces that I envision will continue to make the theory of Culture Care Diversity and Universality highly relevant, and one of the most promising and significant theories in nursing to advance, transform, and soundly establish nursing as a discipline and profession in the twenty-first century. The three areas I will discuss include: (1) rapid and intense multicultural changes in the world with the demand for transculturally based research nursing knowledge and skills; (2) the marked and rapidly growing interest in and focus on culture care as the essence and unifying focus of nursing; and (3) the major shift to qualitative research methods to discover unknown epistemic and onto-logic dimensions of nursing knowledge that will ultimately support and legitimize a dynamic, relevant, and transculturally based discipline of nursing. In this chapter, I take the position that, in the future, the theory of Culture Care will be a major nursing theory to establish and legitimize the *globalization of nursing with transcultural comparative care knowledge and practices.* Culture Care theory will become increas-ingly meaningful as an intellectual and clinical challenge in all areas of nursing education, research, and practice. It will be the new way to know people, the new way to teach, and the new way to practice nursing. It also will be important for new modes of transcultural con-sultation, comparative research projects, and administrative practices. Most importantly, it will help the public, multidisciplinary colleagues, and consumers of nursing services to value nursing as a transcultural caring science and a humanistic discipline and profession.

RAPID AND INTENSE MULTICULTURAL
WORLD CHANGES

Recent worldwide developments reveal that the world is changing and will continue to change rapidly into the twenty-first century. The fall of the Berlin Wall, the consequences of the Persian Gulf War, the violence in South Africa, the multiple natural disasters, and loss of many lives in India, Africa, South America, and the Philippines due to economic, political, and cultural forces make one keenly aware that there are many future changes to anticipate. For, indeed, what happens today influences tomorrow. Accordingly, nurses need to consider how they can meet these changing human needs of people worldwide in the future. How can nurses promote and maintain well being, positive lifeways, prevent accidents, and deal with changing environments and movements of people to new territories or countries. Such changes and others call for building on and envisioning new caring patterns, new knowledge, and new approaches to assist people in changing lifeways. It calls for different ways to care for culture groups never seen or known before in one's lifespan as well as helping people undergoing major transitions.

Quite frequently, nurses are able to respond quickly to accidents and disasters, and handle physical needs of people, but they are somewhat slower to respond to major emotional crises, cultural and social losses of dear family members, friends and others, and worldwide disasters. Such major changes and losses call for *transcultural care knowledge* and a *strong caring ethos* to guide nurses' thinking and action modes. The critical question is how can we best prepare nurses in the future with a transcultural caring ethos to guide their humanitarian work with worldwide changes? A caring ethos of ethical and moral awareness will be extremely important for nurses to function successfully in transcultural, sociopolitical, and legal contexts related to multicultural crises and changes. International disasters often leave nurses feeling especially hopeless and inadequate to respond to such overwhelming conditions. No doubt, such transcultural uncertainties will continue in the future, and nurses will need to anticipate ways to prepare themselves as they go to function in worldwide disasters or with unknown cultural groups nationally and internationally. Such changes and others will occur more rapidly and with greater potential consequences than ever before in the history of nursing and humankind. For there will be technologic and scientific changes in the uses of space, land, ecologies and the ocean in which new nursing knowledge and skills will need to be developed for nurses to function successfully in these arenas of action. Here as elsewhere, caring differences and similarities will need to be studied and responded to with respect to such changes. There also will be multicultural differences in language, values, and practices that will challenge the nurse in working with people of different cultures.

Intense and frequent multicultural experiences will prevail not only on a macro or global perspective, but also on a micro or local (home) community basis. Nurses will encounter many more cultural strangers living next door to care for, or with, in the home or neighborhood hospital. New kinds of local and national businesses will be owned and operated by foreign cultural leaders. New kinds of foods, human conditions, and lifestyle activities will prevail among different cultures. Clients will speak different languages, act differently, and have different expectations of nurses and other health personnel. The impact of multicultural communication, new electronic equipment, worldwide audiovisual programs, and many other kinds of new technologies along with rapid and intense transportation modes will make the nurse realize the tremendous influence of these forces on nursing care. This will be realized especially as one travels and works in different cultural contexts and sees different "have" and "have not" cultures in the above areas cited. Relevant to the study of these rapid changes in an intense multicultural world and their impact on nursing care, education, and practices is the theory with research findings of Culture Care Diversity and Universality.

With culture changes intensifying to a point rarely seen in the long history of human kind, the nurse will be challenged to become keenly sensitive to and knowledgeable about culture care practices. Caring for cultural strangers and for people who are in transition, shock, or trying to adjust to new changes in their lives will make transcultural nursing an imperative focus in all aspects of nursing. Nurses will be expected to function with many different cultural groups in any typical day or night in the hospital, home, or in a new kind of nursing service. As such, nurses will be expected to have general knowledge of *many* cultures, but also *specific* knowledge of several cultures. Most unicultural values, norms, and practices in nursing education and service will be gradually replaced by multicultural values and practices. Nurse clinicians working in urban hospitals will be expected to know, understand, and work with clients from many different cultures in any typical day or night by the year 2000. Both commonalities (or universals) and diversities within cultures can bring nurses closer to people with a caring humanistic focus. In rural areas, where cultural diversity will not be manifest, nurses will nonetheless tend to be more homogenous and firm in their beliefs, values, and lifeways concerning health and nursing care. The solidarity of some rural cultures will require that the nurse's knowledge and skills be different than those required in large heterogenous hospitals and urban centers. Nurses will need to respond openly, appropriately, knowingly, and creatively to these different cultural groups and especially to their particular health care concerns or problems. The nurse will look for theories and research findings to understand, interpret, and work with many different cultural representatives. Different patterns of client needs will become apparent to the nurse if he or she takes time to listen and hear "their stories" of what keeps them well or how they become ill. Most importantly, the professional nurse of tomorrow will not be only an efficient or competent nurse technician, but will be compassionate, sensitive, and competent to handle diverse caring needs of clients. The nurse will try to avoid professional ethnocentrism, strong prejudices, and cultural imposition practices (Leininger, 1978, 1988). Nurses will find that the Sunrise Model and the tenets of the Culture Care theory will be extremely helpful in providing holistic care and nursing care that identifies and respects similarities and differences among clients. Culturalogical health care assessments also will help the nurse acquire new insights and become a competent nurse to support culturally congruent care practices.

In the future, there will be a marked increase in focus on the nurse's responsibility to preserve clients' cultural rights. Respect for human rights largely derived from one's cultural values, beliefs, and practices, will be imperative. If client's cultural rights are not respected and protected, the nurse can anticipate open confrontations, cultural conflicts, legal suits, and other kinds of unfavorable consequences. To protect the nurse from such difficulties, he or she will need to practice culture-specific care, with the client's culture values and beliefs cognitively known, respected, and considered in nursing decisions and actions (Leininger, 1988, 1990). To guide nurse's decisions and actions in identifying cultural differences and similarities of client rights will be transcultural care knowledge generated from Culture Care theory. Moreover, culture care knowledge will be essential in guiding nurses as expert witnesses in legal cases where cultural rights have been violated or neglected, and which is already becoming evident today.

By the year 2010, one can predict that clients from diverse cultures will carry a "Transcultural Health Card," or what I call a "Pink Card," which they will use to enter a foreign or new culture, and particularly as they travel, migrate to, or live temporarily in a new location. The "Pink Cards" will be used to gain quick access to health care services and will have client computerized data for transnational uses. The card will provide basic information to nurses, physicians, and other licensed health care personnel about clients from another culture. A brief ethnohealth history with past and current care practices, medical treatments, medications and other data thus will be available to health personnel in order to facilitate client's entry into a familiar or different health care service. Many clients as "Pink Card" holders will be culture strangers to the nurse in their first contact. The nurse will be expected to understand and respond appropriately and sensitively to these strangers. Culture-specific and some general knowledge of the client's culture will be essential to facilitate the nurse's approach, assessment, and direct nursing care practices. The three modes from the Culture Care theory will be used to make sound judgements and decisions from the "Pink Card" and from other clinical data obtained with the use of the Sunrise Model and with a focus on providing holistic nursing care services derived from the theory.

By the year 2010, nurses will be expected to speak and to read two or more languages in nursing. Already many Canadian, European, Scandinavian, and nurses from other cultures speak several languages, and so have a "headstart" on most nurses in the United States. Ethnolinguistics and the use of nonverbal or gestural communication will be essential to know and respond to client's nursing care needs. Thus, nurses will be required to know several languages, especially the language(s) in the countries where employed. English will not be used in all countries. Of course, the theory of Culture Care emphasizes the importance of language in different environmental contexts and with respect to ethnohistorical and other social structure factors.

After the turn of the twenty-first century, more nurses will be certified in transcultural nursing in order to provide safe and congruent care to clients from different cultures. Certification will be especially important as nursing shifts to transcultural care and to functioning with people of diverse cultural backgrounds worldwide. Certification will be necessary before being employed in many countries to assure that the nurse is reasonably knowledgeable and culturally safe to serve people in the culture. Nurses will experience a greater urgency to be prepared to serve people of different cultures and to have "holding or suspended" generic (folk) and professional knowledge of the people. Knowing and creatively blending professional nursing practices with generic folk care knowledge will be the new challenge in practice and for certification examinations. Certification will protect nurses from legal suits, cultural care negligence, culture care imposition practices, and unsafe practices. Certification in transcultural nursing, which began in 1987 by the Transcultural Nursing Society for worldwide and certification practices, will gradually be adopted by nursing organizations and will become large scale and a worldwide and competitive certification business by several organizations by the year 2020. As home health care services increase and nurses become primarily *care facilitators* (rather then primary caretakers), they will need to be certified to provide responsible care. Culture care test items for certification will come largely from research generated from the use of Culture Care theory, which will provide substantive and culture-specific knowledge with universal and diverse professional knowledge.

In the future, nurse leaders with doctoral preparation will be expected to deal with global or worldwide culture care education practice issues, policies, and practices of different countries. This shift from largely unicultural to multicultural practices will be difficult. Today, still less than 3 percent of the nearly 60 doctoral programs in the United States focus on transcultural care research, theory, and practices (Leininger, 1990). By the year 2025, over 50 percent of professional nurses will have master's and doctoral preparation in nursing, and transcultural nursing with a care focus will be imperative for these leaders to function in global nursing education and practice services.

Due to the present critical shortage of well-prepared transcultural nurse educators, researchers, and practitioners, however, preparation of transcultural nurses will be difficult. Doctoral preparation in comparative care and health will be essential to establish the credibility of nurses and to ensure effective consultant work in unfamiliar cultures. Graduate nurses without preparation in differentiated culture care will find themselves greatly handicapped in research, education, and practice, and will encounter intercultural stresses and other transnational problems. Unquestionably, transcultural exchange programs and consultant services will demand cultural knowledge, ethical commitments, and professional competencies in the host cultures. In becoming competent exchange scholars, consultants, or practitioners, doctoral and master's prepared nurses will be required and the use of Culture Care theory and research findings will be most helpful to these nurses (Leininger, 1978, 1989). While graduate prepared nurses will increase their interest and work in many different countries, their credibility will be recognized mainly with transcultural knowledge and competencies defined largely by culture and in their language. Again, transcultural care knowledge and skills will be essential to prevent cultural backlash, ethnocentrism, cultural conflicts, and legal problems in international work. Most importantly, it will make nurses work more satisfying.

During the intense and growing multiculturalism era of the twenty-first century, nursing service administrators also will be seeking nurses prepared in culture care and with transcultural nursing preparation. Demands for transcultural nursing faculty will far exceed the supply until nearly 2020 (Leininger, 1989). Nursing faculty in many academic centers will be needed in order to prepare students for intense multicultural health care services. The present cliche of faculty and nursing service personnel focusing mainly on "client awareness" or "becoming culturally sensitive" will be extended to prepare nurses to become highly knowledgeable and culturally competent in care practices. Moreover, the new generation of nursing students will continue to demand transcultural care knowledge to assure quality care to clients of different cultures (Leininger & Watson, 1990). Mentorship and the use of Culture Care theory in research and action-research will gain in importance here. Faculty who are unable to teach and mentor students in transcultural clinical and community work also will find themselves greatly handicapped in the future. Knowledge of culture care concepts, principles, theoretical ideas, and research findings will be essential for nurses to pass local and the worldwide certification examinations and to function competently and safely with clients. Both nursing faculty and service personnel will rely on such knowledge in practice.

In the near future, many nurses will critically examine extant nursing theories to determine the extent to which different nursing theories help nurses to study and explicate culture care and health knowledge. Nursing theory critics will reevaluate nursing theories to assess their ethnocentric biases, beliefs, uses of language, values, and philosophic orientation. Although some nurse theorists recently have begun tagging on the terms *culture* and *culture care* to their theories, their conceptual insights are superficial and not well integrated in their theories. The adequacies or inadequacies of nursing theories to study multicultural phenomena in diverse cultures will become problematic for many students who are using most of today's nursing theories. The long-range credibility and usefulness of any nursing theory will rest largely with the conceptual and theoretical emphases from a worldwide culture perspective in order to generate meaningful and useful nursing knowledge. Currently, there are nursing theories with limited or questionable culture care theoretical orientations to facilitate explication of culture care phenomena. For example, Orem's (1980) self-care deficit theory provides only a tacit and superficial focus on culture care and with limited emphasis to explicate "other-care" or "other-culture-care" phenomena or patterns. During my three decades of care research, however, I have found many cultures that do not value "self-care," "dependent care," or "self-care deficit" concepts as discovered in China, Philippines, and several cultures in the Pacific Islands, unless they are highly acculturated to Western ideologies. More cultures in the world tend to espouse "other-care" rather than "self-care" ideologies, and these cultures want and expect to be cared for by others when they come to the hospital or clinic, or for home care. Self-care is often not what is desired or expected except as a last resort or in dire circumstances. Often, it is a struggle for minority and oppressed cultures to obtain funds for health care when they enter a hospital, and many are baffled with the dominant Anglo-American middle class emphasis on "self-care" practices such as those in the United States. It is apparent that Orem's self-care theory fits mainly those culture values of middle- and upper-class Anglo-Americans in which self-reliance, independence, and autonomy characterize the culture (Leininger, 1988). In this light, I would think that Orem's self-care deficit/dependent theory will have less relevancy and usefulness in the future and especially in non-Western cultures unless substantially modified. Orem's theory of self-care in the United States, which seems to be a popular and driving force in nursing curricula and some clinical practices, will need to be reevaluated for its usefulness transculturally and especially with minority and oppressed cultures. Orem's theory, however, is not alone in this concern about the full inclusion of culture care in nursing theories.

Another example of theory reevaluation for relevancy uses in transcultural contexts is Roger's "unitary science of man" (Rogers, 1970). This theory, which focuses on unitary man, space, and energy and other related abstract phenomena, may be very difficult for nurses to use in some cultures that are cognitively oriented to concrete and practical daily life experiences, poverty conditions, oppressive political forces, very limited education, and virtually no technologies. For nurses to use Roger's theory to conceptualize such cultures in an abstract way may be extremely difficult and viewed as impractical, impossible, and non-relevant to these cultures. Moreover, nurses may have considerable difficulty in interpreting findings in relation to the theory and in "testing" it in their cultural context and frame of reference. But, of course, there are other nursing theories that will require reevaluation and certain modification to become transculturally relevant to different cultures drawing on ethnohistorical factors, dominant values, and environmental contexts. I predict we will see only a few theories that are sufficiently comprehensive to be used transculturally in the future, and several nursing theories will become extinct.

Still another example of theory reevaluation involves Whall and Fawcett's (1991) book on family theory development in nursing, which offers no cultural theory or conceptual reference to consider families from a transcultural perspective. The absence of a theoretical cultural focus to study families reveals how much education is yet needed to help nurse theorists value, understand, and realize the importance of culture care in nursing. Today and in the future families of all types will use their culture values, beliefs, and lifeways to guide their behavior. Failure to account for this very substantial aspect of family life theoretically is more than telling. It involves a "blind spot" in nursing theory that the Culture Care theory can "cure." In general then, nursing theories will be reexamined and selected for their actual or potential relevance to a culture. Only those culture theories that are not ethnocentric will be used by nurses in the future. By the year 2010, culture care as the long standing and major missing domain in nursing and in nursing theories will be recognized and in demand by nurses.

As more nursing faculty, clinicians, students, administrators, and others learn about and use the theory of Culture Care Diversity and Universality, they will discover a number of these important features and strengths of the theory. First, the theory of Culture Care has been thoughtfully constructed and refined over the past three decades to discover transcultural nursing care phenomena that is grounded or "rooted in" diverse cultures. It is a theory that offers a broad and comprehensive means to study human beings and culture care. It is a theory that can be used in any culture or subculture in the world to discover cultural care differences and similarities in a systematic and rigorous systematic way. The nurse also can focus on one culture or several cultures depending on his or her interests, research skills, and holding knowledge of the culture. It is a theory that supports comparative culture care whether at one point in time (synchronic) or over several time periods (diachronic) to study culture care and related nursing phenomena.

Second, the theory of Culture Care is comprehensive, holistic, and broad in scope, and yet can explicate specifics of an individual, family, group, community, or institution under study. It is a theory that is used to focus on dimensions, but it is also used to study total cultures, incorporating the broadest conceptual and theoretical perspective. *Discovering the totality of how a culture knows and experiences caring from their emic perspective* is important in today's nursing world. Worldview, social structure (including the religion, kinship, economics, politics, cultural values, education, and technology), language expressions, environmental context, ethnohistory, and the folk and professional health care practices of any culture are the multiple factors studied that influence care. These dimensions are some of the most important aspects to get at the totality of human lived experiences of any culture, and to focus on actual or potential care factors that influence human well being or health. The theorist also can choose a particular focus, such as an individual, a family, a special group culture, a community, or an institution, when using the theory and Sunrise Model. Human care factors tend to be "nested" into social structure and other factors identified in the theory. To prevent a partial or fragmented view of culture care behavior, I deliberately chose these multiple influencers or dimensions to help the nurse extend his or her perspective beyond the traditional biopsychosocial individual viewpoint. The theory also lends itself to intracultural variabilities as well as to external contrast among several cultures for similarities and differences among cultures about human caring and health. And since the theory can be used to discover synchronic or diachronic care and related phenomena, the findings can provide longitudinal comparative time perspectives. The discovery, however, of the totality of lived experiences of people and the multiple forces that influence people care (or caring) related to well being and health can provide new knowledge about individual, group, and institutional culture care.

Third, the theory of Culture Care was designed to be used primarily from an inductive *emic* generating knowledge focus with the ethnonursing method and within the qualitative paradigm. The inductive qualitative focus is used to "tease out" the largely covert, invisible and often embedded epistemic and ontologic care data for nursing's discipline knowledge. This contrasts sharply with deductively derived knowledge in which research has *a priori* assumptions and specific hypotheses to test. My research has shown that generic care is embedded in the Sunrise Model components which need to be explicated knowledge to guide professional care practices. The theory of Culture Care with the use of the Sunrise Model can guide the nurse researcher to examine very specific phenomena, but also abstract symbols, spirituality, worldview, subjective, and other often vague aspects. Such comprehensiveness and specificity helps the nurse researcher to become aware of the many dimensions that can actually or potentially influence care or caring for nursing practices. While it is possible to use the theory from a hypodeductive quantitative perspective with different purposes and goals, this has not been as fruitful for reasons already stated. Nonetheless, quantitative studies also may be pursued.

Fourth, the theory of Culture Care should not only be used to generate abstract, philosophical, spiritual, and existential knowledge of human care or caring, but also knowledge to guide nurses in their actions and thinking. The three modes of action and decision (seen in the lower part of the Sunrise Model) generate specific knowledge to know how best to serve the client(s) for culturally congruent care. As a consequence, culture-specific care knowledge is being generated and used to improve or initiate a new culture care that is tailored to fit the clients' needs or conditions.

Fifth, the theory is important to generate knowledge of human care patterns and value themes that are congruent with the cultural lifeways, beliefs, and meanings to individuals and groups. The theory also generates knowledge that is non-congruent care to cultures which can lead to culture conflicts, stress, and potential legal suits. This latter point is extremely important today, and will be more so in the future with anticipated multicultural conflicts of a continuous and serious nature. Some culture groups are already in action to protect *their* cultural values by so called "cultural defenses." Some minorities and oppressed cultures who have been rather silent for years are becoming active such as the Mohawk Indians and other Indians in Canada. Today, many cultures are defending and making known their cultural identity, autonomy, values, and legal rights. They are willing to defend specific culture care rights as well. Minority and oppressed cultures in the United States, Great Britain, Africa, South America, and Eastern Europe will become more active in supporting their cultural identity values and rights. Clients of these diverse cultures who have experienced cultural oppression, offenses, imposition practices, or cultural conflicts in health care will become more determined to protect their rights—a trend that will become an active pursuit well into the twenty-first century. I have observed that cultural values, beliefs, and practices of many cultures worldwide are becoming stronger in their cultural identities since 1980 with local collective group actions. Nurses of tomorrow will realize these trends and the importance of the Culture Care theory in discovering such culturally constituted, ground values in human health care and nursing situations.

As more nurses give care in the home, they will be especially vulnerable to legal suits as families assess care needs in their own natural cultural context. The twenty-first century is already anticipated to be a highly legitious era in the Western world with a marked increase in numbers of lawyers, cultural group migrations, and strong cultural identities. Most importantly, nurses in acute-care centers and long-term care institutions will realize the importance of multiple factors influencing culture care identity needs and culture-specific nursing practices. In order to provide congruent and satisfying care, Culture Care theory data again will be sought to obtain culture value data of individuals, families, and groups. New culture-specific nursing care guidelines will be taught and established in diverse health contexts to help the nurse work with clients or families of specific cultures. For example, Laotian parents usually do not permit the nurse to touch the head of a child because it is sacred until the parents perform certain cultural rituals. After these rituals, health professionals can touch and work with the child for surgical or for other reasons. But if cultural violations occur, one can predict avoidance and negative attitudes toward health personnel and even legal suits. In general, minority cultures who have in the past often been very polite, kind, and deferent will be less willing to acquiesce to health personnel wishes. Likewise, dominant cultures also will assert their culture rights. Of course, some present-day dominant cultures will become the minority cultures of tomorrow requiring nurses to change nursing practices. While some nurse anthropologists fear dealing with cultural diversities and want to stress only commonalities because of the increased distance between nurse and client, I firmly contend we must work with both diversity and commonality factors in client care.

CULTURE CARE: THE ESSENCE AND CENTRAL PHENOMENON OF NURSING

During the past decade, there has been a tremendous groundswell of interest and research focused on human care as the central phenomena of interest to many nurses (Aamodt, 1976, 1978; Leininger, 1988, 1990; Leininger & Watson, 1990; Watson, 1985, 1987, 1988). Because nurses are discovering anew or rediscovering care as a significant way to help people, this trend will steadily increase during this decade. Nurses also are aware that quality of care services can make a difference in healing and well being. By the twenty-first century, care knowledge and practices should be firmly established as the central, dominant domain of nursing.

The active stance of the National League for Nursing to support human care as central to nursing curricula, theory development, and clinical services through recent publications has been most encouraging (Bevis, 1990; Gaut & Leininger, 1991; Leininger & Watson, 1990; Moccia, 1989; Watson, 1989). This support from a major nursing organization is becoming a significant force in transforming nursing education by freeing it from conventional medical ideologies focused on cure. In other countries too—Finland, Australia, Japan, Korea, and Africa—there are movements to promote and focus on human care from a transcultural perspective. These trends in nursing and in several societies will be significant to make culture care an integral part of thinking and action in health care. Gradually, nursing service administrators will combine their interest in preparation of nurses in care with their efforts to make care a highly marketable service in a variety of different contexts (Valentine, 1990). Care will become *context specific* as well as having universal features to guide nurses in teaching clinical services. Quality of care will take on some entirely new and different meanings as care knowledge and practices from different cultures are established. The present cliches and metaphors about "quality of care" in nursing will be far different and be more meaningful in the future than they are today. Care performance services reflecting high levels of nursing skills will become greatly valued—without such care, client's well being or health may be jeopardized. The theory of Culture Care and the ethnonursing method will be used to discover fully the essence, nature, and expressions of human care among clients and staff of different backgrounds. Western nurses also will shift from past emphases on individualism and dyadic nurse–patient interactions to some broader conceptualizations of care that are focused on institutions, communities, cultures, and subcultures. This trend will be extremely important in preventing illnesses and in maintaining patterns of well being with clients in their natural living contexts.

In the very near future, one can predict that the current concepts of *person, environment, health,* and *nursing* will no longer be upheld. Instead, *human care, environmental contexts,* and *well being (or health)* will become of major interest to most nurse researchers and new theorists. The idea of a metaparadigm and the use of logical positivism for developing theories and testing them will change as qualitative paradigmatic investigations and other new paradigms provide different ways for nurses to discover nursing phenomena. Linear and casual thinking will be less valued and used as nurses employ different theories with the qualitative paradigm to conceptualize and study nursing phenomena. Nurses from other countries will express competing theories and models to challenge nurses in the United States and to show the value of culture-specific theories in nursing. Most importantly, traditional disease-symptom medical model content and practice areas such as medical-surgical, maternal child, psychiatric mental health nursing, and community health will have changed as they no longer will be viewed as nursing domains or units of study and practice. Instead, *human care* transculturally, *health,* (or wellness), and *environmental* (ecologic) *contexts* will be the dominant academic and clinical nursing units with lifecycle and other creative relationships for teaching, research, and practice.

During the next century, there will be a significant increase of knowledge not only about human caring and healing, but with rich, comparative transcultural nursing data. Comparative education in all nursing specialties and general arenas at the master's, doctoral, and post-doctoral levels will occur. Nursing education and clinical practices will be radically transformed by the year 2020 to support *differentiated culture care nursing education and practices*. Not all schools of nursing will be experts in *all* cultures, but the faculty prepared in certain areas will prevail in certain schools. Scholars will focus on patterns of transcultural care with clients from numerous, different cultures in the world. While comparative culture care will be the challenge to all health personnel, it will apply especially to nurses who will remain as first-line care providers or facilitators to clients. Due to new research findings and variable study contexts, the meaning of health and illness in different cultures will change. Many new and largely unknown aspects of differentiated cultural living, dying, and celebrating of life-cycle events will begin to be incorporated into nursing education, administration, and clinical practices.

Far more emphases will be given to nurses *learning outside of the classroom and to learning from multicultural experiences in diverse and similar cultures worldwide*. The latter will emphasize discovering different care patterns related to being cared for or being a caregiver in different environmental and cultural contexts. Classroom lectures and learning about medical diseases, symptoms, and treatments will markedly decrease to newer dimensions related to healing, prevention, and health with human care as the powerful force influencing well being. Learning about universal and diverse culture care ethos, moral, and ethical imperatives will become a major area of qualitative study and teaching in nursing worldwide. Research findings from Culture Care theory will be used to greatly expand nurses' awareness of different care modalities to influence healing and well being or to prevent illnesses. The importance of nurses as exquisite caring specialists gradually will prevail. The traditional community health or public health nursing service will focus more on specific rural and urban environments to identify preventive care and health maintenance nursing care practices. Community health nursing will change with long-term field placements similar to current anthropological and transcultural nursing experiences to gain in-depth knowledge about cultures and subcultures in communities and ecological niches. Nurses will soon focus on *action research* to generate and use new knowledge discovered as soon as possible in client care. Culture care knowledge of specific subcultures and cultures in different environmental contexts will be identified with care and health policies derived from most components conceptualized in the Sunrise Model such as social structure, worldview, environmental context, and ethnohistorical data. The body of transcultural nursing care knowledge with principles and specific research findings will be heavily drawn upon by nurses working in urban and rural environments. Most importantly, the largely invisible and complex phenomena of human caring today will become much more visible, known, and used by nurses. The care constructs identified in Chapter 11, along with the theory, will be some of the new body of knowledge in nursing with differentiated and in-depth meanings and guidelines to serve clients in different environments or ecological settings.

A significant nursing development in the future will be the *globalization of human care.* The idea of global care to help people survive, grow, and be responsive to the many others living beside them will be analogous to current worldwide environmental protective agendas. Global care will help people realize that they are living in one large *world culture* with many smaller cultures, subcultures, groups, and institutions embedded within it. Care will be promoted in health care institutions, but also in governments, organizations, businesses, and many areas for marketing, public relations, and as "good business" emphases. A worldwide care agenda will be used to guide intercultural relationships in all spheres of living, business, and health services to support human survival, prevent crises, promote national growth, and for promoting peace and reducing conflicts. Nurses will have the opportunity to make significant contributions to the globalization of care. By 2020, when this trend becomes fully evident nurses will be more knowledgeable and competent in transcultural nursing to make their contribution noteworthy. The globalization of care will prove a powerful force to lead to a new world caring ethos for the well being, health, and peace of the human race.

USE OF QUALITATIVE PARADIGM METHODS: THE "TURNING TIDE" IN NURSING

Early in the twenty-first century, nurses will have come to value and use qualitative paradigmatic research methods in nursing—the major turning point in nursing history and in the development of nursing knowledge. A significant shift in nursing from the past heavy reliance on experimental, quasiexperimental, and other quantitative studies clearly will be evident. As one of the first nurses to initiate this cultural movement in the 1950s and early 1960s with the use of ethnography, ethnonursing, and other qualitative methods in nursing, it will be rewarding to see this trend greatly expand in nursing and the health sciences. Many young nurses of the new research generation as advocates of the qualitative paradigm and its concomitant methods will see the advantages of naturalistic and humanistic research methods to study care and health phenomena. This new generation of researchers will draw on the past efforts of qualitative researchers' thinking and work (Leininger, 1985; Lincoln & Guba, 1985; Munhall & Oiler, 1986; Reason & Rowan, 1981; Morse, 1989; Watson, 1985).

Graduate nursing programs will shift from past heavy emphasis on quantitative research to greater use and valuing of qualitative paradigmatic methods. Faculty and research mentors well prepared in such methods will conduct sound and credible research, and especially related to culture care meanings, lived experiences, metaphors, and symbolic referents. Because of the complexity of qualitative research methods and with nearly 20 major qualitative methods available, schools of nursing (master and doctoral) will offer expertise in three to four methods depending on faculty skills and experiences. However, in the master's program, students will need an overview of all major qualitative methods; in doctoral programs, students will select and learn the major method they will be using. Because theories developed and traditionally taught with the quantitative paradigm are already different from those developed and examined with the qualitative paradigm, teaching and research will follow the qualitative or quantitative paradigm. Research mentorship will be extremely important in qualitative nursing research so that the people's lived experiences, human conditions, values, life aspirations, and other aspects will gain full explication. Qualitative research findings will reveal some entirely new knowledge on which to establish the discipline of nursing, including a wealth of transcultural care knowledge of diverse and similar cultures in the world.

Past emphases on controlling, directing, prescribing, "case managing," and being interventionists will be modified to nurses functioning as expert care *facilitators* and as coparticipants in helping people of diverse and similar cultures. As nurses learn how to be facilitators, enablers, supporters, and assume other major care roles as they work closely with people with different care needs and cultural heritage, new rewards and satisfactions in nursing will flourish.

With the use of qualitative paradigmatic research, nurses will become more confident of their abilities and more definitive in their leadership in patterns and structural ways of caring for clients. Nursing administrators, clinicians, and educators will use the philosophy, principles, and characteristics of the qualitative paradigm to guide them in their new ways of functioning. As qualitative paradigm features are highly congruent with the nature and practice of nursing, new and unexpected discoveries will be forthcoming. Gradually, other health disciplines will value and discover the advantages of using qualitative methods in therapeutic contexts. However, medicine will cling largely to its "double-biund" studies and other quantitative research methods congruent with medicine's curing ethos and its ability to control and regulate human behavior. By the use of qualitative research methods to improve people care—ethnonursing, phenomenology, grounded theory, life histories, ethnohistory, narratives, metaphors, constructionism, philosophical inquiry, and others—nursing will gain a highly positive public image. Nursing knowledge of the twenty-first century will be emically people-centered and less based on past professional *etic* ideas. Transcultural care knowledge will help all nurses and the public see the vital importance of entering into and learning about the people world be it in South American street urchins, oppressed African-Americans, Finish coastal lifeways, feminist abuses, or the life of rural Vietnamese now living in an urban context. This new nursing knowledge will have quite a different focus from past traditional nursing curricula and teaching modalities. If nurses truly enter the people's world of learning and experiencing, it will bring us close to consumers.

By the year 2020, nursing will have at last become recognized as a transcultural nursing profession and discipline with knowledge and skills to serve people in most places in the world. While the theory of Culture Care will have gained a major status as the theory to establish human caring knowledge and practices, variant spin-offs from the theory via the many different interests of nurses will all contribute to the prevailing major theory. Both *universal* and *diverse* care practices will be established largely by the use of nearly 20 different qualitative research methods. While considerable nursing leadership will have been given to help nurses value qualitative research, the efforts to establish the structure, epistemic, and ontologic base of nursing for differentiating humanistic from scientific nursing care will have occurred. For the first time in nursing, humanistic care will have gained credence and meaning equal to that of scientific nursing care. As a result, the science of caring or caring and nursing science will be differentiated to reflect different emphases in humanistic and scientific care. A new structure of nursing knowledge will become evident for the discipline's knowledge.

While many feminists theories and research studies will become evident, gradually some nurse researchers will begin to focus on new male culture ways of knowing and expressing human caring. This then will help nurses put into perspective gender differences and similarities to advance male and female roles and their contributions to nursing knowledge and practices. Female nurses' past fears of identifying with care as "too soft, domestic, and feminine," as expressed in the 1960s and discussed in Chapter 1, will be reversed to deeply valuing care as extremely important domestic (generic) and professional care knowledge and practices. Male nurses will study culture care with renewed and new interests and to identify their gender contributions to humanistic and scientific care. Already some studies on male protective care patterns are becoming evident as well as nurturant care given by males. Out of transcultural gender research will come valuable insights about nurses, clients, and cultural institutions in diverse countries in the world.

PRACTICAL USES OF THE THEORY
OF CULTURE CARE

As stated earlier, some nurse theorists hold that theories are only abstractions of phenomena and can serve only that purpose. I restate my position here that theories generate *abstraction and practical knowledge* for ultimate uses in nursing, and the theory of Culture Care reflects this stance. In the future, more nurses and users of the theory will find it has many practical benefits with the goal of improving nursing care practices by deliberate inclusion of culture care knowledge. In addition, the theory can lead to culture-specific care knowledge and practices related to professional and generic (folk) health care. Insights about these two major systems of diverse cultures related to *emic* and *etic* are extremely important in establishing and building the epistemic and fundamental knowledge base of nursing. Unquestionably, as professional and generic care knowledge and practices are brought close together, clients will be able to receive meaningful and congruent nursing care practices. This knowledge of generic and professional care also is needed to prevent intercultural health hazards, reduce cultural value conflicts, reduce major gaps in health care services, and prevent cultural imposition practices. Generic care knowledge remains largely unknown to nurses today, yet it is what most cultures believe important for quality care services. Such data can be used by the nurse in many creative ways, but especially in relation to the three modes of culture care action or decisions which are part of the care theory and whose goal is to provide culturally congruent care. Professional nurses will be encouraged to use knowledge learned in schools of nursing, but may find they need to alter past knowledge to be acceptable to and congruent with the client's cultural values and lifestyle.

Generic and professional knowledge I and other transcultural nurses have discovered is beginning to be valued and used by some nurses as first-line thinking to help people obtain congruent care practices that are easily accessible, of limited cost, well known, and used and valued by specific cultures. Generic care practices, considered familiar and safe by culture groups, will continue to be used in the future to ease pain or discomforts, and often before professional care practices. Generic care often is effective in healing modes with culture-bound illnesses. Today, as nurses learn from different cultures about differences between generic and professional care, they will gain a new appreciation for appropriate uses of their professional beliefs and practices. For example, the Navajos of Southwestern United States have a ritual folk "blessing ceremony" for young infants that includes giving recognition to the young child by extended family members of the Navajo community. The care constructs of *respect for, attention to,* and *centering on* the Navajo child during the ceremony are significant caring modes that sustain and promote well being. When these care constructs are used with the Navajo child, the family feels they are valued, loved, and an integral part of the Navajo community from birth until death. In addition, a piece of the umbilical cord is often placed in the Navajo home as a symbol that the newborn child will always want to return to the Navajo homeplace and land. Of course, there are numerous other examples that show how generic folk care is beginning to be understood and respected in professional nursing practices. Such generic care constructs will become a central focus and integral part of professional nursing practice in the future.

A practical and significant part of the care theory will be to design and synthesize nursing care practices from abstract or concrete data, from worldview, social structure, environment, and ethnohistory for the three modes of action or decisions of concern: (1) culture care preservation or maintenance, (2) culture care accommodation or negotiation, and (3) culture care repatterning and restructuring (Leininger, 1988a). These modes of nursing require thoughtful reflection and the use of culturally based knowledge to design congruent and meaningful nursing care services. This aspect of the theory is one of the most creative features of nursing and most valuable to clients. For example, nurses may need to include generic folk foods such as ground chili for the elderly Mexican-American in order to help the client get and stay well. A mode of cultural care accommodation is selected here to facilitate the client's recovery from illness. Another example concerns a nurse who was caring for an African-American client with severe hypertension. This nurse used the care construct of *concern for* as a major focus to repatterning and restructuring the African-American's family lifeway which helped the client to avoid salt and pork, and to rely on the local cultural care rituals of daily activity. Consequently, the client responded well to the therapy—blood pressure and other health problems were no longer evident. The nurse should always work closely with the family or significant individual(s) to decide which of the three modes are appropriate, and then work with the individual to implement care plans. Positive results have been forthcoming from the practical use of the three modes of nursing action and decision (Leininger, 1978, 1988), and they also are being used by other health professionals in treatment plans. Indeed, findings from the Culture Care theory are giving new ways to help clients and families.

As more nurses learn about and use the theory, they will find that the Sunrise Model will be invaluable to assess clients and provide guidelines for holistic nursing care practices. Nurses are realizing that what people want most is a choice of what to include or exclude in nursing care practices, based on clients own values, beliefs, and goals. Transcultural nurses also are helping other nurses and students to learn about different cultures, and to use the theory in discovering ways of becoming sensitive and skilled in identifying cultural values, beliefs, and patterns of care with the use of the Sunrise Model. Accordingly, clients respond favorably to nursing care when their values and beliefs are recognized and respected by nurses in their actions and judgements.

The theory of Culture Care is especially practical and important to studying human care and caring transculturally as it provides a *comparative* focus that makes nurses become keenly aware of differences and similarities that must be recognized to care for or with clients. It is these comparative knowledges about care that will make a major difference in nursing's body of discipline knowledge. As nursing will at last recognize the importance of differentiated knowledge to be used for different cultures, nursing also will use universal commonalities and diversities in nursing education and practice. These comparative perspectives provides different contrasts of care and health knowledge to support nursing's claim as a discipline and profession. In this light, the theory of Culture Care involving a comparison of diversities and universalities is unique among extant theories. Constructed explicitly to study culture care as a universal phenomena involving specific cultural diversities, this new body of comparative culture care will be a major force in improving client care and in stimulating nurses toward new ways of thinking and practice. Knowing how to use both diversities and commonalities with clients can bring nurses close to clients and improve care practices. Presently, the *Journal of Transcultural Nursing*, first established in 1988, has become a major publication by which the study of transcultural care diversities and universalities as well as other research related to transcultural nursing can take place in the public domain.

In sum, through the lens of Culture Care theory, the future of nursing looks exceedingly promising. The change of nursing from largely a unicultural profession to a multicultural perspective is fundamental. It is helping to make culture care the essence of nursing. The · following futuristic directions seem especially inevitable:

·1.   By the year 2010, transcultural nursing with a human care diversity and universality focus will become the arching framework of nursing. Transcultural nursing care will be a highly valued philosophy and a mode of nursing education, research, and practice. Transcultural care knowledge will lead to major changes in every aspect of nursing as nursing establishes a new body of nursing knowledge to guide curricular, teaching, and practice modes. It will shift nursing content in schools of nursing from a *unicultural* to a *multicultural* focus and lead to different approaches to work with students, faculty, and clients of diverse cultures. The theory of Culture Care, established in the early 1960s, will have been a strong impetus for these changes to occur.

2. Schools of nursing and institutes will become identified with *cultural areas or regions* to serve cultural groups in their particular communities. Accordingly, nursing curricula, teaching, and research *areas* will be developed with faculty cultural experts and community resources to support transcultural nursing care practices. Transnational exchanges of students and faculty will markedly increase worldwide and will become a competitive enterprise among schools of nursing and universities. Schools of nursing prepared in transcultural care will be highly valued for well planned and implemented cultural changes.

3. All major national and international nursing organizations will need to move beyond the present focus on "culture sensitivity" to in-depth knowledge and competency skills in comparative culture care. Accreditation of nursing schools and the certification of nurses in transcultural nursing with a care focus will be important by 2020. Closely related to this trend will be the growing demand for faculty, nurse clinicians, and nurse researchers prepared in transcultural nursing with a human care focus. All faculty will be expected to be transculturally focused and to value and appreciate theories such as Culture Care Diversity and Universality. Clinical nursing practices will markedly shift from largely Anglo-American to multicultural care practices to meet rising societal and consumer demands to receive congruent care practices and to avoid cultural imposition practices and legal suits.

4. The NANDA classificatory system of nurses and others that has been built largely on Western culture values will no longer be relevant or useful in the next century, the system being far too culture-bound, ethnocentric, medically symptom-based to meet diverse cultural group needs (Leininger, 1990). The current medical emphases of nurses in the United States on NANDA classificatory trend also will be viewed as inadequate as nurses become more knowledgeable about diverse cultures and the offensive imposition practices with some nursing diagnoses. The inadequacy of this system will be realized with nurses recognizing differences between culturally based generic health practices and professional *etic* practices.

5. By the year 2010, many cultural groups and institutions with particular values, beliefs, and lifeways will regulate and control the quality of care by governing councils and policies. Culture leaders who represent community constituents will largely develop, implement, and evaluate health care practices that are culturally acceptable to the people. Health care policies will be strongly influenced by cultural groups at all levels and organizational norms. Culture care safety will be emphasized with "quality of care" to protect people.

6. Funding for transcultural nursing and worldwide cooperative nursing care research studies will be soon recognized as imperative with the globalization of nursing care, but also with worldwide health care practices and use of the "Pink Card." Countries will recognize the importance of transcultural care and will want to support transcultural research. Although this trend is becoming evident in Canada, Europe, and Scandinavia, it remains rather limited in the United States. Of special interest is the fact that Culture Care theory will be used as a model by many disciplines to study transcultural health care. The theory goals will be slightly modified to fit specific disciplines. The Sunrise Model, already being used by many disciplines, will be used more in the future by many health researchers and clinicians. Nursing theories will be fewer in number and will be "synthsized theories" from several current theories to guide nursing research and practices.

The new differentiated nursing care services will be based on culture care competencies of nursing staff serving clients from many different cultures in the world. This will involve a new philosophy of services based on transcultural nursing care models rather than on medical ideologies and practices.

The theory of Culture Care will continue to stimulate nurse researchers, theorists, clinicians, and educators into new and futuristic directions that are barely perceptible today. To see some of my lifelong efforts, dreams, and predictions become a reality will be more than rewarding. What I said in 1960 should come true: "Someday all people in the world will be served by professional nurses prepared in transcultural nursing and using research findings generated from Culture Care theory."

REFERENCES

Aamodt, A. (1978). Sociocultural dimensions of caring in the world of the Papago child and adolescent. In M. M. Leininger (Ed.), *Transcultural nursing theory and practices.* New York: John Wiley & Sons.

Gaut D., & Leininger, M. M. (1991). *Caring: The compassionate healer.* New York: National League for Nursing.

Leininger, M. M. (1977). The phenomena of caring: Caring the essence and central focus of nursing. *American Nurses' Foundation Nursing Research Report, 12*(1), 2–14.

Leininger, M. M. (1978). *Transcultural Nursing: Concepts, theories, and practices.* New York: John Wiley & Sons.

Leininger, M. M. (1988). *Care: Discovery and uses in clinical and community nursing.* Detroit: Wayne State University.

Leininger, M. M. (1989). *Transcultural nursing trends in schools of nursing in U.S.A.* Unpublished manuscript. Detroit: Wayne State University.

Leininger, M. M. (1990e). Issues, questions, and concerns related to the nursing diagnosis cultural movement from a transcultural nursing perspective. *Journal of Transcultural Nursing.* Memphis, TN: University of Tennessee Press, Summer Issue, 2(1), 23–32.

Leininger, M. M., & Watson, J. (1990). *The caring imperative for nursing education.* New York: National League for Nursing.

Lincoln, G., & Guba, Y. (1985). *Naturalistic inquiry.* Beverly Hills, CA: Sage Publications.

Moccia, P. (1988). At the faultline: Social activism and caring. Nursing Outlook, 36(1), 32–33.

Morse, J. (1989). Qualitative nursing research: A contemporary dialogue. Beverly Hills, CA: Sage Publications.

Munhall, P. L. & Oiler, C. J. (1986). Nursing research: A qualitative perspective. Norwalk, CT: Appleton-Century-Crofts.

Orem, D. (1980). Nursing: Concepts for practice. New York: McGraw-Hill.

Reason & Rowan, (1981). Human inquiry: A source book of new paradigm. New York: John Wiley & Sons.

Rogers, M. (1970). An introduction to the theoretical basis of nursing. Philadelphia: F. A. Davis.

Valentine, K. (1985). Advancing care and ethics in health management: An evaluation strategy. In M. M. Leininger (Ed.), Care: Discovery and uses in clinical and community nursing. Detroit: Wayne State University, 151–169.

Watson, J. (1985). Nursing: Human science and human care. Norwalk, CT: Appleton-Century-Crofts.

Watson, J. (1987). Nursing on the caring edge. Metaphorical vignettes. Advances in Nursing Science, 10(1), 10–18.

Watson, J. (1988). Human caring as moral context for nursing education. Nursing and Health Care, 423–426.

Wenger, A. F., & Wenger, M. (1988). Community and Family Care Patterns of the Old Order Amish. In M. M. Leininger (Ed.), Care discovery and use in clinical community nursing. Detroit: Wayne State University.

Whall, A., & J. Fawcett (1991). Family theory development in nursing: State of the science and art. Philadelphia: F.A. Davis.

Appendix A

SOME PUBLICATIONS ON LEININGER'S CULTURE CARE THEORY

Alexander, et al. (1989). Madeleine Leininger: Culture care theory. In A. Marriner-Tomey, (Ed.), *Nursing theorists and their work*. St. Louis: C. V. Mosby.

Brenner, P., Boyd, C., Thompson, T., Marz, M., Buerhaus, P., & Leininger, M. M. (1986). Care symposium: Considerations for nursing administrators. *Journal of Nursing Administration, 16* (1), 25-30.

Cohen, J., (1991). Two portraits of caring: A comparison of the artists. *Journal of Advanced Nursing, 16*, 1-4.

Gates, M. (1991). Transcultural comparison of hospital and hospice as caring environments for dying patients. *Journal of Transcultural Nursing, 2*(2), 3-16.

Leininger, M. M. (1967). The culture concept and its relevance to nursing. *Journal of Nursing Education, 6*, 27-37.

Leininger, M. M. (1969). Ethnoscience: A promising research approach to improve nursing practice. *Image: Nurse Scholarship, 3*, 22-28.

Leininger, M. M. (1970). *Nursing and anthropology: Two worlds to blend*. New York: John Wiley & Sons.

Leininger, M. M. (1972). *Using cultural styles in the helping process and in relation to the suculture of nursing*. Nursing papers at the Illinois Psychiatric Institute, May 13-14, Chicago, 1971.

Leininger, M. M. (1976). Towards conceptualization of transcultural health care systems. In M. M. Leininger (Ed.), *Transcultural health care issues and conditions*. Philadelphia: F. A. Davis, 3–22.

Leininger, M. M. (1973). An open health care system model. *Nursing Outlook, 21*(3), 171–175.

Leininger, M. M. (1976). Caring: The essence and central focus of nursing. *American Nurses Foundation, Nursing Research Report, 12*(1), 2, 14.

Leininger, M. M. (1978). *Transcultural nursing: concepts, theories, and practices*. New York: John Wiley & Sons.

Leininger, M. M. (1983). Cultural care: An essential goal for nursing and health care. *Journal of Nephrology Nursing, 10*(5), 11–17.

Leininger, M. M. (1984). Cultural care: An essential goal for nursing and health care. *EDTNA Journal III*, 7–20.

Leininger, M. M. (1985). Transcultural nursing care diversity and universality: A theory of nursing. *Nursing and Health Care, 6*(4), 209–212.

Leininger, M. M. (1988). Leininger's theory of nursing: Culture care diversity and universality. *Nursing Science Quarterly, 2*(4), 11–20.

Leininger, M. M. (1988). Cultural care theory and administration. In B. Henry (Ed.), *Dimensions of nursing administration*. Boston: Blackwell Scientific Publications, 19–34.

Leininger, M. M. (in press). The future of nursing: Differentiated nursing practices with use of nursing theories.

Luna, L. (1989). Transcultural nursing care of Arab muslims. *Journal of Transcultural Nursing, 1*(1), 22–27.

Luna, L., & Cameron, C. (1988). Leininger's theory of culture care diversity and universality. In J. Fitzpatrick & A. Whall (Eds.), *Conceptual models of nursing: Analysis and applications*. Norwalk, CT: Appleton & Lange.

Rosenbaum, J. (1990). Culture care of older Greek-Canadian widow's within Leininger's theory of culture care. *Journal of Transcultural Nursing, 2*(1), 37–48.

Symanski, M. E. (1991). *Use of nursing theories in neonatal intensive care setting: Challenges for the future*. MD: Aspen.

Wenger, A. F., & M. Wenger (1988). Community and family care patterns of the old-order Amish. In M. M. Leininger (Ed.), *Care: Discovery and use in clinical community nursing*. Detroit: Wayne State University.

Wenger, A. F. (1991). Role of context in culture specific care. In L. Chinn (Ed.), *Anthology of caring*. New York: National League for Nursing, 95–110.

Wooldridge, P., Schmitt, M., Skipper, J., & Leonard, R. (1983). *The current status of practice theories in nursing*. St. Louis: C.V. Mosby, 107–114.

Appendix B

A PARTIAL LIST OF KNOWN RESEARCH STUDIES USING LEININGER'S CULTURE CARE THEORY

Berry, A. (1989–1991). *Culture care theory in the study of Mexican-American mother's and maternal care.* Detroit: Wayne State University. (Doctoral Field Study)

Bohay, I. (1989). *Ethnonursing: A study of pregnancy and childbirth in the Ukrainian culture within Leininger's culture care theory.* Detroit: Wayne State University. (Master's Thesis—MSN)

Burns, G. (1987). *Ethnocare of the homeless in large urban communities.* Detroit: Wayne State University. (Master's Field Study)

Cameron, C. (1986). *Relationship between select health beliefs and value and health practices of Philippine elderly.* Detroit: Wayne State University. (Post-Master's Field Study)

Cameron, C. (1990). *Health status of elderly Anglo-Canadian wives providing extended caregiving to their disabled husbands within Leininger's theory.* Detroit: Wayne State University. (Doctoral Dissertation)

Carvell, H. (1987). *Culture care in a Belgium hospital in Europe.* Detroit: Wayne State University. (Master's Field Study)

Enteshary, F. (1989–1991). *Culture care theory and loneliness of African-American's in a community context.* Detroit: Wayne State University. (Master's Field Study)

Finn, J. (1988). *Ethnonursing: A study of generic and professional care practices of mothers and infants within Leininger's theory of culture care.* Detroit: Wayne State University. (Post-Master's Field Study)

Gates, M. F. (1988). *Care and cure meanings, experiences and orientations of persons who are dying in hospital and hospice settings.* Detroit: Wayne State University. (Doctoral Dissertation)

Gates, M. F. (1991). Transcultural comparison of hospital and hospice as caring environments for dying patients. *Journal of Transcultural Nursing, 2*(2), 3–16.

Gelazis, R. (1988). *Well-being and humor in Lithuanian Americans.* Detroit: Wayne State University. (Post-Master's Field Study)

Gonclaves, L. (1988). *Ethnonursing study of elderly in a nursing home setting.* Detroit: Wayne State University. (Post-Doctoral Field Study)

Leininger, M. M. (1978). *Transcultural nursing: Concepts, theories and practices.* New York: John Wiley & Sons. (Gadsup research 1960–62)

Leininger, M. M. (1978). Early Gadsup childhood caring behavior with nursing theory implication. In *Transcultural nursing: Concepts, theories, and practices.* New York: John Wiley & Sons.

Leininger, M. M. (1981–1991). *Study of ten cultures in urban community using culture care theory and ethnonursing method.* Detroit: Wayne State University. (Includes Italian, Mexican, Appalachian, Chaldean, Arab-Muslims, African-American, Greek-American, North-American Indians, and homeless. (Post-Doctoral Research)

Leininger, M. M. (1985). Southern rural black and white American lifeways with focus on care and health phenomena. In *Qualitative research methods in nursing.* Orlando, FL: Grune & Stratton, 195–217.

Leininger, M. M., & Luna, L. (1985–1991). *Culture care of Arab Muslims in urban context with action ethnonursing research.* Detroit: Wayne State University.

Leininger, M. M., & McFarland, M. (1991). *Culture care in an urban nursing home with African and Anglo-Americans.* Detroit: Wayne State University.

Luna, L. (1987). *Ethnonursing and ethnographic: A study of Arab-Americans in an urban U.S. city.* Detroit: Wayne State University. (Post-Master's Field Study)

Luna, L. (1989). *Care and cultural context of Lebanese-Muslims in an urban U.S. community: An ethnographic and ethnonursing study conceptualized within Leininger's theory.* Detroit: Wayne State University. (Doctoral Dissertation)

McFarland, M. (1987–1989).*Culture care theory and ethnonursing mini-study of care experiences in residential nursing homes and Mexican-American communities.* Detroit: Wayne State University. (Post-Masters Field Study)

Morgan, M. (1988–1989). *Ethnonursing: A study of care in a hospital context using Leininger's theory of culture care.* Detroit: Wayne State University. (Post-Master's Field Study)

Pak, M. (1984). *A Study of Korean and American nurses' perception of caring.* Detroit: Wayne State University. (Master's Field Study)

Panfilli, R. (1984). *Ethnocaring perceptions, values, beliefs, and practices of selected Mexican-Americans in a large urban community.* Detroit: Wayne State University. (Master's Field Study)

Perez, T. (1986–1987). *Ethnonursing: A study of Cheppewa Indians in Canada and culture care needs using Leininger's culture care theory.* Detroit: Wayne State University. (Master's Field Study)

Riveria, J. (1986). *Ethnocare: A study of Tuscany (Italians) beliefs, values, and practices with Leininger's care theory.* Detroit: Wayne State University. (Master's Field Study)

Rosenbaum, J. (1987). *Ethnonursing study of grief with Greek-American widows with culture care.* Detroit: Wayne State University. (Post-Master's Field Study)

Rosenbaum, J. (1990). *The meaning and experience of cultural care, cultural care continuity, cultural health and grief phenomena of older Greek Canadian widows.* Detroit: Wayne State University. (Doctoral Dissertation)

Rosenbaum, J. (1990). Culture care of older Greek-Canadian widows within Leininger's theory of Culture Care. *Journal of Transcultural Nursing, 2*(1), 37–48

Scott, J. (1987). *Use of Leininger's theory and care of Afro-Americans in Chicago.* Chicago: Xavier College. (Master's Thesis)

Spangler, Z. (1985). *Ethnonursing study of care with Philippine urbanites and using Leininger's theory.* Detroit: Wayne State University. (Post-Master's Field Study)

Spangler, Z. (1991). *Nursing care values and practices of Philippine-American and Anglo-American nurses using Leininger's theory.* Detroit: Wayne State University. (Doctoral Dissertation)

Stasiak, D. (1991). *Ethnonursing: A study of Mexican-American in urban cities.* Detroit: Wayne State University. (Master's Field Study)

Wenger, A. F. (1986). *Health and care phenomena among Soviet-Jewish immigrants in the acculturation process: A mini-ethnonursing study.* Detroit: Wayne State University. (Post-Master's Field Study)

Wenger, A. F. (1988). *Phenomenon of care in a high-context culture: The Old Order Amish.* Detroit: Wayne State University. (Doctoral Dissertation)

Wenger, A. F., & Wenger, M. (1988). Community and family care patterns of the old-order Amish. In. M. M. Leininger (Ed.), *Care: Discovery and use in clinical community nursing.* Detroit: Wayne State University.

Appendix C

SOME NURSES USING THE THEORY
IN DIFFERENT COUNTRIES

Anderson, M. *Integrity and care.* University of Uppsala, Uppsala, Sweden (Research Project—post-graduate study in progress, Wayne State University, 1988)

Brink, H. *Cultural care assessment to improve client care with students.* University of Pretoria, Pretoria, South Africa. (Wayne State University visitor, 1988).

Cianciarullo, T. I. *Family-centered culture care.* Sao Paulo, Brazil, South America (Teaching and research project).

Gaston, C. (1986). *Cultural care of the Greeks in Australia* (Visiting student, Detroit: Wayne State University, 1985-1986)

Gonclaves, L. *Culture care variabilities with elderly in Brazil villages.* St. Caterina, Florinapolis, Brazil, South America (Teaching and research project).

Grund, G. *Culture care theory in schools of nursing.* University of Lund. Lund, Sweden (Teaching project).

Gualda, D. M. *Family centered culture care.* Sao Paulo, Brazil, South America. (Visiting post-doctoral student at Wayne State University, 1987) (Teaching and research project).

McNeil, J. (1989-1991). *Culture care theory with AIDs victims in West Africa.* World Health Organization Project (in progress).

Meriläinen, Pirkko. (1987-1991). *Culture care and health of coastal Finish villages.* University of Kuopio, Kuopio, Finland (in progress).

Anita v. S. *Culture care theory in a Helsinki hospital.* Helsinki, Finland (in progress).

Index

427